Somatovisceral Aspects of

CHIROPRACTIC

An Evidence-Based Approach

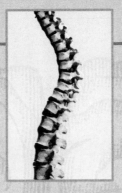

Somatovisceral Aspects of
CHIROPRACTIC
An Evidence-Based Approach

Charles S. Masarsky, DC
Marion Todres-Masarsky, DC
Vienna Chiropractic Associates, PC
Vienna, Virginia

with 75 illustrations

CHURCHILL LIVINGSTONE

A Harcourt Health Sciences Company
New York   Edinburgh   London   Philadelphia

CHURCHILL LIVINGSTONE
A Harcourt Health Sciences Company

The Curtis Center
Independence Square West
Philadelphia, Pennsylvania 19106

Library of Congress Cataloging-in-Publication Data

Masarsky, Charles S.
  Somatovisceral aspects of chiropractic : an evidence-based approach
/ Charles S. Masarsky, Marion Todres-Masarsky.
    p. ; cm.
  Includes bibliographical references and index.
  ISBN 0-443-06120-3 (hardcover)
  1. Chiropractic. 2. Spinal adjustment. 3. Autonomic nervous
system—Physiology. 4. Viscera—Innervation.
  [DNLM: 1. Chiropractic—methods. 2. Autonomic Nervous
System—physiology. 3. Cervical Vertebrae. 4. Dislocations—therapy.
5. Evidence-Based Medicine. 6. Viscera—physiology. WB 905.9 M394s
2001]   I. Todres-Masarsky, Marion. II. Title.
  RZ242 .M375 2001
  615.5′34—dc21

                                                    2001023483

Editor-in-Chief: John A. Schrefer
Associate Editor: Kellie F. White
Associate Developmental Editor: Jennifer L. Watrous
Project Manager: Linda McKinley
Senior Production Editor: Julie Eddy
Designer: Julia Ramirez
Cover photo: provided by Photodisc

SOMATOVISCERAL ASPECTS OF CHIROPRACTIC: AN EVIDENCE-BASED APPROACH   ISBN 0-443-06120-3

CONTRIBUTORS

Joel Alcantara, BSc, DC
Assistant Professor
Research
Life Chiropractic College West
San Lorenzo, California

Claudia A. Anrig, DC
Private practice
Fresno, California
Postgraduate Faculty, Life Chiropractic College
    West
San Lorenzo, California
Postgraduate Faculty, Palmer College of
    Chiropractic
Davenport, Iowa
Postgraduate Faculty, Parker College of
    Chiropractic
Dallas, Texas

James E. Browning, DC
Private practice
Director, Pelvic Pain and Organic Dysfunction
    Treatment Center
Suttons Bay, Michigan

Carl S. Cleveland, III, DC
President
Cleveland Chiropractic College
Kansas City, Missouri
Los Angeles, California

Edward E. Cremata, DC
Postgraduate Faculty, Life College of
    Chiropractic West
Postgraduate Faculty, Los Angeles Chiropractic
    College
Research Associate, Gonstead Clinical Studies
    Society
Private practice
Fremont, California

Darryl D. Curl, DDS, DC
Attending lecturer, UCLA School of Dentistry
Diplomate American Board of Orofacial Pain
Diplomate Board Status American Academy of
    Pain Management
Orofacial Pain Clinic
Los Angeles, California
Norco, California

Cheryl Hawk, DC, PhD
Associate Professor
Palmer Center for Chiropractic Research
Davenport, Iowa

Christopher Kent, DC, FCCI
Postgraduate Faculty
Life Chiropractic College West
San Lorenzo, California
Cleveland Chiropractic College
Kansas City, Missouri
Ramsey, New Jersey

Everett Langhans, DC
Director, Quad City Board of the National
    Arthritis Association
Director of Chiropractic Studies
Centro Universitario Feevale
República Federativa do Brasil

Charles S. Masarsky, DC
Co-Editor, *Neurological Fitness*
Postgraduate Faculty, Life Chiropractic College
    West
San Lorenzo, California
Postgraduate Faculty, Cleveland Chiropractic
    College
Kansas City, Missouri
Private practice
Vienna, Virginia

Marion Todres-Masarsky, DC
Co-Editor, *Neurological Fitness*
Private practice
Vienna, Virginia

William S. Rehm, DC, HCD (hc)
Founding President and Director Emeritus,
    Association of the History of Chiropractic
Private practice
Baltimore, Maryland

Anthony L. Rosner, PhD
Director of Research and Education
Foundation for Chiropractic Education and
    Research
Brookline, Massachusetts

William J. Ruch, DC
Adjunct Faculty & Research Associate
Department of Clinical Sciences
Life Chiropractic College West
San Lorenzo, California
Private practice
Oakland, California

John L. Stump, DC, OMD, EdD
Private practice
Fairhope, Alabama

Steven T. Tanaka, DC, DACAN
Private practice
Watsonville, California

Dedicated to our mothers, Lillian Weber and Eleanor Masarsky, and to the memory of Philip Masarsky.

At the beginning of this new millennium, the chiropractic profession enjoys the highest public visibility and patient utilization rate in its over 100-year history. This increased awareness may be attributed in part to various studies demonstrating the outcome effectiveness and patient satisfaction using spinal adjustment procedures in the management of back and neck pain. Doctors of Chiropractic, the primary providers of the spinal adjustment, are now fast emerging as the leaders in conservative and cost-effective management of pain from spinal origin.

History records, however, that the origins of the chiropractic profession do not lie solely in the treatment of musculoskeletal conditions; from the beginning, practitioners observed an association between altered spinal function and autonomic dysfunction. The attention directed to the demonstrated effectiveness of spinal adjustive procedures in the management of musculoskeletal conditions has, however, monopolized both research funding and personnel. Thus the chiropractic profession has not fully explored opportunities for research associated with the somatovisceral manifestations of spinal dysfunction.

This text, *Somatovisceral Aspects of Chiropractic: An Evidence-Based Approach,* by Charles S. Masarsky and Marion Todres-Masarsky, provides a theoretic foundation for discussion and understanding of the anatomic and functional mechanisms that link conditions of the spine and autonomic function. These mechanisms provide a rational basis for the clinical correlations observed in chiropractic practice and suggest an important role for chiropractic spinal adjustment in the management of visceral function.

As the chiropractic profession continues its emergence into mainstream health care and as opportunity for multidisciplinary health care partnerships expands, the importance of research exploring the role of chiropractic spinal adjustments in the management of autonomic function and systemic health will increase. This text serves as a reference resource fundamental to future somatovisceral disorders research and clinical practice.

Carl S. Cleveland, III, DC
President
Cleveland Chiropractic College
Kansas City, Missouri
Los Angeles, California

PREFACE

Somatovisceral Aspects of Chiropractic: An Evidence-Based Approach explores the autonomic and systemic implications of chiropractic methods of health care. The chiropractic research literature, biomedical sources, and osteopathic contributions are discussed from the point of view of the vertebral subluxation complex (VSC) clinical model. The organization of this book is intended to be especially useful to chiropractic students and field practitioners, but this book should also find readership among those involved in the profession's legal and policy arenas.

The text opens with an exploration of the topic from a variety of historic outlooks. Chapter 1 focuses on the intraprofessional forces that placed somatovisceral considerations in and out of the chiropractic "closet" during its first century. Chapter 2 considers the chiropractic concept of health care in relation to other healing arts, both Eastern and Western. In Chapter 3 the American judicial system serves as history's stage, providing further insight into the societal forces affecting the evolution of chiropractic as a full-fledged health profession.

A general clinical orientation to the topic is next. Chapter 4 is a practical review of the autonomic neuroanatomy of the VSC. Chapter 5 relates the phenomena of referred pain and referred tenderness to the chiropractic analysis. Chapter 6 provides clinical assessment tools that go beyond musculoskeletal pain to address such issues as emotional balance, vitality, and global well-being. Chapter 7 identifies methods of instrumentation and imaging that help characterize autonomic aspects of the VSC.

The text goes on to consider the influence of the VSC on specific regions and systems of the body. Chapter 8 provides a systematic study of the lower sacral nerves' influence on pelvic organic function. Chapters 9 to 11 are concerned with the health of the alimentary canal, the cardiovascular system, and the respiratory system. Chiropractic involvement with headache is too often viewed as a strictly musculoskeletal concern; Chapter 12 places this subject in a broader context. Chapter 13 focuses on disorders of vision, hearing, and balance. The influence of the VSC on endocrine physiology is explored in Chapter 14.

Infants and children are often brought to chiropractic practitioners with nonmusculoskeletal presentations. Unfortunately, chiropractic management of the pediatric patient has often been a flash point for medical and media critics, the insurance industry, and even small sectors of the chiropractic profession itself. This controversy has dissuaded too many clinicians from making what may be their most important contributions to the long-term health of their patient populations. Therefore Chapter 15 reviews somatovisceral literature relevant to the pediatric patient.

Chiropractic aspects of neuroimmunology, central nervous system function, and emotional health, among other topics, are the concerns of Chapter 16.

Chapter 17 attempts to relate the philosophic implications of the topic to the profession's scientific future.

An extensive glossary is offered, as well as questions to guide the study of each chapter.

The somatovisceral aspects of the VSC have too often and for too long been given short shrift within the profession while attention has been lavished on the musculoskeletal aspects. This reflects an artificial division between the neurology of the musculoskeletal system and the neurology of the viscera. Nature does not recognize this sharp division. Instead, the natural world has produced a nervous system that is a wonder of integration. Under the influence of this master integration system, smooth and striated muscle, activity and stillness, thought and emotion all contribute to the texture of life in a whole being.

The authors believe that the chiropractic profession can move beyond the back pain "box" and make unique contributions to the general health and global wellness of the public. To make these contributions, the profession needs no help, just no interference. Holding onto the artificial somatic/visceral division is a major source of interference within the profession. It is hoped that this volume will help to correct the fixation on the somatic/ visceral divide. If this can be done, the public will have access to a profession more worthy of the nervous system it serves.

Charles S. Masarsky, DC
Marion Todres-Masarsky, DC

ACKNOWLEDGMENTS

The authors gratefully acknowledge the invaluable assistance of the Manual, Alternative, and Natural Therapy Indexing Service (MANTIS) in conducting many literature searches required for the production of this textbook. We are also grateful for the support of the Foundation for Chiropractic Education and Research (FCER), which funded the MANTIS searches. For encouraging us in this endeavor from the beginning, we thank Daniel Redwood, DC, Joseph Keating, PhD, Lisa Killinger, DC, Norman Strutin, DC, Ruth Sandefur, DC, and Patrick Gentempo, DC. Our thanks goes to Trent Bachman, DC, who assisted us in locating literature on the respiratory aspects of chiropractic. We are grateful indeed for the help of Alana Callender, MS, and Dana Lawrence, DC, who guided us through the process of gaining permission to reproduce copyrighted illustrations, which was unfamiliar territory for us. Our thanks also goes to David Walther, DC, who graciously granted permission to reproduce new illustrations before publication. Special thanks must be given to our assistants, Helga Yunker and Merina Khatrichettri, who endured seemingly endless requests to photocopy, collate, and otherwise wrestle the material that appears in this textbook.

Finally, we gratefully remember the late A. Earl Homewood, DC, who never stopped reminding the profession of the importance of the somatovisceral aspects of chiropractic. Although his physical absence precluded any direct contribution to this textbook, his inspiration is one of the factors that made it possible.

MAKING THE MOST OF THE STUDY GUIDES

You will find a group of questions following each chapter in this text. We want you to think of these questions as study guides.

Several kinds of questions exist. Some use phrases we think are important to trigger your memory and solidify certain concepts and some will ask you simply to retrieve facts. Some are designed to encourage you to relate the chapter information directly to chiropractic philosophy and experience and some will require you to go beyond the presented material and search your own thought processes. For some, no concrete answer exists, but we are hoping the workout will get those neurons firing and juices flowing now and for the future.

The questions will often ask you to relate material from one chapter to that discussed in another, and we expect that they will often send you back to the text to reread pages, paragraphs, and lines. We do not expect you to absorb everything in this book on the first, second, or even fifth reading.

Many people worked on this book and you will see some differences in vocabulary and even in approach to chiropractic. Even with those differences, we all come together on the basic concepts of chiropractic; on the promise of our art, science, and philosophy; and on the tremendous potential of the gifts we can bring the world. If we have done our job well, you will finish this text agreeing with us and adding your own personal perspective too.

We would like to offer you three "grand unifying" questions. Ask them of yourself after each chapter, at the end of each semester, and sometimes, at the end of each work day:

1. What does this mean in terms of the chiropractic paradigm?
2. Why is it important? Or is it? If it isn't, why is it off-base?
3. How could I design a research project to test this idea or explore this hypothesis? How can I be sure to maintain the integrity of my project so that my work meets its potential and is understandable to the world at large?

We hope you learn as much reading this book as we have in compiling it.

The Authors

CONTENTS

15   Somatovisceral Involvement in the Pediatric Patient
Marion Todres-Masarsky, DC, Charles S. Masarsky, DC, Claudia A. Anrig, DC, Steven T. Tanaka, DC, Joel Alcantara, DC

16   The Somatovisceral Interface: Further Evidence
Marion Todres-Masarsky, DC, Charles S. Masarsky, DC, Everett Langhans, DC

17   Neurologic Holism: Chiropractic's Scientific Future
Charles S. Masarsky, DC, Marion Todres-Masarsky, DC

CHAPTER 1

Introduction: Somatovisceral Considerations in the Science of Tone

Charles S. Masarsky, DC • Marion Todres-Masarsky, DC

Autonomic Function and the Chiropractic Identity Crisis

In 1996, the Association of Chiropractic Colleges (ACC) published a consensus document, which included the following statement on the role of the subluxation in the chiropractic paradigm[1]:

> Chiropractic is concerned with the preservation and restoration of health, and focuses particular attention on the subluxation.
>
> A subluxation is a complex of functional and/or structural and/or pathological articular changes that compromise neural integrity and may influence organ system function and general health.

This position statement, signed by the presidents of 16 chiropractic colleges in the United States and Canada, hopefully represents a turning point in the profession's long identity crisis with regard to autonomic function. Although the general health aspects of chiropractic can claim a solid pedigree in the profession's history, a distinct movement has occurred in the past several decades towards limiting the field to the management of musculoskeletal pain.

For years, musculoskeletal pain relief has been seen by the profession as the "coin of the realm" in its quest for legitimacy. Narrowing the profession's focus to musculoskeletal pain made licensure possible in Canada's Ontario province.[2] In Australia, intense pressure has been placed on practitioners who mention nonmusculoskeletal pain in their advertising, despite supportive research findings and the widely held belief among

the nation's practitioners that chiropractic care can improve visceral function.[3,4]

Concerning the British chiropractic profession's effort for legitimation, Baer notes the following[5]:

> Like chiropractic in other countries, British chiropractic has evolved from a heterodox health system that claimed to be a complete alternative to biomedicine, to one that has increasingly come to accept a more limited niche in health care as a manual musculoskeletal specialty.

In the landmark 1979 report on chiropractic in New Zealand, the Commission of Inquiry noted that much of the medical opposition to chiropractic had to do with claims that adjustments could influence the course of systemic and visceral (type O) disorders.[6]

This international struggle to control the public's external opinion of the profession has created a parallel identity crisis within the profession. Today, one can find vocal advocates of a professional identity that positions chiropractic as a unique system of health maintenance. This identity suggests a "parallel" profession that is cooperative with but distinct from the current orthodox allopathic establishment.

The more recent push from the chiropractic profession to position chiropractic as an alternative form of pain control (a complementary profession adjunctive to orthodox allopathic medical care) has been readily observable in the United States, which is home to the majority of the world's doctors of chiropractic. This promotion has largely come from within the profession and has focused on winning the hearts and minds of chiropractic students and practitioners.

During a personal communication that we had with Wiehe, a former president of the American Chiropractic Association (ACA) Council on Diagnosis and Internal Disorders, he maintained that during the 1960s and 1970s the chiropractic educational facilities became silent regarding non-musculoskeletal conditions[7]:

> Finally, at least two chiropractic college presidents, whom I will never name, confided in me. They told me that it was now an unwritten rule that the profession from an educational standpoint would make no reference to chiropractic treatment of internal disease.

During this same time, Barge, a former president of the International Chiropractors Association (ICA), recalled pressure from his local state association[8]:

> I can so clearly remember being told by the Wisconsin Chiropractic Association (in the late 1960's) to stop lecturing on the chiropractic care of infectious conditions. . . . The WCA told me to be silent on controversial subjects, to stick to back pain and the musculoskeletal domain. They said we need to get a 'foot in the door,' so to speak; we need to be included in Medicare, worker's compensation, and other third-party plans.

According to the Panel on Chiropractic History of the Council on Chiropractic Education (CCE), the desire for chiropractic to fit into the professional culture of the biomedical research establishment might have been an important factor in generating the pressures noted by Wiehe and Barge[9]:

> For the first 75 years of its history, chiropractic emphasized the visceral importance of the spinal adjustment. About 1975, following the NINCDS Conference in Bethesda, MD, the emphasis changed to biomechanical problems with emphasis on back pain. At least one generation of chiropractors has been educated in the musculo-skeletal format with inadequate exposure to the importance of the autonomic nervous system.

The strong wish for access to the greater scientific community and research grant money by chiropractic professionals and the role of the 1975 conference on the research status of spinal manipulation sponsored by the National Institute of Neurological and Communicative Disorders and Stroke (NINCDS) was further emphasized in a recent interview with Vear, a prominent retired chiropractic educator who participated in the conference[10]:

> I remember going to Bethesda, Maryland to meet with Dr. Murray Goldstein, Director of the National Institutes of Health, to have first hand information on what chiropractic colleges must do to meet the changing standards and be credible when seeking NIH research grants. His response was a wake up call for those colleges who did take NINCDS seriously.
>
> One of the first things to change was a reduced emphasis on visceral clinical problems and an increased focus on pain syndromes, particularly of the lumbopelvic area. Literally, we were 'throwing out the baby with the bathwater' in our quest for research grants, for which purpose pain syndromes are easier to study and document.

To summarize, during the 1960s and 1970s, significant sectors of the chiropractic political and academic leadership tacitly orchestrated the public perception that chiropractic is an analgesic performed by hand. Those who contradicted this perception were often attacked and ostracized.

This limited analgesic role for the profession has been institutionalized considerably by the insurance industry. Medicare carriers in the United States do not consider a chiropractic diagnosis complete unless it includes a musculoskeletal pain component.[11] Similar requirements are commonly encountered in private insurance and managed care organizations.

Because of such intense political and economic pressure, the ACC's unambiguous stance that chiropractic's concern with subluxation encompasses the visceral as well as the somatic arena has to be understood not only in the context of contempory research but also in relation to the profession's earliest intellectual foundations.

Autonomic Function as an Aspect of Tone

The concept of tone was the foundation of early chiropractic science and practice. *Tone* was understood to be the rate or intensity of function of any tissue or organ, reflecting the status of that tissue or organ's innervation[12]:

> Life is the expression of tone. In that sentence is the basic principle of chiropractic. Tone is the normal degree of nerve tension. Tone is expressed in functions by normal elasticity, activity, strength and excitability of the various organs, as observed in a state of health. Consequently, the cause of disease is any variation in tone.

D.D. Palmer's method of chiropractic analysis (nerve tracing) demonstrated that the concept of tone was not restricted to the musculoskeletal arena. Nerve tracing was the use of digital pressure to follow a line of hypersensitive tissue from an uncomfortable body part to the spine or vice versa. A nerve trace to a particular spinal segment was assumed to represent disturbed tone in the indicated spinal nerve. The chiropractor would suspect disturbed neurologic tone as a cause of dysfunction in all tissues, somatic or visceral, innervated by the indicated nerve. Originating a nerve trace from a patient's nauseated stomach or painful kidney was believed to be as legitimate as nerve tracing from a patient's sore shoulder or painful hip.

Nerve tracing data correlated with autonomic neuroanatomy was systematized into the Meric system of chiropractic analysis.[13] This development was already underway when Mabel Palmer published *Chiropractic Anatomy* in 1918 and reached maturity by the time R.W. Stephenson published *Chiropractic Textbook* in 1927. In Meric analysis, a clinical problem is considered in terms of the *zone* (the body section innervated by a particular pair of spinal nerves) in which it occurs. All tissue of a particular type within a zone is termed a *mere*. For example, a zone's muscle tissue is its *myomere;* its visceral tissue is its *viscemere.*

When a patient's symptoms included stomach complaints, the Meric chiropractor would recognize the involved organ as part of the viscemere corresponding to the fifth through eighth thoracic vertebrae. The results of nerve tracing and the palpation of "taut and tender fibers" would indicate the precise subluxated vertebra requiring adjustment. Once x-ray technology was available, a radiographic examination would often serve as a tie-breaker if the nerve tracing and palpation data were ambiguous.[14]

By the early 1920s, many chiropractors used the back of the hand to palpate for *hot boxes,* or areas of increased temperature along the spine. Fascinated by this analytic method, Dossa D. Evins, a 1922 graduate of the Palmer School of Chiropractic, developed the Neurocalometer, the first chiropractic heat-reading instrument. It consisted of two thermocouple probes and a galvanometer, which indicated left-to-right thermal asymmetry as the examiner glided the instrument up or down the spine. Persistent thermal asymmetry was assumed to be a sign of disturbed vasomotor tone, consistent with the presence of vertebral subluxation.[15]

Clearly, assessment of autonomic tone was an integral part of chiropractic analysis from the earliest years of the profession. This took the form of nerve tracing, Meric analysis, and vasomotor assessment by instrument or by hand. Disturbed tone was considered the most readily observable manifestation of *dis-ease.*

Dis-ease was understood as a failure of organisms to adapt optimally to internal and external stressors because of loss of contact with the inherent organizing principle, or innate intelligence, found in every living organism.[14] The traditional chiropractic concept of dis-ease has much in common with the more recent biomedical concept of *dysponesis*. Similarly, the concept of innate intelligence originated from the ancient idea of *vis medicatrix naturae,* or the healing power of nature.[16]

Dis-ease, both at the local tissue level and at the level of the organism as a whole, was seen as the most important consequence of the vertebral subluxation. Therefore the assessment of tone was not merely perceived as a clinical decision-making tool but also as a window into a patient's overall state of ease or dis-ease.

Modern Developments in the Science of Tone

By the early 1990s, a revived interest in the chiropractic concept of tone had occurred, as evidenced by a provocative paper by Donahue.[17] Although Donohue is distinctly uncomfortable with such concepts as innate intelligence and dis-ease, he sees much value in the concept of tone for today's chiropractic profession[17]:

> Tone, besides being a 'traditional' concept, has a uniquely chiropractic appeal because it is a

dynamic and animated metaphor, pregnant with research possibilities. . . . Tonal measurements can surely help us create a unique system of chiropractic diagnosis.

This sentiment was recently repeated by Leach, who proposed that the modern nerve compression and neurodystrophic hypotheses were derived from Palmer's concept of tone.[18]

These hypotheses are presented as integral aspects of the neurologic component in Cleveland's recent review of the vertebral subluxation complex (VSC).[19,20] Nerve compression is cited as a potential cause of hyposympatheticotonia; the effects of this hypotonic sympathetic function can include inappropriate vasodilation; and neurodystrophy involves immunosuppression as a result of disturbed axoplasmic transport.

Cleveland also discussed facilitation (hypertonia) of the visceral pain pathways because of subluxation, leading to simulated visceral disease by pain referral. Thus the most widely discussed clinical and theoretical model in chiropractic to date, the VSC, is firmly based on D.D. Palmer's concept of tone. When considering the neurologic component of the VSC, autonomic implications are inescapable.

Two aspects of the neurologic component of the VSC model discussed by Cleveland are critically important. One is the possible disturbance of the anterior, lateral, or posterior horn of the spinal cord. Clearly, dysfunction of the spinal cord implies disturbance of tone throughout the body.

The other critical aspect is the concept of abnormal articular nociception and mechanoreception (joint dysafferentation) leading to hypertonic or hypotonic autonomic function (somatoautonomic reflexes). This somatoautonomic reflex activity is viewed as a possible source of systemic errors in energy expenditure (dysponesis).

One possible reason for this dysfunctional somatoautonomic reflex activity may come from the fact that the sympathetic nervous system responds to the energy requirements of posture and locomotion. This phenomenon has been a central interest in the osteopathic research conducted by Korr. Korr refers to this phenomenon as the *ergotropic function* of the sympathetic nervous system.[21] The tonicity of this ergotropic function is a response to afferent signals from the musculoskeletal system. If subluxation causes dysafferentation, ergotropic activity will be based on erroneous information. In other words, sympathetic activity can be altered by *illusory* changes in musculoskeletal demand.

Without cord involvement and ergotropic dysfunction, subluxation might be seen simply as a disturbed joint, with effects neatly isolated to a limited sector of the musculoskeletal system. With ergotropic function and cord dynamics accounted for in the VSC model, the subluxation is expected to affect the nervous system in a way that puts dys-

STUDY GUIDE

1. Define subluxation.
2. What is meant by type M and type O in chiropractic?
3. Why would you define chiropractic as a parallel rather than an alternative health care profession?
4. Name one major effect of the NINCDS conference on the chiropractic profession.
5. What is tone in terms of chiropractic?
6. Nerve tracing was a precursor of what system of chiropractic analysis?
7. What is a viscemere?
8. Who invented the Neurocalometer and why was it considered important?
9. Define dis-ease. Differentiate it from disease.
10. What, according to chiropractic philosophy, is the organizing principle in every living organism?
11. What is dysponesis? If you have to use another source for your definition, cite it.
12. Name a potential cause of hyposympatheticotonia.
13. Name something that could cause disturbance of tone throughout the entire body.
14. Describe ergotropic function in terms of appropriate tone.
15. What would cause illusory changes in the musculoskeletal system?

functional demands on heart rate, breathing, lymphatic flow, glucose catabolism, adrenal function, and virtually every other aspect of physiology. With this perspective, the concern of chiropractic clinical assessment becomes systemic rather than local and holistic rather than reductionistic.

Our organizing principle in this textbook is the VSC model, with its broad perspective. From this perspective, the study of the effects of vertebral subluxation on systemic function is part of normal chiropractic research, and the assessment of autonomic tone is a legitimate activity in chiropractic clinical assessment. We offer this work in the hope that it will be viewed it as a modern contribution to D.D. Palmer's "science of tone."

REFERENCES

1. Association of Chiropractic Colleges: Issues in chiropractic. Position paper #1. The ACC Chiropractic Paradigm, Chicago, July, 1996, Association of Chiropractic Colleges.
2. Coburn D: Legitimacy at the expense of narrowing of scope of practice: chiropractic in Canada, *J Manipulative Physiol Ther* 14:14, 1991.
3. Polus BI, Henry SJ, Walsh MJ: Dysmenorrhea: to treat or not to treat, *Chiropr J Austral* 26:21, 1996.
4. Jamison JR, McEwen AP, Thomas SJ: Chiropractic adjustment in the management of visceral conditions: a critical appraisal, *J Manipulative Physiol Ther* 15:171, 1992.
5. Baer HA: The sociopolitical development of British chiropractic, *J Manipulative Physiol Ther* 14:38, 1991.
6. The Government Printer: *Chiropractic in New Zealand,* p 27, Wellington, New Zealand, 1979, The Government Printer.
7. Wiehe RJ: Personal communication, August 17, 1990.
8. Barge FH: Chiropractic's greatest tactical error, *Dynamic Chiropr* 18:45, 1993.
9. Association Notes: The roots of somato-visceral clinical treatment, *Chiropr Hist* 11:7, 1991.
10. Vear H: Neurological fitness interview, *Neuro Fit* 7(1):4, 1997.
11. X-act Medicare Services: *Medicare part B reference manual,* p F-1, Camp Hill, Pa, June, 1997, X-act Medicare Services.
12. Palmer DD: *The chiropractors adjustor: the science, art and philosophy of chiropractic,* p 7, Portland, 1910, Portland Printing House.
13. Peterson D, Wiese G, editors: *Chiropractic: an illustrated history,* St Louis, 1995, Mosby.
14. Stephenson RW: *Chiropractic textbook,* Davenport, Iowa, 1948, Palmer School of Chiropractic.
15. Kyneur JS, Bolton SP: Chiropractic equipment. In Peterson D, Wiese G, editors: *Chiropractic: an illustrated history,* p 262, St Louis, 1995, Mosby.
16. Phillips RB et al: A contemporary philosophy of chiropractic for the Los Angeles College of Chiropractic, *J Chiropr Humanities* 4:20, 1994.
17. Donahue JH: Palmer's principle of tone: our metaphysical basis, *J Chiropr Humanities* 3:56, 1993.
18. Leach RA: *The chiropractic theories: principles and clinical applications,* ed 3, p 28, Baltimore, 1994, Williams & Wilkins.
19. Cleveland CC: Vertebral subluxation. In Redwood D, editor: *Contemporary chiropractic,* p 29, New York, 1997, Churchill Livingstone.
20. Cleveland CC: Neurobiologic relations. In Redwood D, editor: *Contemporary chiropractic,* p 45, New York, 1997, Churchill Livingstone.
21. Korr IM: Sustained sympatheticotonia as a factor in disease. In Korr IM, editor: *The neurobiologic mechanisms in manipulative therapy,* New York, 1977, Plenum Press.

CHAPTER 2

Health Care Paradigms in Perspective

John L. Stump, DC, OMD, EdD

Health Care Paradigms in Perspective

Because a belief is common or even accepted by a majority of people does not make it a final and exclusive truth. Although allopathy is currently highly regarded by the Western world, medical doctors have only enjoyed this esteemed position since the commissioning of the Flexner Report less than 100 years ago. This report, which led to a procrustian standardization of health care practices in this country, was ordered not by any health care profession but by big industry.

Many other more holistic health paradigms have been successful not only in maintaining life but also in enhancing it, some for thousands of years. Although all models are different, they are united in the concept that the capacity for good health comes from within. They often depend on an internal network along which a vital force must be free to travel unencumbered. They also tend to recognize the role lifestyle plays in achieving and maintaining optimum health. Rather than concentrating on an isolated body part, these systems recognize the involvement of the entire body, often concentrating on the spine or other central pathways. In these systems, the somatovisceral connection is seen as obvious, a very different perspective than allopathy, which continues to view this connection as controversial.

In this chapter, I discuss several of the world's larger health care paradigms, including allopathy, and encourage you to place them in perspective.

Mechanism and Vitalism: Newton and Einstein

The technologically oriented biomedical perspective that has dominated Western medical practice for decades maintains a rich historical legacy in the rationalist tradition of medical thought and concomitant allopathic approaches to healing.[1-4] It does this in the vacuum of Western hubris, ignoring the wealth of information from great societies all around the world, despite increasingly easy access to this information, certainly over the last century.

The biomedical model assumes that disease may be fully accounted for by quantifiable somatic variables independent of social, psychological, and behavioral dimensions of pathology.[5,6] It does this with the seeming assumption that although we still have a few things to learn, our way of thinking is absolutely accurate and all variables have been accounted for.

In his classic analysis of medical thought from 450 BC to 1914 AD, *Divided Legacy*, Coulter[7-9] documented the perennial relationship between two opposing paradigms: the Rationalist (mechanistic) and Empirical (vitalistic) approaches to therapeutic methods. Historically, rationalist methods have been concerned with isolatable physiologic processes governed by the laws of logic, and empirical approaches have emphasized the whole organism and its interaction with its environment.[10]

The most profound influences on contemporary Western medical philosophy, theory, and practice have been those associated with rationalist doctrines.[7-9] Coulter reports that the rationalist view first emerged in recorded history in a body of Greek writings traditionally referenced as *Group III of the Hippocratic Corpus* (Airs, Waters, Places, The Sacred Disease, Nature of Man, Regimen in Health, Breathes, and Regimens I-IV). The major precepts of the rationalist doctrine are as follows[7]:

> The internal processes of the body are knowable 'a priori.' Medical doctrine is a body of logically coherent theory reflecting the essentially logical structure of the human organism, the aim of medical diagnosis is to discover the (specific) disease, and the aim of therapeutics is to counteract or oppose this cause by the appropriate "contrary" medicine. The emphasis on 'contrary,' or opposition, leads to an interpretation of symptoms as being in and of themselves harmful, morbific phenomena.

In other words, illness is an assault on the body that comes from the outside in as opposed to a weakness in the organism allowing for a destructive static in the system causing it to go awry, with the symptoms indicating that this has happened.

The French mathematician Descartes ushered in the Western scientific revolution in the seventeenth century. His introduction of analytic, reductive reasoning formed the basis of a new philosophy of science that overrode older Western concepts such as the bodily humours and became the philosophy of modern Western medicine. Descartes considered the human body a machine, comparing a healthy man to a well-made clock. Descartes' dedicated followers engaged in the following[11]:

> (The followers) administered beatings to dogs (as part of their research) with perfect indifference and made fun of those who pitied the creatures as if they felt pain. They said the animals were clocks; that the cries they emitted when struck were only the noise of a little spring that had been touched, but that the whole body was without feeling.

He also built a firm division between mind and matter asserting, "There is nothing in the concept of body that belongs to the mind; and nothing in that of the mind that belongs to the body."[12] This mechanistic view of nature led to the fixed and absolute physical laws devised by astronomer and mathematician Isaac Newton, who outlined the cause and effect method of explaining the material, or visible universe. This logic formed the basis of the scientific method as it is known today.

The Newtonian view is based on early models of mechanistic behaviors that came from observations of (visible) nature. Acceleration and gravity were analyzed by Newton from his supposed observation of a falling apple. Early Newtonian laws enabled scientists to make predictions on the way mechanical systems would behave.[13]

The Cartesian-Newtonian mechanistic view of life is only one approximation of reality. In many other systems, pharmacologic and surgical approaches would be considered incomplete because they ignore the vital forces that animate and vitalize the biomechanics of living organisms. They ignore the ghost in the machine. In a machine, the underlying principle is that the function of the whole can be predicted by the sum of its parts. Humans, unlike machines, are more than the summation of a cluster of chemicals. In other paradigms, all organisms are dependent on a subtle vital force that creates synergism and harmony in the unique structural organization of the organism.[13] It is this unique vital force that makes the whole organism greater than the sum of its parts.

Another unique principle that distinguishes the vitalistic view from the mechanistic belief occurs when the vital force leaves the organism at death. The physical (structural mechanism) slowly degrades into a disorganization of collected chemicals.[13] When people are considered to be only like machines, modern medicine becomes obliged to keep the machine running. Its purpose is defined as avoiding death, rather than enriching life.[12]

The Asian model, based on vitalism, may help the Newtonian-Einsteinian separation to become whole again. Eastern philosophy is based on the premise that all life occurs within the cycles of nature, explained in the early Chinese literature as the *Tao*. Objects within this foundational system are interlinked and relate to each other, much like the Einsteinian viewpoint of vibrational medicine, which sees human beings as a physical and cellular system in dynamic interplay with complex regulatory energetic fields, all interrelated to the universe around them.[13]

The theoretical model of a matter and energy relationship is an important revelation that was being used and taught by D.D. Palmer in the late 1800s in his practice of magnetic healing. This same model is explained in Gerber's *Vibrational Medicine*[13]:

> The healer's energies differ from conventional magnetic fields in that they are not only quali-

tatively different in their effects, but also quantitatively different in that the magnetic fields associated with healers are exceedingly weak, yet they have powerful biological and chemical effects.

Einstein's equation predicts the existence of a faster-than-light energy referred to by physicist William Tiller[14] as *magneto-electrical energy.* This is apparently similar to the energy emitted from the hands of today's healers using manual therapies.[13]

The Empirical Perspective

According to Coulter,[7] the ancient Greek view of health that was established by the earliest writings of the Hippocratic Corpus (Coan Prognosis, Epidemics I and III, Prognosis, Aphorism, and Regimens in Acute Disease) was clearly empirical because it emphasized the importance of a dynamic equilibrium between the bodily humours. It also underscored the establishment of a harmonious relationship between the body, the individual's living habits, and all the environmental influences (e.g., quality of water, air, and food). Within this perspective, sickness represented a disruption of this intricate linking of factors. In his essay, "Neo-Hippocratic Tendency of Contemporary Medical Thought," Castiglioni promotes the essence of this view as follows[7]:

> This Hippocratic conception considers man as an indestructible part of the cosmos, bound to it and subject to its laws: it may be called, therefore, a universal, cosmical, unitarian conception. Disease, according to it, is a general fact which strikes the whole organism and has its origin in a perturbation of natural harmony.

Empirical doctrines have traditionally included a strong vitalistic belief in the innate curative powers of the individual and have stressed the importance of the quality of the doctor-patient relationship.[7] Their observation of symptom patterns led them to the conclusion that the organism can manifest sickness and disease in an infinite number of different ways, each of which represent a different dynamic pattern taken by the body's innate healing power in its effort to affect a cure.[7]

Homeopathy

Hahnemann, credited by some as the father of modern experimental pharmacology,[3,15] invented the term *allopathy* to describe the orthodox medical tradition of his time and to distinguish it from his own system of health care that he called *homeopathy.* He composed a set of rules for testing drugs and from his experimentation he formulated the basic laws of homeopathy. Hahnemann hypothesized that people became ill in unique ways and that individuals could be cured when administered minute doses of substances that when given in large doses to healthy individuals would produce the unique patterns of symptoms. From his point of view, similar medicines were thought to affect the reactive and curative power of the individual, the vital force. Hahnemann's concept of vital force underscored his belief that an interrelationship existed between spiritual and material aspects of life.[15] He theorized that disease, rather than being an entity with a specific knowable cause, represented an impairment of the spiritual vital force as follows[9]:

> Disease . . . considered as it is by the allopath, is a thing separate from the living whole, from the organism and its animating vital force, and hidden in the interior, be it of ever so subtle a character, is an absurdity, that could only be imagined by minds of a material stamp. No disease . . . is caused by any material substance, but . . . everyone is only and always a particular, virtual, dynamic derangement of the health.

The vital force could be affected by a multiplicity of internal and external influences. Consequently each disease was different for each person and could not be classified with respect to a single cause. In other words, the disease process for an individual was inimitable and only revealed by a unique pattern of signs.

Qi Hua

Qi Hua means *mutations of energy.* The classic example is the cycle of seasons, with the transformation from one season to the other, or the cycle of days and nights. In every modification of substance or essence, a Qi Hua has occurred, or a transformation of energy inherent in the substance has taken place. Water and ice are physically different even though the chemical formula H_2O identifies them both. When water is transformed into ice or vice versa, a Qi Hua has taken place. The law of Qi can be applied to the cyclic change in all nature. With a change of Qi Hua, a body can go from health to sickness and back.

To illustrate this fundamental principle in a practical manner, Chinese philosophy presents the Tao as an undifferentiated whole. It is both the unity of all things and the way the universe works. Out of this oneness Yin and Yang emerge. Both are ideal and complementary and antagonistic to each other. They are a symbolic representation of the universal dynamic of change, rather than a static picture. The Yin and Yang model is also used to differentiate aspects of a process. Within the magnetic field of fundamental opposition and creative tension, each aspect depends on the other. Neither of these states can exist in an absolute or static condition because both are in a perpetual state of dynamic transformation, continually blending with each other in greater or lesser proportions. Some Yang always exists in Yin and some Yin always exists in Yang.

Humankind cannot escape the general law by which we are governed because we too reflect the cyclic variations of our environment. In health, weak points still exist and in sickness, some aspects of health still occur. A person is more active (Yang) during the day and summer and more reposed during the night and winter (Yin). The organs of the body also follow the variations of the energy changes, as when cardiac rhythm increases during the activity of day and slows at night, with rest. Thus, the ancient Chinese philosophy reflects the relatedness of all things to each other; up does not exist without down.

Yin and Yang also describe the human process. The stages of life include conception to birth (Yang), growth, maturity, decline, and death (Yin). Chinese philosophy views a healthy life as one that contains an even balance of the forces of Yin and Yang. Maintaining a perfect balance is felt to result in perfect health of mind, body, and spirit. An imbalance of these polar characteristics and energies causes a shift in the equilibrium of the organism that ultimately crystallizes into patterns of disharmony and illness in the physical body. Energetic dysfunction at the physical level may be reflected by imbalances in the paired meridians or Chings of the body.[13]

Acupuncture

Around 1558 BC, the Shang dynasty advanced the healing method known to us as *acupuncture* with the development of porcelain and metal needles to be used in practice. The earliest existing medical treatise in China is Huangdi Nei Jing (Canon of Medicine), as compiled in the Warring States period (475-221 BC). It summarized the current medical knowledge and that of the ancients passed through history.[16] In one of the great classics, "ShiJi" (Historical Records), Pien Chueh, a famous doctor, writes[17]:

> Huang Ti speaks to Chi Po: I who am chief of the great people and who should receive taxes from them find myself afflicted by not being able to collect them because my people are sick. I desire, therefore, that the employment of remedies cease and that only needles be used. I order that this method be transmitted to all future generations and that the laws concerning it be clearly defined so it will be easy to practice it, hard to forget it and that it will not be abandoned in the future. Besides this, the actual modalities are to be accurately observed so that the way to research will be opened.

Empirical until that time, acupuncture obtained the status of a science by declaration of the Yellow Emperor to his physician. Succeeding generations began to write treatises illustrated by anatomic drawings that related points along lines that are called *meridians* or *ching*. In the Sung dynasty (420 AD) the emperor Wei Teh ordered a bronze statue to be cast, on which all the known acupuncture points were located. Dating from that epoch are treatises establishing the relationships between the 12 basic meridians and the human organs that are divided into 5 tsang (heart, liver, spleen, and kidneys) and the 6 fu (stomach, gallbladder, large and small intestines, bladder, and the functional organs known as the *triple heater*). To these original 11, the functional organ of the pericardium and heart protector was later added (Academy of Traditional Chinese Medicine).

The meridians distribute the subtle magnetic energies of Qi or Chi (Ki in Japan; Prana in India), which provide sustenance and organizations for the physical-cellular structure of each organ system of the human body. Although the subtle energies that the Chinese refer to as *Qi* are hard to measure, evidence for some types of electromagnetic energy circuits exist, which involve the meridians and acupuncture points.[13]

The meridians can be viewed as electrical circuits that act as conduits for the passage of Qi and the connection of acupuncture points to the internal organs and their function. For health and wellness of the individual to exist, optimal energy should occur in these meridians and they should all be balanced with respect to one another. A characteristic rhythmic flow used by the Qi energy exists as it passes across the basic meridians that supply energy to the internal organ structures. This energy flow reflects the basic biologic rhythms and cycles of the subtle energies of nature. These well-defined cycles and energies as described by the Asian masters are a reflection of the cyclic energy interaction between humans and the universe.

Diagnosis or evaluation by the practitioner is thus the process of determining what, how, and why particular events occur so that the location of an energy blockage or imbalance is revealed. It is a process of discovery in which decisions are made according to different frames of reference and orders of complexity from the most general parameters of Yin-Yang to the very specific ones of meridian and Qi imbalance. The art of the practitioner, like that of an investigator, is in capturing the essence of the individual and the cause and nature of illness within the framework of the specific environment and world. The practitioner also is concerned with eliminating the energy blockage or imbalance within the individual so that harmony and balance may be restored to the energy system. This results in health and homeostasis and is similar to a chiropractor removing a subluxation in an individual.

Ayurveda

Ayurveda is a very ancient form of health care based in India and practiced there and around the world today. It is concerned with the balance of energy centers, referred to as *chakras,* from the Sanskrit meaning *wheels.* They are said to resemble whirling vortices of subtle energies.[18] According to

Leadbeater and other authorities of Yogic philosophy, chakras are somehow involved with absorbing the higher energies and transforming them to a usable form within the human body.

From a physiologic viewpoint, the chakras appear to be involved with the flow of higher energy frequencies by specific subtle energy channels into the cellular structure of the physical body. At one level, they seem to function as energy transformers, stepping down energy of one form and frequency to a lower level of energy. This energy is, in turn, translated into harmonial, physiologic, and ultimately cellular changes throughout the body. At least 7 major chakras appear to be associated with the physical body and possibly more than 360 exist in the human body.[13]

In the Hindu and Yogic literature, this unique energy system that activates the energy of the chakras and assists in awakening the higher consciousness is referred to as the *Kundalini.*[19] The Kundalini is visualized as a coiled serpent (the Sanskrit translation of the word kundalini), which lies dormant in the coccygeal region at the first major chakra, an area recognized not only in gross neurology but also in many chiropractic techniques as an area of major importance to the well-being of the individual. The kundalini, similar to a nerve impulse or power surge, is always poised to move into action; however, in most individuals this energy is dormant. When its power is unleashed in a coordinated manner, for example in meditation, yogic asanas, or the martial arts, the kundalini energy rises slowly in the spinal column, activating the sequential chakras as it moves up.[19] The energy then moves throughout the body, giving and distributing life force as it is transmitted across the network of the body.

Hidden in all energy is the working of a conscious will. It manifests in nature as the working of intelligence through the movement of energy. The life energy is called *Prana,* meaning the primal breath, or life force. It is the first of three vital forces. The second force of the triad is perceived as the *principle of light* or *radiance.* Energy is light. The third of these forces is seen as a principle of cohesion. In all manifestations, this is a common unity. An affinity of forces exists in which all energies are ultimately linked in one great harmony. This cohesiveness is seen not only as a chemical property but also as a conscious intent.

According to Ayurveda, three primary life

forces, or three biological humors reside in the body. In Sanskrit, these are called *vata, pitta* and, *kapha*. They correspond primarily to the elements of air, fire, and water, functioning somewhat like the Chinese elements of fire, earth, metal, water, and wood. When out of balance, the elements are the causative forces in the disease process.[20]

Chiropractic

The following statement was central to a meeting of all presidents of U.S. chiropractic colleges, plus Canadian Memorial Chiropractic College (CMCC). In a profession often beleaguered by conflicting opinions about the most basic aims, duties, and expectations of its members, the ACC statement very solidly declares a basic foundation on which the profession is to be built (ACC, 1996):

> A subluxation is a complex of functional and/or structural and/or pathological articular changes that compromise neural integrity and may influence organ system function and general health.

Although the origin and evolution of chiropractic is deeply rooted in ancient healing practices, when movement of the spine was first used to correct health problems is not known. In the far East, around 2700 BC, Kong Fou is responsible for what is probably the first written account of manipulation.[21] Ancient civilizations from Babylonia (Iraq) to Central America and Tibet practiced manipulative therapies.[22] Egyptologists relate that the replacing of displaced vertebra was practiced by the ancient Egyptians many years before Christ. Evidence exists to show that early Greek physicians employed this method of curing disease.[23,24] In Europe and the American West, in particular, practitioners known as *bonesetters* flourished.

D.D. Palmer founded chiropractic as a separate and distinct healing art in 1895 in Davenport, Iowa. He readily stated that he was not the first to use manipulation for the correction of human ailments.[25] but he did claim to be the first to use the spinous and transverse processes of vertebrae as levers. During this time he was practicing as a magnetic healer and this art seemed to him to be a natural advancement of his art.

Magnetic therapy in which the patient's body is stroked so as to increase its magnetic flow was then practiced by many lay healers and physicians, much as Reiki and therapeutic touch are now practiced. Palmer learned the technique from Paul Castor and originally opened an office in the 1880s.[20]

Little is stated in the literature concerning the practice of magnetic healing, yet recent studies by Dr. Justa Smith have shown that healers can accelerate the kinetic activity of enzymes in a fashion similar to the effects of high intensity magnetic fields,[13] This shows that the energetic fields of the healer's hands were able to repair ultraviolet damaged enzymes in a manner similar to that of magnetic fields. The experimental evidence from the previous study suggests that the energies of healers appears to be magnetic in nature. This is a fascinating revelation when one considers that as far back as the eighteenth century, Franz Anton Mesmer's experiments were referred to as working with *magnetic healing*.[13] These magnetic fields could not be measured then as they can now. It is hoped that researchers will further investigate this phenomenon for the possible advancement of noninvasive health care.

Substantial controversy exists about whether D.D. Palmer and Andrew Still, the father of osteopathy, borrowed each other's new healing modality. Even more dispute appears concerning whether Palmer first studied osteopathy with Dr. Still.

Although osteopathy attempts to restore health by following the *rule of the artery*, chiropractic has always recognized the primacy of the nervous system and the need to keep it free of interference. This interference is known as the *vertebral subluxation complex*, which consists of areas of the spine where deranged motion or positioning of one or more vertebrae causes dis-ease within the living system. The nerve energy transmitted is electrical and has a clear relationship to acupuncture and Ayurveda regarding a force that vitalizes the network, or the hologram of the living body. The philosophic assumption is that an intelligence occurs in the universe that is seen in living organisms as Innate Intelligence, the organizing factor in life. The vertebral subluxation complex (VSC) interferes with the full transmission of this force, allowing the body to fall into dis-ease and eventually into recognizable illness and decline.

Practicing chiropractors also recognize principles stating that limitation of matter exists and that, most important in the world where chemical pharmaceuticals are often used for their quick action and ability to mask problems, all things take time, particularly the reversal of damage.

D.D. Palmer's son, Dr. B.J. Palmer, was known as the *developer of chiropractic* and acquired the Palmer School of Chiropractic that was founded by his father shortly after his discovery and established a clear philosophy that future chiropractors would use to guide their studies. B.J., an Orientalist by avocation, specifically and heavily emphasized not only the concepts of the VSC but also the need for specificity in removing blockage wherever found.

A question remains whether D.D. Palmer knew that the ancient texts of the far East maintained proof that the spine was a main channel of energy and that between practically each spinal vertebra a specific acupoint existed that could be used to heal a sick organism.[12,16] His conscious mind probably did not know the answer but, in view of the unified field theory espoused by Einstein and the recent work of physicist and theorist William H. Tiller, PhD,[13] his unconscious mind perhaps knew.

Chiropractic and the Other Paradigms

Some connection exists between chiropractic and the other paradigms discussed previously.

Chiropractors associated with the International College of Applied Kinesiology have long recognized a place for meridian therapy as a modality accompanying the chiropractic adjustment. They also accept several systems of reflexes, among them stress receptors, neurolymphatics, and neurovasculars, which work along no visible tracts but can be demonstrated to strengthen muscles and participate in physiologic change.

In 1987, the *American Journal of Acupuncture* published a paper by Philip Shambaugh, DC in which he discusses the balancing of the bladder meridian as a possible mechanism by which a particular low-force contact at the sacral apex may work. He further hypothesizes that a weak form of electromagnetic energy from the chiropractor's finger may be operating in this case. The area of the contact in this paper is very close to the coccyx, near the reputed seat of prana. The technique employs auxillary contacts going up the sides of the spine that Shambaugh believes relate

to points along the bladder meridian, which run bilaterally parallel to the spine.

In *Low Back Pain . . . Mechanism, Diagnosis and Treatment*, ed 5, James Cox, DC recommends goading bladder points BL24 and BL35, parallel to the lumbar spine, before and after flexion and distraction of the low back. He recommends BL49 to relieve the pain of sciatica. Although Cox's reasons for stimulating these points are not those of the ancient Chinese in conducting energy flow from one area to another, even Cox's cookbook approach recognizes a possible relationship between the two paradigms.

Nothing mentioned earlier is intended to suggest that chiropractors should become acupuncturists or Ayurvedic doctors. Certainly any and all of these systems can involve a lifetime of study on its own without achieving anything near perfection. I believe the paradigms are related through their holistic approach to balancing powerful forces to achieve whole body health. Recognizing this greatly alters the perspective of most systems in terms of a normal or rational approach to health care, with roots in human history.

Allopathy

Although advances in the medical sciences have been important in the control and eradication of a host of infectious diseases associated with viral and microbial pathogens, the shift in research today suggests that microbes are simply adapting to the attempt at eradication.[26] The failure to isolate a single biologic pathogen as a cause for each chronic disorder, in the manner of Koch's Postulates, forces the reexamination of the basic assumptions of the mechanistic medical view.[26-28]

The iatrochemists of seventeenth century Europe used the contrary properties of acids and alkalines in their medical treatments (the establishment of pharmaceuticals), while their interomechanic colleagues viewed the human organism as a hydraulic system and ascribed diseases to obstructions in the veins and arteries. They selected medicines based on their ability to dissolve those obstructions.[7] Similarly, the Cartesian revolution in the late seventeenth century led to a view of the body as an intricate machine. This notion readily fostered a rationalist view of disease existing because of a breakdown of the machine and of the doctor's task being to repair the machine.[12,29] When in the late nineteenth century bacteriology developed as the principle mechanistic discipline, diseases were reinterpreted as the products of pathogenic microorganisms, or germs. Medicines that could "kill the germ in vitro were thought to remove the associated disease in vivo"[7] and became the major emphasis in allopathy.

The term *allopathy* (from the Greek *alloin pathos* or unlike disease) was invented by the German physician and theorist Samuel Hahnemann (1775-1843) and used to describe the orthodox medical tradition of his time and to distinguish it from his own system of medical practice, which he termed *homeopathy* (from the Greek *homoin pathos* or similar disease). Since that time, the term *allopathic medicine* has been used interchangeably with *regular medicine, orthodox medicine, scientific medicine,* and *rational medicine.*[1,3,9] Weil concludes the following[3]:

> In Western, urban society, allopathy is the only form of medicine taken seriously. Backed by vast sums of money and the intellectual prestige of great universities, decked in all the trappings of modern laboratory science and supported by an impressive record of clinical success, allopathic medicine experts have an influence on our lives and thinking equal to that of law and religion.

The premise of allopathic medicine is its principle of treating illness, as opposed to the patient, primarily through methods structured to oppose or reduce the symptoms of malady and sickness. This idea is readily seen in the approach to healing by the use of antibiotics to eliminate certain microorganisms believed to be causally related to the symptoms of the illness. Antiinflammatory medications, antihypertensives, anticoagulants, and antidiuretics are also used to eliminate specific symptoms.

The center of contemporary allopathic practice is the widely accepted *germ theory* of disease that states that certain microscopic entities, because of their association in space and time with certain manifestations of sickness, are specifically causative of disease.[3,30] Scientists working within the allopathic paradigm are currently searching for pathogenic bases for chronic and degenerative conditions.

A primary contributor to the previously mentioned paradigm was Robert Koch, a 1905 Nobel Laureate and author of Koch's Postulates.[26] This allopathic dictum asserts that one must clearly and unquestionably reproduce the symptoms of the disease in an organism under controlled conditions. This was required to establish the causal relationship between a given microbe and a particular disease. To prove that an organism or agent caused a disease, Koch, who discovered the pathogen believed to cause tuberculosis, stated that a scientist had to do the following:

Identify the presence of the agent in every case of the disease.

Isolate the organism and grow it in the laboratory.

Show that the laboratory-grown sample caused the disease when it was injected into animals.

Reisolate the organism or toxin from the ailing laboratory animals.

Following this line of reasoning, infectious disease can presumably best be treated through allopathic methods intended to coerce these organisms out of existence.

The assumption that particular organisms directly cause certain disease states is the issue here. Although the observation and consummation of Koch's Postulates have been used to logically deduct a causal relationship between the presence of specific organisms in the body and the occurence of various physical symptoms of a disease, the experimental rigor required to demonstrate such effects in the laboratory arguably severely compromises the relevance of the data to the world and does no more than establish a correlative association between these observations.[26]

The allopathic position may be questioned when the workings of immunity are observed.[31,32] According to this view, many exogenous and endogenous factors patterned over time determine whether a particular disease will occur in a specific organism. Although some infectious agents usually produce a disease state, most fail to do so because a particular organism at a certain point in time may be capable of withstanding the specific demand. Disease may be said to occur by reciprocity of the host organism. This was observed by Claude Bernard when he wrote the following[33]:

> Illnesses hover constantly above us, their seeds blown by the wind, but they do not set in the terrain unless the terrain is ready to receive them.

D.D. Palmer wrote the following in 1910[25]:

> Health is the condition of the body in which all the functions are performed in a normal degree. If they are executed in too great or too little measure, just in that proportion will there be disease.

The issue is also raised that serves to underscore the active, participatory role of the organism in the disease process, not that the organisms attack the host but that something happens in the host that permits a breakdown of the immunity or the symbiotic relationship and harmonious balance between the host and the microbes in and around the host. Weil[4] writes the following:

> While antimicrobial agents have been considered the 'wonder drugs' of the 20th century, clinicians and researchers are now acutely aware that microbial resistance to drugs has become a major clinical problem . . . a variety of solutions have been proposed. The pharmaceutical industry is attempting to develop new agents that are less susceptible to current resistance mechanisms. In the inpatient setting, strict adherence to infection control procedure is essential. Health care workers need to understand that antimicrobial resistance is an accelerating problem in all practice settings that can directly compromise patient outcomes.

Linear thinking dominates Western medical philosophy and postulates that events occur in a series, similar to a line of billiard balls into a pocket, with one shot triggering reaction in a spatiotemporal sequence. Allopathy emphasizes a single cause that initiates a specific disease or pathologic event. Conversely, Eastern medicine teaches that if the doctor or individual recognizes an existing pattern of disharmony and reorganizes it into a harmonious pattern, the initiating cause will disappear because the conditions in which it materialized stop and no longer exist.

This interactive position represents a challenge to the present-day Newtonian mechanistic view-point of life and reality. The foundation for this scientific thinking originated in Aristotle's empirical materialism, which enjoyed renewed attention during the Rennaissance. According to Aristotle, reality came to mean that which could be substantiated materially. Matter was understood to be fixed and unchanging on any level, therefore real.[12]

The Near Past, the Present, and the Near Future

Around the same time B.J. Palmer was developing his school and modern chiropractic's place in the health care delivery system, something happened that had a much broader effect on practitioners of the chiropractic paradigm than any intraprofessional controversy.

About the same time B.J. Palmer was working to strengthen the new profession, general anarchy was occurring in American health care. A wide variety of philosophies and practices competed for the favor of the American public. Even in cases where practitioners had some professional education, schools and approaches varied widely, from "science-based" curriculum at prestigious universities, to many small proprietary schools, to apprenticeships. Graduates of all these systems called themselves *doctors*. Graduates of institutions such as Harvard, Yale, and Johns Hopkins had more status and an advantage in the marketplace over the graduates of less well-known and backed institutions, but legally little difference existed.[22]

Concluding that the system was in chaos, that many schools delivered substandard educations, and that in general a problem existed with the public's respect for and expectations of the medical profession, the Carnegie Foundation for the Advancement of Teaching published a report entitled *Medical Education in the United States and Canada*. This survey, known as the *Flexner Report* after its author, was a defining event in the history of American health care.[30]

The Flexner Report recommended a system of standardized training, licensing, and regulation. Subsequently, schools that met the Flexner standards were accredited and others were disqualified. Although this might be seen as a great advance in consumer protection, it was also a huge boon to Newtonian-oriented practices, while nonallopathic forms of health care were discounted and became more disorganized trying to get their messages heard. The Flexner Report, the product of a culture of industrialism and mass production standards, was urging a young, culturally insecure nation to apply those same standards to health care that they would to a factory product coming off the assembly line. Implicit in this recommendation is the suggestion that people are similar to clocks and fixing them is very mechanical, probably necessitating the products of other burgeoning factories.

From this point on, only graduates of the newly accredited schools were granted the medical doctor (MD) degree and allowed to apply for membership in the American Medical Association (AMA), which, because of the huge amounts of money and political power backing it through the older, prestigious schools, their graduates, and their industrial alliances, soon came as close to being a governmental agency as a private institution could come. Acceptable health care practices became those that conformed to what were considered the standards of Newtonian science, while the philosophies, concepts, and practices associated with unaccredited schools, despite their merit and pedigree, were in many cases ostracized into extinction, not the least of which was organized homeopathy.

Schools specializing in curricula such as osteopathy, chiropractic, homeopathy, and naturopathy and healing methods less known in the comparatively new nation could scarcely have been accredited by the standards established by the Flexner Report; therefore they were deemed unscientific and unacceptable. In addition to the economic problems created by this procrustian approach in terms of developing schools and practices and in obtaining much needed financing for research, the situation established by the Flexner Report made it almost impossible to become licensed in a world where the unlicensed practitioners, particularly the ones who were successful, were ever in danger of being arrested and imprisoned for practicing medicine without a license, regardless of the paradigm under which they were operating.

Although some groups such as the homeopaths all but disappeared and others such as the os-

teopaths altered their basic philosophies in the name of acceptance, chiropractors fought for their place in health care. Although the practice of chiropractic is now legal in every state, the perceived need among some doctors of chiropractic (DC) for acceptance as part of the medical community has led to great disagreement not only in terms of basic philosophy but also in terms of great confusion among clinicians and the public as to appropriate scope of practice. The ACC declaration is a start, but every student and practicing chiropractor needs to recall the story of the Flexner Report when the concept of standards of care is confused with standardization. The chiropractic community should avoid situations in which we cannot work within our paradigm to restore health to a world in increasing jeopardy from applying crisis methods to daily problems.

The reason philosophy and history of other concepts of health care and our own are important in chiropractic textbooks is worth considering. In most cases, everything we have learned about health and health care has been based solely on allopathic theory. Many people will live and die without any idea that this is only one of many systems and that it has risen to preeminent status in the Western world largely through the twin powers of finance and politics. The older and more basic concepts of health care are firmly secured in the idea of living beings as carefully balanced energic entities existing in synchronicity with the natural world. Quantum physics and research in high-energy particle physics have shown us that at the particle level, all matter is energy.[34]

People have a definite chemical structure that is certainly capable of being out of balance. However, the electromagnetic frequencies of our cells and the organization of those forces governs those chemical functions and processes. A mechanical aspect to our being certainly exists but surely no true student of science, let alone philosophy or history, could seriously ignore the knowledge of the past and the discoveries of modern physics and claim that at our core we are strictly well-designed machines.[35] Hopefully, this chapter will encourage you not to disparage linear concepts such as allopathy but see them in perspective as you prepare to practice a more holographic kind of health care delivery.

STUDY GUIDE

1. What is the Flexner Report and who commissioned it?
2. What is mechanism in terms of health care? Describe basic rationalist doctrine.
3. Describe the work of Descartes and Newton in promulgating the above theory.
4. What is vitalism? Discuss this in terms of Einstein and vibrational medicine and of D.D. Palmer and magnetic healing.
5. Discuss the Hippocratic concept of health.
6. Describe classical homeopathy.
7. What is Qi Hua? Explain this in terms of chiropractic.
8. Relate the acupuncture bladder meridian to the spinal nerves. How do they differ?
9. What are the chakras? Does anything exist in chiropractic or in standard neuroanatomy that relates to or coincides with them? What is Kundalini?
10. "Hidden in all energy is the working of a conscious will." Describe this in terms of vitalism, mechanism, and principle I.
11. What is the ACC's definition of subluxation?
12. Name three ancient civilizations with a history of using some form of purposeful spinal movement to improve health.
13. Working backwards, relate chiropractic to magnetic healing. How does this relate to the research of Justa Smith?
14. Although osteopathy and chiropractic may share some techniques, the philosophies differ. What is the philosophical basis of each paradigm?
15. Discuss the possible effects of disturbed movement at the coccyx in terms of chiropractic, ayurveda, and acupuncture.
16. What are Koch's Postulates and how might they relate to chiropractic philosophy?
17. Discuss immunity in terms of allopathy and chiropractic.
18. Discuss standards of care versus standardization. How do each of these affect the ethical, effective practice of chiropractic, acupuncture, homeopathy, osteopathy, and allopathy? Is it possible to establish one set of standards that would suit all of the above?
19. Why is it important for the general public to know about the existence, durability, and philosophy of all of these forms of health care?

REFERENCES

1. Grossinger R: *Plant medicine: from stone age shamanism to post-industrial healing,* Garden City, NY, 1980, Anchor Press.
2. Vithoulkas G: *The science of homeopathy,* New York, 1980, Grove Press.
3. Weil A: *Health & healing: understanding conventional and alternative medicine,* Boston, 1983, Hough Mifflin.
4. Weil A: *Spontaneous healing,* pp 40-67, New York, 1995, Ballantine Books.
5. Borysenko J: *Minding the body, mending the mind,* pp 9-27, New York, 1988, Bantam Books.
6. Wilcher CC et al: Beyond the mechanical subluxation: the science, art and philosophy of comprehensive chiropractic, *Digest of Chiropractic Economics 36* (2), 18-26, 1993.
7. Coulter HL: *Divided legacy: a history of the schism in medical thought,* vol I, Washington, 1977, Wehawkin Book Company.
8. Coulter HL: *Divided legacy: a history of the schism in medical thought,* Vol II, Washington,1977, Wehawkin Book Company.
9. Coulter HL: *Divided legacy: a history of the schism in medical thought,* Vol III, Washington, 1977, Wehawkin Book Company.
10. Pelletier KR: *Holistic medicine,* New York, 1979, Dell.
11. Masson JM, McCarthy S: *When elephants weep: the emotional lives of animals,* p 18, New York, 1995, Bantam Doubleday Dell Publishing Group.
12. Beinfield H, Korngold E: *Between heaven and earth . . . a guide to chinese medicine,* pp 3-33, New York, 1991, Ballantine Books.
13. Gerber R: *Vibrational medicine,* pp 40-43, 172, Sante Fe, 1988, Bear & Company.
14. Tiller W: Creating a new functional model of body healing energies, *J Holist Health* (4): 102-114, 1979.
15. Lyddon WJ: Emerging views of health: a challenge to rationalist doctrines of medical thought, *J Mind and Behav* 8 (3): 365-371.
16. Mann F: *Acupuncture: the ancient art of healing & how it works scientifically,* pp 1-5, 16-17, New York, 1973, Vintage Books.
17. Ping WW: *Chinese acupuncture,* Sussex, England, 1962, Health Science Press.
18. Leadbeater CW: *The chakras,* Wheaton, Ill, 1927, Theosophical Publishing House (reprint).

19. Frawley D: *Ayurvedic healing: a comprehensive guide,* Salt Lake City, 1989, Passage Press.
20. Rosenfield I: *Alternative medicine,* New York, 1996, Random House.
21. Haldeman S: *Modern developments in the principles and practice of chiropractic,* New York, 1980, Appleton-Century-Crofts.
22. Leach RA: *The Chiropractic theories, a synopsis of scientific research,* p 24, Baltimore, 1986, Williams & Wilkins.
23. Janse J, Houser RH, Wells BF: *Chiropractic principles and technic,* Chicago, 1947, National College of Chiropractic.
24. Palmer DD: *The adjuster,* Davenport, 1910, Palmer College.
25. Palmer DD: *The science, art & philosophy of chiropractic,* pp 15, 33-35, Portland, 1910, Portland Printing House Company.
26. Garrett L: *The coming plague,* pp 30-52, New York, 1994, Penguin Group.
27. Karoly P: *Measurement strategies in health psychology,* pp 3-45, New York, 1985, John Wiley & Sons.
28. Levy MR, Dignan M, Shirreffs JH: *Essentials of life and health,* p 8-22, New York, 1988, Random House.
29. Engle GL: The need for a new medical model: a challenge for biomedicine, *Science* (196): 120-136, 1977.
30. Janiger O, Goldberg P: *A different kind of healing,* pp 23-24, New York, 1994, Putnam Books.
31. Jemmott JB, Locke SE: Psychological factors, immunologic meditation, and human susceptibility to infectious disease: how much do we know? *Psych Bulletin* 95: 78-108, 1984.
32. Locke SE, Colligan D: *The healer within,* New York, 1987, Penguin Books.
33. Jaffe DT: *Healing from within,* p 19, New York, 1980, Knopf.
34. Capra F: *The Tao of physics,* Boston, 1991, Shambhala.
35. Castiglioni A: Neo-Hippocratic tendency of contemporary thought, *Med Life, XLI* 2:115-145, 1934.

CHAPTER 3

History of Legal Conflict

William S. Rehm, DC, HCD (hc)

The chiropractic profession came into a legal atmosphere that largely equated healing the sick with the practice of medicine. In such a climate, no distinction was made for technical or philosophic uniqueness. In choosing to become unique practitioners, the early chiropractors decided to clash with an adversary armed with the authority of the state.

In these circumstances, survival depended on gaining a public constituency and judicial and legislative recognition of the value of chiropractic as a separate and distinct health profession. Current disputes over whether chiropractic is to offer a unique form of total health care or a more limited role as a therapeutic modality can be cast from historic reflection on the struggle for survival.

Nineteenth Century Medicine

Early Problems

As the nation emerged from its colonial period into the era of Jacksonian expansionism, medicine had not yet recognized its considerable inadequacy. As Starr[1] observed, "The failure of doctors to establish any effective authority within the profession or in society at large profoundly affected their relationship with patients."

Because no standard existed for either medical education or its institutions, the profession intuitively adopted a caste system for ranking doctors. On the top rung were the so-called *elite* whose tenure was never questioned. They occupied the top rung for no particular distinction other than family name and wealth. They were generally the best-educated, had a collegiate background, and garnered credentials from better medical schools, often European. Occupying the middle rung were the *majority,* whose background and education were average. With perhaps 2 years of classwork plus apprenticeship, their medical diploma was not highly regarded by the elite. The last rung were the *autodidactics,* as Starr calls them. Their training consisted of a few months in a commercial school and apprenticeship, if any. This class of people were also known as *irregulars* and included the sectarians (homeopaths, eclectics, and others). They were generally disdained equally by the two higher groups. The considerable inequality between those who practiced medicine was so great that doctors cannot be said to have belonged to any particular social class, leading to increased social strain.[1]

Nineteenth century medicine had yet another serious flaw—it was too unspecialized. Except for the upper strata of society, those in need of medical care faced hard choices. As the population shifted away from the cities, the alternative for the lower class was often the undertrained, even self-styled doctor. A notable exception, especially in rural areas, were the bonesetters. Although they were few in number and were regarded contemptuously by regular practitioners, the unique talents of these folk healers were highly prized and greatly sought after by the public.

For the genuinely poor, their only real access to medical care was the charity hospital found in most larger cities, which was a carryover of rehabilitated Jacksonian consciousness of the plight of the American Indian. Because the poor areas were rarely attended by socially prominent physicians, if serious medicine was practiced there it was the exception. This undoubtedly contributed to the feeling that, as George Bernard Shaw[2] said, "The medical profession was an organized conspiracy against the common man."

Encouraged by the self-serving stratification of physicians by class, medicine's professional authority was virtually nonexistent. Just as the elite did not identify with the interests of other practitioners, professional organization languished. Without leverage over individual doctors, the orientation of all was "competitive rather than corporate."[1]

Consolidating Authority

The first effort to unify doctors came in 1846, in New York City, where a small group of concerned younger physicians discussed ways to rein in the seeming chaos within medicine by proposing standards for training, adopting a code of ethics, and constructing a platform for scholarly discourse. Thus the American Medical Association (AMA) was created.

However forthright the objectives of the AMA, it failed miserably for much of the half-century. The fiercely independent medical schools fought any notion of oversight and doctors continued their natural inclination to solve problems individually. "The forces pulling the profession apart prevailed over the common interests that might have held them together."[1]

Not the least of medicine's concerns was the rise of sectarianism. According to Gibbons,[3] the public began to turn on doctors:

> The public favored the alternative schools because of the acceptance of dissent in the new republic. 'As much as anything,' quoting Duffy, 'it was the public's decision to turn to the herbalists, homeopaths and other medical sects eschewing heroic practices which literally forced orthodox physicians to reconsider their position.'

As orthodoxy recognized in the growth of the dissident movement their own failures, these very divergents, with the sweet sense of acquittal, would help bring about stability in the profession. Submitting to public pressure, especially in New York, the AMA relaxed all sanctions against the dogmatic sectarian practitioners and allowed them into the association.

The surrender of orthodoxy still carries with it a remnant that even today causes most medical doctors (MDs) to bristle: the term *allopath*. It had

been coined by the followers of Hahnemann to remind regular medicine that it too had an exclusive dogma—cure by opposites, the reverse of homeopathy.[1]

Although many felt uneasy, the new accommodation allowed regulars and sectarians to focus their attention on mutual self-interest—protection against competition.

Gaining Control: Medical Licensing Laws

The concept of physician licensing soon gained new support, even though it was once scorned by the most successful as unnecessary and insulting and was feared by the less secure as a Trojan horse. In the 1870s and 1880s, the first statutes were minimal in their requirements. Only a medical school diploma was required. As state licensing evolved, the AMA was given authority to approve schools and reject diplomas. Finally, all candidates would have to not only acquire an acceptable diploma but also complete a state-approved examination. (In West Virginia, this would lead to the first, but unsuccessful, court challenge of licensing authority.) By 1901, no state existed without a licensing statute.

In 1919, the AMA declared that although states have the right to protect the public, they cannot judge any profession's claims of legitimacy as follows[4]:

> The Supreme Courts hold without exception, from the Supreme Court of the United States to that of the youngest state, that the sole justification for the enactment of medical practice acts is the protection of the public from incompetent and unscrupulous persons; that the state has the right to enact laws creating any reasonable standards for this privilege that the object of such laws is not the protection or the benefit of physicians but the protection of the public; that it is not the function of the state to decide scientific questions of the relevant value of one school or method of practice as compared with another; but to establish and enforce reasonable regulations for the protection of the public; that the qualifications and conditions enacted must be reasonable and must be the same for all those who desire the same privilege; and that the function of examining boards is to test the qualifications and knowl-

edge of the applicant in order to determine whether he may be entrusted with the treatment of the sick without public danger.

Wardwell describes an interesting dilemma: Although the AMA willingly ceded some regulation of the profession, neither the state nor the courts had authority to evaluate competing claims of more than one school or method of practice. Left to state regulatory agencies, the question then became,[4] "Which schools are to be represented on these boards and given power to administer the licensing machinery?" This was often a purely political decision.

The First Challenge

The courts and the legislatures now supported the medical profession. The first crucial test to licensing authority occurred in 1888, when the issue came before the U.S. Supreme Court in the legal case, *Dent v. West Virginia*.

In this case, the state had refused to recognize the credentials of Frank Dent, an eclectic physician, under the 1882 medical statute requiring the applicant to possess a degree from a reputable medical college, pass an examination, or prove that he had been in the state for the previous 10 years. Dent had been practicing for 6 years.

The Court's unanimous opinion, which would become a precedent in such matters, held that although every citizen had the right to follow any lawful calling: the state had the right to protect society by imposing conditions for the exercise of that right, as long as they are imposed on everyone and were reasonably related to the occupation in question. In their decision, the Court said that "reasonable" meant excluding persons from medical licensure who did not qualify to the letter of the law.[1,4,5]

Chiropractic Confronts Medical Domination

The first state laws governing healing, which usually excluded dentists and clergy, recognized only a generic medicine. By definition, medicine was assumed to be inclusive and, therefore, all practitioners were assumed to be similar. Existing statutes made no provision at all for technical or philosophic uniqueness. As the new alternative schools of osteopathy and chiropractic made their appearance in the latter nineteenth century, states had no way of distinguishing their claims to autonomy. "An appeal to state legislatures for separate licensing seemed to be the only safe route to survival."[5]

The founder of chiropractic, D.D. Palmer, was unequivocally opposed to licensure. He believed that because he was the discoverer and had established the principles of chiropractic and its standards of training, no one else should have the right to judge.

Early in 1905, Minnesota chiropractors Dan Riesland and Solon Massey Langworthy of the American School of Chiropractic (ASC), had successfully shepherded a chiropractic licensing bill through the Minnesota legislature, then to await only the governor's signature. But Palmer personally intervened, persuading the governor to veto the profession's first licensing act. Palmer's reaction was as follows[6]:

> Too bad—after Riesland had spent the winter and some cash, when the fruits of his labor were about to fall into his hands—for 'Old Chiro' to stick his foot in the bill and upset the school proposition.

A number of D.D. Palmer's earliest followers modified his vitalistic concepts for a mechanistic approach to chiropractic as a spinal speciality.[5] The most important of these early dissidents were Solon Massey Langworthy, Oakley Smith, and Minora Paxson of the ASC. The ASC's therapeutic philosophy was that spinal compression at the intervertebral foramina or spinal windows contributed to failing health and could be relieved and even reversed through mechanical stretching, or spinal traction. This was a fundamental departure from Palmer's belief of hand-fixing.

In 1904, the ASC had also implemented a more vigorous curriculum of 20 months as opposed to Palmer's course of 4 months or less and began publishing the profession's first serious journal, *Backbone*.[7] That Langworthy and his associates would be anathema to Palmer and that he would so vigorously oppose a licensing law based on teachings contrary to his own is not a surprise.

Palmer had assumed a proprietary right of ownership, believing that his accumulated knowledge in the various fields of healing he had studied created an entirely new field of practice, both in theory and application.[8]

Osteopathy's Rebuke

Gibbons wrote the following[3]:

> Inevitably, the two manipulative schools came into conflict with each other, while the regulars pointed disdainfully at the 'new sectarians' who had rejected, they declared, the fundamentals of science and the biological truths that now fueled a medicine flush with power, influence, and increasing public favor.

When D.D. Palmer announced his discovery in his 1897 broadside *The Chiropractic,* osteopathy immediately assumed a belligerent attitude. The *Journal of Osteopathy* denounced him as the following and threatened legal action[9]:

> (Palmer is a) fake Magnetic Healer in Iowa who issues a paper devoted to his new system; and until recently made up his entire publication from the contents of the *Journal of Osteopathy* . . . It is to shut off such frauds from the use of Osteopathic literature that the *Journal* has been copyrighted.

Osteopathy had also assumed a right of ownership of manipulative healing. Only later, Lerner suggests, did they realize that they had no such rights under law; they realized that the only way to gain protection was through special laws that at the same time would prohibit others from engaging in similar practice.[9] Thus, osteopathy would also become chiropractic's legislative adversary.

Gibbons concluded the following[3]:

> Surgery, obstetrics, and materia medica soon became standard at the Kirksville (Mo.) mother school and at others that had mushroomed across the country. The 'Old Doctor' (A.T. Still) protested about the 'medicalization' of his osteopathy but, by the time he died (in 1917), few osteopaths would claim to be 'drugless' physicians using spinal manipulation only.

In time, osteopathy would become indistinguishable from medicine, in both scope and philosophy.

Is Chiropractic Medicine?

The answer to the above question of whether chiropractic is medicine ultimately depended on legal interpretation, but in 1906, Palmer preferred jail rather than submit to the argument. "Chiropractors have no desire to practice medicine, surgery or obstetrics," was his only defense.[10] However, chiropractic came to recognize the necessity of legislative protection for its survival and, disagreeing with Palmer, declared that the profession must be established as a separate and distinct branch of the healing arts. In contrast, D.D. Palmer did not believe that chiropractic was a branch of healing.

The Wisconsin Case

Japanese-born Shegataro Morikubo, a 1906 Palmer School graduate, seemed unlikely to be indelibly linked with shaping the early history of chiropractic, yet became the central figure in a courtroom drama that would establish chiropractic legal defense for decades.

On July 22, 1907, the State of Wisconsin brought charges against Morikubo for violating statutes in medicine, surgery, and osteopathy. The reason for Morikubo being targeted was clear. The state had brought a case against him it felt could be won quickly. He was a newcomer in the city of La Crosse and had openly advertised his illegal services. The La Crosse *Tribune's* subtle racism as seen by the use of the pejorative word *Jap* to describe Morikubo, made his situation seem ominous.[11]

Quick to respond to Morikubo's plea for assistance, Dr. B.J. Palmer, D.D. Palmer's son, arrived in La Crosse within a day to arrange a legal defense. Having assumed the presidency of the Palmer School of Chiropractic (PSC), Palmer was also secretary of the new Universal Chiropractors' Association (UCA), formed in Davenport, Iowa a year earlier to represent the Palmer Infirmary, then under indictment in Iowa. The Morikubo case would be the UCA's first trial under fire.

Palmer's first task was to find a local attorney to represent the client at his arraignment and devise a trial defense. It would not be a difficult search.

Tom Morris, senior partner of the La Crosse firm of Morris and Hartwell, was a household name in Wisconsin. He had served as the La

Crosse County district attorney from 1900 to 1904 and was currently serving in the legislature. At the arraignment, Morris pled his client "not guilty of violating any state law" and agreed to a trial date of August 13, 1907, which was only 3 weeks away.

It was obvious to Morris that the state seemed to have the advantage. Legal precedent existed on which to build the case because the only other chiropractor ever arrested for practicing medicine without a license, Palmer, had chosen not to defend himself. Morris also realized that he would have difficulty explaining why the founder was on record as opposing any state regulation of chiropractic.

The salvation of this case would not be the expert testimony of B.J. Palmer, who had never before testified in a legal defense, but in the scholarly writings of S.M. Langworthy, the arch enemy and chief rival of both D.D. Palmer and B.J. Palmer.

A 1906 textbook, *Modernized Chiropractic*, coauthored by Langworthy, Smith, and Paxson, and the only current published work explaining the theory and practice of chiropractic, provided a working formula to save the profession[12]:

> Many of the most learned authorities in the medical ranks maintain marked differences in their pathological hypotheses, but because of such differences it does not follow that they are of different schools. That which is the real foundation of a "separate school of healing" is its philosophy, its practice, the science and art, all of which is peculiar to itself.

As Langworthy indicated, for Palmer to announce the discovery of a new science was not enough; the new science should be supplemented with its own philosophy. *Modernized Chiropractic* purported to establish for the first time the ideas of "a correct philosophy, a well-developed technique, and a reliable and extensive system of correction."[13] Through Langworthy, Morris would be able to define the philosophic and technical differences between chiropractic and any other healing art. He could present evidence that the brain and not the blood, as the osteopathic and allopathic philosophies stated, was the source of the "unseen power in the body." Langworthy's meticulous demonstration of the spinal windows and the interconnections of the autonomic nervous system

and possible aberrations of health and well-being would allow Morris to explain the effects of the chiropractic adjustment as opposed to other spinal techniques.[13]

When the trial began and the indictments were read, Morris asked the court to dismiss the charges of practicing medicine and surgery without a license because Morikubo obviously used only spinal manipulation. Not suspecting a trap, the prosecution agreed. Morris would now be able to show convincingly that chiropractic and osteopathy were vastly different and, therefore, his client could not be barred from practice.

The prosecution became increasingly defensive as Morris pushed his argument that only chiropractic recognized the supremacy of the nervous system, as Langworthy had first stated in his 1904 journal. To refute the state's expert witness testimony that D.D. Palmer had pilfered Still's osteopathy, Morris produced the sworn affidavit of A.P. Davis, DO, DC, who had studied under both founders, renouncing the charge. Morikubo and B.J. Palmer were effective as they demonstrated that the techniques of chiropractic spinal adjustment were unique.

After 2 days of testimony, a jury of 4 deliberated for less than 30 minutes. On August 15, 1907, Morikubo was acquitted.[13]

Although the Morikubo verdict did not lead directly to legalization of chiropractic in Wisconsin, it served to lessen the hostility of the law. An informal state registration would require chiropractors to post signs in their offices advising the public that, "This office is not licensed in Wisconsin," until a separate licensing board was established in 1925.[14]

Kansas v. Hall

The Kansas Board of Medical Registration & Examination was created in 1909 to replace a loosely charged board appointed by the governor 8 years earlier to nominally register the state's growing number of medical practitioners. Exempting only dentists and ordained ministers, the previous medical practice act specified that "all healing is the practice of medicine."[15] Thus the sectarian practices of osteopathy and chiropractic would be subject to the law. The new statute grandfathered in osteopaths already in practice but allowed no such accommodation for the dozen or so chiropractors operating in Kansas at the time. In fact, few state lawmakers were even aware of the profession. As far as the medical board was concerned, chiropractic was part of osteopathy, an interpretation to be upheld by the state supreme court in 1911.[15]

Irving B. Hall, a 1910 graduate of the PSC, had settled in the open Western prairie of Scott City, the county seat and center of a scattered population numbering about 2000. He began practice as the only chiropractor in a four-county area. His reputation quickly grew, and the resentment of Scott County's three medical doctors became apparent.[15]

On December 22, 1910, *The Scott Republican* announced that the three physicians had formed a county medical society for "the protection of their rights and interests, and the elevation and strengthening of the medical profession of Scott County."[15] The press notice also advised that the society would assist the State Board of Medical Registration & Examination in the "vigorous prosecution of any and all violators of the state law."[15] As warned, in January 1911, the secretary of the Scott County Medical Society filed three warrants against I.B. Hall, the county's only chiropractor.[15]

Hall was not the first doctor of chiropractic (DC) to face prosecution in Kansas. Under the previous law, virtually every known chiropractor in the state had been either warned or arrested, some choosing to leave rather than accept prosecution. This trial, however, would attract inordinate attention.

The defense was handled by Tom Morris, the same attorney who had so successfully defended Morikubo in Wisconsin. The firm of Morris & Hartwell, now chief counsel of the UCA, had by now become the chief defenders for many a beleaguered chiropractor in trouble with the law.

In a boisterous, hot, and overcrowded courtroom, with sympathies decidedly on the defendant's side, opening arguments began on April 20, 1911. Reportedly, about 100 spectators who could not be seated listened to the proceedings at open windows.

The state's case consisted of testimony from three reluctant witnesses, to show that the defendant had performed medical services, and two of the three members of the Scott County Medical Society. Testifying for the defense were Hall and the so-called *big three* of the UCA team: Dr. B.J.

Palmer; Dr. Alfred Walton, a graduate of Harvard Medical School and the PSC; and Dr. Lee W. Edwards, a graduate of the University of Nebraska medical department and the PSC. Similar to the Morikubo case, Hall's defense was constructed to show that he could not be in violation of any state law because no evidence existed that he had made a medical diagnosis or claim. The charge of practicing osteopathy was also spurious because the theory and practice of chiropractic was demonstrably unique from osteopathy, as was shown in the Wisconsin trial.

Trying his first case since being elected, the county prosecutor seemed bewildered by the well-prepared defense argument. After closing statements on the second day, the jury took 30 minutes to return a verdict for acquittal.[15]

The Hall trial became a touchstone for chiropractic in Kansas as it clearly demonstrated the public's feelings that the profession had a right to exist on its own merits, separate and distinct. Still, the profession remained in a curious predicament. The Kansas Supreme Court's reaffirmation of the law relative to the practice of osteopathy caused the *Stafford Courier* to ponder the following dilemma[16]:

> The law recognizes medicine, surgery and osteopathy, but does not specifically recognize chiropractic. The court held that the law included chiropractors, but there is no way (they) can get licenses to practice. . . . Until the court handed down its decision, the chiropractors held that they did not come under the present law. But when the court held that they were under the jurisdiction of the board, the board refuses to give them licenses and they are not permitted to practice without licenses.

Hall's highly publicized acquittal became a ready-made public relations tool for the chiropractic profession. In June 1911, the Kansas Chiropractic Association (KCA) presented the following petition to Governor Stubbs signed by 10,000 Kansas citizens imploring him to support chiropractic legislation in the next legislative session and to end state-supported oppression against the profession[17]:

> The monster bill that has been circulated asks that Gov. Stubbs issue an executive order permitting chiropractors to practice in Kansas

pending the next session of the legislature, when the amendment can be made to the existing laws. In addition to this petition, Gov. Stubbs is receiving dozens of letters on the subject from every part of Kansas.

The overwhelming support for legislation could not be reversed.

Legislation and Enactment: Kansas, 1913-1915

In 1913, Kansas became the first jurisdiction anywhere to officially legalize chiropractic but appointing a board of examiners would become the next serious controversy. The new chiropractic law had specified that board appointees must have reputably practiced in the state for 2 years. Practicing "reputably" would mean *legally,* something the attorney general, who made no secret of his disdain for chiropractic, would insist could not be done: "It is not possible for the governor to find persons in Kansas who have the qualifications prescribed by the Act."[15] The resulting stalemate effectively deadlocked the executive branch.

Further confounding the dilemma, the attorney general ruled that because the chiropractic law was unenforceable, an amendment carefully placed into the 1913 legislation exempting chiropractors from the medical law was null and void and that the state's chiropractors were subject to prosecution under the laws of 1909. The KCA appealed the ruling to the supreme court. All either side could do was wait for the court's opinion, although this did not stop the medical board's threats.

Despite the temporary forced truce, one more legal skirmish unfolded. The State Board of Osteopathic Registration & Examination, which the current legislature had made an independent entity, believed it had authority to prosecute chiropractors for infringement into its field of practice. One action was filed but was dismissed.

The high court's long-anticipated decision was not announced until the last days of the 1914 session. It agreed with the state's argument that all chiropractors in practice without a license from the medical board were violating the law and therefore none were legally eligible for appointment to the new chiropractic board. Concurrently, the clause in the new medical practice law ex-empting chiropractors was ruled to be valid. The insertion of that clause had proved to be a brilliant strategy on the part of the KCA as it averted disaster for the profession in Kansas. All that was now necessary to legally seat a chiropractic board was to wait the prescribed 2 years. Credit for plotting the successful KCA legislative approach would go to their Oklahoma neighbor, the legendary Willard Carver, LLB, DC.

As expected during the 1915 legislature, the medical interests did their best to void the chiropractic law, but on March 19 it was overwhelmingly ratified. A board of chiropractic examiners could now be seated. Although Kansas and North Dakota were the first two states to pass chiropractic legislation in 1913, Arkansas, which passed its law in 1915, was the first state to actually issue chiropractic licenses.

The great Kansas debate, however tumultuous, was settled in the most orderly way possible, through the mundane process of the law. Despite the highly charged emotional atmosphere, the early Kansas chiropractors practiced as competent professionals, winning the case for chiropractic with thorough planning, calm, and reason.

Lessons from Oklahoma

One of the most extraordinary exercises of political chicanery occurred in 1917, when chiropractic activist and private citizen Willard Carver was jailed for contempt of the Oklahoma senate. This remarkable saga began in 1908, during the first legislative session of the forty-seventh state.

As Jackson[18] recounts, the legislature had explicitly defined what constitutes the practice of medicine and granted enforcement authority to a board of physicians. Unlike osteopathy, which was recognized and defined with limited privileges, chiropractic had received no mention in the proposed law. The newly formed Oklahoma Chiropractic Association (OCA) received legislative help from Carver and succeeded in having the medical bill amended to gain exemption from prosecution for chiropractors. He later accomplished this in Kansas as well. Simultaneously, an OCA-sponsored chiropractic bill seemed certain to pass.

When the session ended, the OCA bill became lost in limbo, and the medical bill, now ready for final enactment, was not a part of the chiropractic amendment. Carver charged that a breach had occurred and demanded that either the exemption clause be restored or the medical bill be declared invalid. Through the governor's personal intervention, the bill was correctly repaired and signed into law.[18] Although Oklahoma now had a medical practice act, chiropractors were protected from prosecution. Chiropractors would fail to gain legislation for many years, but the protection clause was a satisfactory beginning.

In 1917, a chiropractic bill again appeared close to success. Legislators also introduced a revised medical practice act in this session, and again the OCA rebutted with a protection amendment, which the medical lobby argued was redundant. Carver and the OCA agreed to concede in exchange for a guarantee of nonintervention on its bill. In the end, however, the bargain proved worthless. While passing the new medical legislation without complications, the senate soundly defeated the OCA bill. Chiropractors would likely be left without protection from prosecution.

An outraged Carver next bought a newspaper advertisement with his own funds, accusing key senators of double-crossing and accepting bribes to defeat the chiropractic bill. Whether his charges had any merit, Carver managed to inform the public of the possibility of legislative malfeasance with a heated controversy reported by every paper in the state.[18]

As expected, the senate leadership acted quickly against Carver, issuing an arrest warrant charging him with contempt of the senate. Without benefit of the sheriff, Carver presented himself to the senate leadership to answer his charges, pleading "not guilty."[18]

Unprecedented in state legislative affairs, a trial proceeded before the entire body. Because he had offered no other defense besides his plea of innocence, Carver was convicted by (senate) resolution. For his perceived insurgence, he was fined $500 and sentenced to 10 days in the county jail. The senate continued its attacks. According to Jackson, "every judge in the state was contacted verbally and warned not to accept any writs from Carver, else they would face impeachment."[18]

Realizing what the profession faced without the benefit of a protective clause in the medical practice act, the OCA was able to acquire more than the 14,000 signatures required to petition the new medical act to referendum. When lobbyists attempted to block the petition, the supreme court ruled the initiative was legal, and the act was placed on the November 2, 1920 ballot for citizens to vote on. The court action also delayed implementation of the medical bill. When the votes were finally counted, the bill was defeated overwhelmingly.[18]

When the 1921 legislature convened, the pretense, rancor, suspicion, and deal-making were gone. Oklahoma's first chiropractic practice act was passed by acclamation on February 21.

Commonwealth v. Zimmerman

Precedent law established in *Dent v. West Virginia* became the most frequently cited opinion for denying an individual a medical license for cause (see p. 21). In 1914, Boston chiropractor J.O. Zimmerman tested this precedent in the Massachusetts Supreme Judicial Court after he lost a lower court appeal of his conviction for unlicensed medical practice. Simultaneously, he challenged the constitutionality of the medical statute that required the chiropractor to be tested in materia medica while exempting osteopaths.

In 1915, the court again relied on *Dent v. West Virginia* when it denied Zimmerman constitutional challenge. The court said further that even if practitioners only engage in analysis, palpation, and spinal adjustment they may still appear to practice medicine[4,19]:

> Although the defendant did not prescribe medicine and testified that he paid no attention to the patient's description of disease or symptoms, yet it is obvious that his purpose is to treat the human body in order to make natural that which he found abnormal in the narrow field of his examination.

The Zimmerman case is an important document for the following two reasons: (1) it became a precedent for legal discrimination against chiropractic and (2) it emphasized that, no matter how illogic its argument, a destructive judicial mindset can be set in motion. Such an antichiropractic mindset was again betrayed in Massachusetts in 1955 when a district court judge who was sentencing a miscreant chiropractor said on the record, "The medical men of this state should be protected."[20] Not until 1968 did the legislature finally approve a chiropractic licensing law.

As difficult as the law once was for chiropractic in Massachusetts, it may have been worse in Louisiana.

England v. Board of Medical Examiners

The vulnerability of chiropractic was demonstrated in the long, bitter, and frustrating confrontation known as *The England case*.

On March 22, 1965, trial testimony in *Jerry R. England et al v. Louisiana State Board of Medical Examiners et al* finally began in the U.S. District Court, nearly 8 years after the action had been filed. The plaintiffs were 40 chiropractors seeking injunctive relief from continued enforcement of the Louisiana Medical Practice Act, which they alleged was unconstitutional.

The critical issues being contested were those decided by the Louisiana Supreme Court in 1927[21] and reaffirmed by the same court in 1951. The following decisions were made[22]:

1. A chiropractor practices medicine and so must obtain certification by diploma and examination.
2. The right to practice medicine is one granted on condition.
3. The state may regulate the practice of medicine and surgery within reasonable bounds, by defining qualifications of the practitioner.
4. A chiropractor is not deprived of liberty and property without due process of law as the Medical Practice Act requires him to first qualify as to materia medica and surgery because, though they are not used in chiropractic, they bear a relation to medicine (generally).
5. The legislature having reasonable discretion as to whether a particular school of medicine should be recognized, a chiropractor is not deprived of equal protection of the law by being unjustly discriminated against because he is not exempt, as are osteopaths, dentists and pharmacists, from qualifying in materia medica and surgery for practice.
6. The legislature is not bound to recognize every school of medicine.

What the state high court had ruled, in essence, was that applying arbitrary standards to chiropractic under the medical practice laws was not unreasonable even while allowing exemptions for certain other groups. Overturning such a faulty opinion, especially in the "enlightened" 1950s, should have seemed a straightforward constitutional matter.

That the England case would require such a withering journey only underscored the difficul-

ties the profession had endured in Louisiana for so many years, a predicament so severe that Dr. Clarence W. Weiant, dean of the Chiropractic Institute of New York, once characterized it as follows[23]:

> We in the other states have long thought of Louisiana as the darkest spot on the chiropractic map, the home of a hopelessly submerged handful of chiropractors foolhardy enough to think they could succeed under utterly impossible conditions.

J. Minos Simon (pronounced Me-nass See-mone), a dynamic New Orleans trial attorney, was hired by the England group in 1955. Simon's plan was to attack the medical examining board based on its arbitrary refusal to recognize a diploma from an approved chiropractic college was unconstitutional.[24] (At the time, the National Chiropractic Association [NCA] and the ICA, as accrediting agencies for chiropractic colleges, published lists of such institutions.) He warned that the task ahead would be difficult and expensive, but even Simon could not foresee the improbable possibility of an 8-year trial.

The suit was filed in the Federal District Court of Eastern Louisiana in May 1957. Although it was not named as a defendant, the Louisiana Medical Society appeared in the complaint as an intervenor. The court agreed that none of the 40 plaintiffs would be subjected to any reprisal from the state for engaging in practice during the duration of the trial. Arrests actually intensified for non-plaintiff chiropractors. Total prohibition against all forms of chiropractic advertising, including in the telephone directory, would continue.[25]

After legal wrangling in various trial and appeals' courts, the U.S. District Court dismissed for the third time the complaint on the grounds that it was without authority to review state law.[26-29]

On January 12, 1964, the U.S. Supreme Court reversed and sent the case back to the state court "on the merits of appellants' Fourteenth Amendment claims."[30] The length of the litigation to this point was not unnoticed by Justice William O. Douglas, who wrote the following[30]:

> This case was started in May 1957, and here we are nearly seven years later without a decision on the merits. This seems an unnecessary price to pay for our federalism.

Jurisdiction had finally been settled, with the England case back were it began in the U.S. District Court of Eastern Louisiana, this time for trial. Exhibits would now be shown and witness testimony would be heard.

The task of the plaintiffs would be to show that the precedent of *Fife v. West Virginia* no longer applied because "enormous progress has been made in the healing arts."[31] The court was unable to rule, without a full evidentiary hearing on the merits, whether chiropractic "is no more entitled to recognition today than it was thirty-odd years ago."[31]

Three days of testimony was heard by the three-judge federal panel. On November 9, 1965, the court denied the complaint and dismissed the England case. The three judges ruled that the Louisiana legislature requiring chiropractors to comply with the provisions of the Medical Practice Act was not irrational or unreasonable.

In denying the complaint, the court seemed to be negatively swayed by chiropractic's own acknowledged shortcomings: lack of educational accreditation, even by the ACA; absence of uniformity in its educational process; and undemonstrated validity of its claims to successfully treat a wide range of conditions, including visceral disease. The following ruling was made[31]:

> If the education obtained in chiropractic schools does not meet the standards of the American Chiropractic Association and the United States Office of Education, it may well be that the legislature of Louisiana felt that in the public interest a diploma from an approved medical school should be required of a chiropractor before he is allowed to treat all the human ailments chiropractors contend can be cured by manipulation of the spine. Other considerations, suggested by the record of this case, possibly affecting the legislative judgment could be stated. Suffice it to say that on this record we are unable to hold that the legislature . . . has acted irrationally and unreasonably. . . . It may well be that chiropractic is a useful profession and that the requirement of a medical education for chiropractors is not in the public interest. But the balancing of the advantages and disadvantages of this requirement is for the legislature.

The trial transcript revealed that the defense was also tough on chiropractic research and unsupported claims to successfully treat a large spectrum of conditions, including systemic disease.[32] The courts, of course, were never expected to decide the merits of scientific and technical claims and did not do so in this case.

In its criticism of chiropractic education, the court apparently failed to recognize that current lack of accreditation was not because of the profession's indifference, but rather a technicality. The Commission on Accreditation of the National Chiropractic Association and the NCA became nonexistent in the 1963 reorganization that created the ACA. During the England trial, a new accrediting mechanism was not yet in place.

If any consolation resulted from the long, frustrating trial in Louisiana, it was the growing grassroots support for chiropractic legislation. In the decade that followed, not only did Louisiana chiropractors gain populist backing but also political clout. In 1974, the Louisiana legislature finally created a chiropractic licensing law. Louisiana was the last state to accomplish this.

Promise and Pitfalls of Legislation

The ultimate purpose of legislative oversight in the healing arts is to serve both the ideals of professional freedom and the public interest. What chiropractic needed, Moore wrote, was friendly licensing laws that allowed "autonomous licensing boards with total independence from state medical and educational authorities."[5]

Osteopathic-style legislation was the model chiropractic wanted to avoid: composite boards, as frequently happened, that permitted control from outside the profession. As chiropractic and medicine were so fundamentally opposed in theory and practice, many viewed composite boards as the road to oblivion. In retrospect, the infamous Stanford Report of 1960 recommended abolishment of the California chiropractic board, closing of chiropractic colleges, and medical upgrading of DCs already in practice, as had been done with osteopathy.[33]

Chiropractors were not always able to secure ideal legislation, which would protect philosophic autonomy[5]:

> Indiana, New Jersey and West Virginia . . . proved to be difficult states for chiropractic applicants because of composite boards with physician members (vastly) outnumbering chi-

ropractors. Colorado, Illinois and Virginia provided no distinct chiropractic board and granted chiropractic licenses only through medical boards without (at one time) chiropractic representation.

A more serious drawback for chiropractic was the insistence on basic science laws, enacted in 21 states and the District of Columbia between 1925 and 1950. These laws, admittedly enacted to exclude chiropractors and osteopaths from licensure,[34] required medical, osteopathic, and chiropractic applicants to pass examinations in the various basic sciences given under the auspices of the state university before they could be admitted to a licensing examination. At first, the laws had their intended effect. However, chiropractic colleges complied with upgraded basic science curricula. By 1980, all such laws were rescinded as redundant and intrusive.

Most chiropractic laws were enacted before 1930 and proved to be justified and agreeable for everyone (Figure 3-1). Only Illinois, Kansas, and Virginia still have composite boards.

Medical Subversion

Despite autonomous statutes, chiropractic was not immune from attempts by organized medicine, and even the state, to subvert the law. One of the more egregious examples occurred in Colorado.

Spears v. Board of Health

A case that may best illustrate power of the state is the 7-year licensing battle in which the Colorado Supreme Court established that the State Board of Health had acted illegally in trying to close Spears Chiropractic Hospital.

The lengthy Spears case began in February 1943, when the newly constructed 200-bed Denver hospital, anticipating an April opening, applied for a hospital license. After first ignoring the application, the board proceeded to cite Spears for numerous alleged building code violations, even though the county had found none. Next, on virtually the eve of the announced opening, the board demanded the chiropractic hospital construct surgical and obstetric facilities to qualify

Before 1920				
Kansas	1913		Maine	1923
North Dakota	1913		Florida	1923
Arkansas	1913		Tennessee	1923
Oregon	1915		Utah	1923
Nebraska	1915		Wyoming	1924
Colorado	1915		Hawaii	1925
Ohio	1915		Wisconsin	1925
North Carolina	1917		West Virginia	1925
Connecticut	1917		Missouri	1927
Montana	1918		Rhode Island	1927
Vermont	1919		Indiana	1927
Minnesota	1919		District of Columbia	1929
Idaho	1919			
Washington	1919		**1930-1939**	
			South Carolina	1932
			Michigan	1933
1920-1929			Delaware	1937
New Jersey	1920		Alaska	1938
Kentucky	1920			
Maryland	1920			
Arizona	1921		**After 1939**	
New Mexico	1921		Texas	1949
New Hampshire	1921		Pennsylvania	1951
Georgia	1922		Alabama	1960
California	1922		New York	1963
Virginia	1922		Massachusetts	1966
Nevada	1923		Mississippi	1973
Illinois	1923		Louisiana	1974

Figure 3-1 Timeline of U.S. chiropractic licensing laws.

for licensure, effectively postponing the opening. With all ancillary demands met, Spears refiled the application. Hearing nothing from the Board of Health, hospital founder Leo Spears, DC proceeded with the newly announced May 1 opening without a license. In response, the board issued a warrant to seize and close the hospital.[35]

On September 27, 1943, after Spears obtained an injunction, the board issued a "provisional temporary permit" for operation of a sanitarium. In 1946, the so-called *license* was revoked. Spears filed for a review of revocation in January 1947, but appealed to the supreme court after it was denied.[35]

In its attack on Spears Sanitarium, the health board alleged that the temporary permit had been violated because minor surgery was performed, medicine and drugs were administered, people with contagious diseases were admitted and treated, and the hospital name was used illegally. In truth, the medical procedures were performed or prescribed by licensed osteopathic physicians, a limited outbreak of scarlet fever was properly quarantined, and the name *hospital* was only used casually.[35] (The signs on the buildings specifically designated *Spears Sanitarium*.)

On July 1, 1950, the Colorado Supreme Court unanimously sided with Spears in a lengthy opinion that supported the following legal conclusions:

1. The state legislature says that chiropractic is a lawful method of treatment and that its practitioners have a legal right to be licensed and to build hospitals.
2. Any rules and regulations the state health board makes governing chiropractic hospitals must be reasonable and not contrary to law.
3. The law requires that permanent licenses shall be issued to hospitals showing a fitness to conduct the institutions, and that they may be revoked solely by reason of not complying with requirements and the act and rules and regulations of the board.
4. The Board of Health did not issue a license in fact to the Spears institution, but merely issued what amounted to an unauthorized provisional permit, not signed by the president of the board or attested to by the board secretary.
5. Conditions of such a permit "are not set up as rules or standards for chiropractic sanitariums generally, but are arbitrary and discriminatory restrictions against the applicant alone."[36]

Regarding the board's contention that practices at Spears Sanitarium unlawful in the state, the court decided the following[37]:

There is not a sentence in the license issued which follows the statute on which it is based. . . . We cannot apply the rule that where the license contains invalid provisions it constitutes a valid license. . . . Instead of pursuing its statutory authority, the Board of Health attempted to usurp the functions of the legislature, and set up law of its own.

The court's decree instructed the Colorado Board of Health to issue Spears a valid hospital license retroactive to September 27, 1943, when the bitter dispute began.[35]

The Wilk Case

In the mid-1970s, Dr. Chester A. Wilk of Chicago and four other chiropractors filed a class-action suit in the seventh U.S. Circuit Court of Illinois charging the AMA and 10 other medical groups of conspiring to violate the Sherman Antitrust Act of the United States by conducting an illegal boycott in restraint of trade directed at chiropractors in an effort to contain and destroy the profession.[38] In litigation for some 16 years before it was fully concluded in the plaintiffs' favor, *the Wilk Case* as it became known, was by far the most important challenge chiropractic had ever mounted against medical domination.

Essentially, trial testimony and evidence revealed that the defendants had conspired to undermine both the public's confidence in chiropractic and proper doctor-patient relationships[39]:

One of the many practices of the AMA that came out at trial was the effort of . . . member physicians to subvert the customary handling of referrals made by chiropractors. The protocol of a referral between health professionals is ordinarily one in which the patient is sent to a specialist who sees the patient, suggests appropriate diagnosis and treatment, and then sends the patient to the referring physician. Instead,

AMA physicians were encouraged to give patients referred to them by chiropractors a 'quack pack,' which was used to discourage the patient from returning to the chiropractor. These clearly anti-competitive activities successfully denied patients both chiropractic services and the advantage of a team containing both medical and chiropractic physicians.

Abundant evidence presented at trial clearly showed that the defendants labeled chiropractic an "unscientific cult" and had pressured physicians into boycotting chiropractors and anyone associated with them. In addition to barring professional dialogue, the boycott extended to closing hospital privileges to chiropractors and the possibility of educational exchange. The AMA argued that their motive was genuine concern for the patient's well-being as follows[39]:

One of the core successes of the Wilk legal team was that they presented enough evidence of the efficacy of chiropractic that the court found the 'patient care defense' objectively unreasonable.

In its verdict for the plaintiffs, the court required the AMA and other defendants to not only rescind their negative policy toward chiropractic but also to implement new policies that did not discourage professional association with members of the chiropractic profession. The Joint Commission on the Accreditation of Hospitals, for example, no longer uses the threat of censure and loss of accreditation to force hospitals to exclude chiropractors from staff privileges. Whether the conspiracy has ended or is merely decentralized is debatable; nothing in the Wilk opinion prevents individual hospitals from choosing not to grant privileges to chiropractors.[39] Perhaps future litigation will occur.

STUDY GUIDE

1. Who were the irregulars in the world of nineteenth century medicine?
2. What did George Bernard Shaw refer to as "an organized conspiracy against the common man" and what prompted the remark?
3. Describe the origin of the AMA.
4. What does allopathy mean?
5. What as the significance for chiropractic of *Dent v. West Virginia*?
6. What was D.D. Palmer's attitude toward licensure and why?
7. Name one of the directors of the ASC. What distinguished their concept of chiropractic from that of D.D. and B.J. Palmer?
8. Describe the significance of the Morikubo case.
9. Is all healing the practice of medicine? Why or why not?
10. What was the first state to officially legalize chiropractic? In what year? What was the first state to actually issue chiropractic licenses? When?
11. What was important about the *Commonwealth of Massachusetts v. Zimmerman?*
12. What was the last state to pass a chiropractic licensing law? In what year?
13. When the Colorado Supreme Court established that the State Board of Health had acted illegally in attempting to close the Spears Sanitarium, what were its conclusions?
14. What was the conclusion of *Wilk v. the AMA* and on what basis?

REFERENCES

1. Starr P: *The social transformation of American medicine*, p 79, New York, 1982, Basic Books.
2. Maple E: *Magic, medicine and quackery* p 163, New York, 1968, AS Barnes.
3. Gibbons RW: The natural health movement, p 1. In Redwood D, editor: *Contemporary chiropractic*, New York, 1997, Churchill Livingstone.
4. Wardwell W: *Chiropractic: history and evolution a new profession*, p 105, St. Louis, 1992, Mosby.
5. Moore JS: *Chiropractic in America: the history of a medical alternative*, p 73, Baltimore, 1993, Johns Hopkins University Press.

6. Lerner C: *Lerner research report (on the early history of chiropractic)*, p 392, New York, 1952, Foundation for Health Research (unpub).

7. Gibbons RW: Solon Massey Langworthy: keeper of the flame during the "lost years" of chiropractic, *Chiro Hist* 1:15, 1981.

8. Lerner C: *Lerner research report (on the early history of chiropractic)*, p 82, New York, 1952, Foundation for Health Research (unpub).

9. Lerner C: *Lerner research report (on the early history of chiropractic)*, p 71, New York, 1952, Foundation for Health Research (unpub).

10. Gielow V: *Old dad chiro: a biography of D.D. Palmer,* p 103, Davenport, Iowa, 1981, Bawden Bros.

11. Jap chiropractic arrested today! Charged with practicing without a license. Jap will test state law, *La Crosse Tribune,* July 22, 1907.

12. Langworthy SM, Smith OG, Paxson M: *Modernized chiropractic,* Cedar Rapids, Iowa, 1906, American School of Chiropractic.

13. Rehm WS: Legally defensible: chiropractic in the courtroom, 1907, *Chiro Hist* 6:5, 1986.

14. Mawhiney RW: *Chiropractic in Wisconsin, 1900-1950,* p 98, Waukesha, Wis, 1984, Roberts.

15. Rehm WS: "Kansas coconuts": legalizing chiropractic in the "first state," *Chiro Hist* 15(1):43, 1995.

16. Chiropractors ask Stubbs for order permitting practice, *Stafford Courier,* June 3,

17. Editorial: *Stafford Courier,* June 18, 1911.

18. Jackson RB: Willard Carver, LL.B., D.C.: doctor, lawyer, Indian chief, prisoner and more, *Chiro Hist* 14(2):13, 1994.

19. Wardwell WI: The cutting edge of chiropractic recognition: prosecution and recognition in Massachusetts, *Chiro Hist* 2(1):55, 1982.

20. Dintenfass J, editor: *Science Sidelights,* quoted from an undetermined issue, 1955.

21. *Louisiana State Board of Medical Examiners v Cronk,* 55 So Reporter 58, 1926.

22. *Louisiana State Board of Medical Examiners v Beatty et al,* 55 So Reporter 761, 1951.

23. Adams PJ: The brief for chiropractic in the England case is available, *J Natl Chiro Assoc* 12:9, 1959.

24. England JR: The England case: a battle for licensure, *Today's Chiro* 6:84, 1995.

25. Adams PJ: Injunctions in Louisiana restrain listings in directories, *ACA J Chiro* 12:27, 1964.

26. *England v Louisiana State Board of Medical Examiners,* 259 Fed Reporter, 1958.

27. *England v Louisiana State Board of Medical Examiners,* 180 Fed Supp 121, 1960.

28. *England v Louisiana State Board of Medical Examiners,* 126 So Reporter 2d 51, 1960.

29. *England v Louisiana State Board of Medical Examiners,* 194 Fed Supp 521, 1961.

30. *England v Louisiana State Board of Medical Examiners,* 375 US 411, 1964.

31. Simon JM: Address to Louisiana Chiropractors' Association, New Orleans, May 1960.

32. *England et al Louisiana State Board of Medical Examiners et al,* US District Court of Eastern Louisiana, 1965 (transcript).

33. Stanford Research Institute: *Chiropractic in California,* Pasadena, Calif, 1960.

34. Gevitz N: A coarse sieve: basic science boards and medical legislation in the United States, *J Hist Med Allied Sci* 43:36, 1988.

35. Rehm WS: Price of dissension: the private wars of Dr. Leo Spears, 1921-1956, *Chiro Hist* 15(1):31, 1995.

36. *Spears Free Clinic and Hospital for Poor Children v State Board of Health of Colorado et al,* July 1, 122 Colo. 147, 1950.

37. Hanna B: Spears wins license suit, *Denver Post,* p 1, July 1, 1950.

38. *Wilk et al v American Medical Association et al,* 895 Fed 2d 352, 1990.

39. Dumhoff H: Chiropractic and the law, p 245. In Redwood D, editor: *Contemporary chiropractic,* New York, 1997, Churchill Livingstone.

Appendix

A Brief Pictorial of Chiropractic

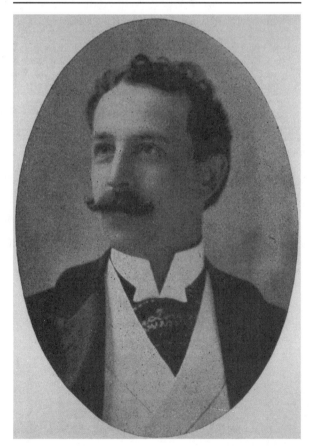

Figure 3A-1 Solon Massey Langworthy, antagonist of the Palmers and rival school founder, shepherded the first chiropractic licensing bill in Minnesota in 1905. His writings would later win the case for Morikubo in Wisconsin. (Courtesy Palmer College of Chiropractic Archives.)

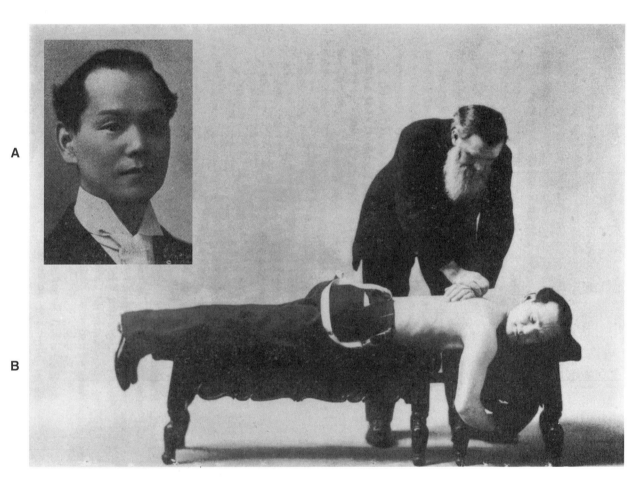

Figure 3A-2 A, Shegataro Morikubo was a significant part of early chiropractic history, as the central figure in a courtroom drama that set the stage for decades of legal defense. **B**, The founder, D.D. Palmer, used "the Jap,"with its racist connotations, in illustrating his 1906 book, *The Science of Chiropractic*. (Courtesy Palmer College of Chiropractic Archives.)

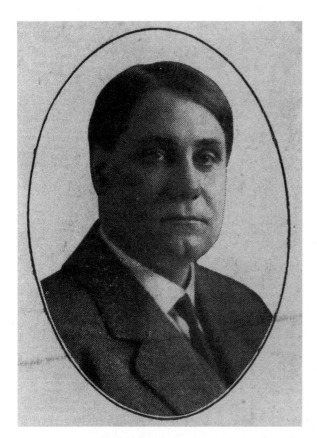

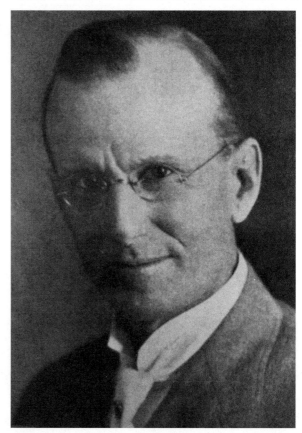

Figure 3A-3 Tom Morris, an "old-timey, small-town barrister," may have influenced the early development of chiropractic as much as the developer, B.J. Palmer. (Courtesy Palmer College of Chiropractic Archives.)

Figure 3A-4 Willard Carver, once D.D. Palmer's attorney, set out on his own educational and philosophic course in 1906 and blazed the trail to recognition in Oklahoma and elsewhere. (Courtesy Palmer College of Chiropractic Archives.)

IN THE
UNITED STATES DISTRICT COURT
EASTERN DISTRICT OF LOUISIANA
NEW ORLEANS DIVISION

CIVIL ACTION

No. 9,292

JERRY ENGLAND, ET AL.,

Plaintiffs,

versus

LOUISIANA STATE BOARD OF MEDICAL
EXAMINERS, ET AL.,

Defendants,

ORIGINAL BRIEF OF PLAINTIFFS.

J. MINOS SIMON,
301 E. Congress St.,
Lafayette, Louisiana;
FLOYD J. REED,
919 Maison Blanche Bldg.,
New Orleans, Louisiana;
RUSSELL MORTON BROWN,
605 Southern Bldg.,
Washington, D.C.;

Figure 3A-5 Civil action case involving chiropractors in Louisiana.

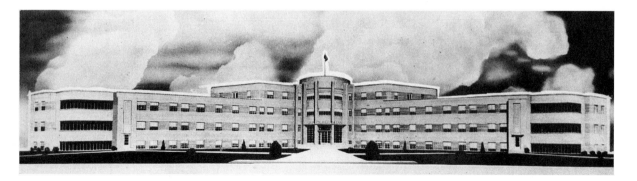

Figure 3A-6 The original building of Spears Hospital in 1943 was dedicated to chiropractic pioneer Willard Carver, D.C. (Courtesy William S. Rehm.)

CHAPTER 4

Autonomic Neuroanatomy of the Vertebral Subluxation Complex

William J. Ruch, DC

In this chapter, I will use the current Western anatomic terminology in describing and classifying the relevant structures of the nervous system. However, the reader will hopefully remember that many different maps can and will be made of this complex territory. A classification scheme that makes sense today may require modification for the knowledge of tomorrow.

Our bodies developed in antiquity, before language. Language brings its underlying cultural assumptions into the task of mapping the complex territory of the body. For instance, the term *somatic* comes from the Greek word "soma," meaning body. This word is separate from the term *psyche* and undoubtedly reflects a European tendency to consider mind and body as distinct entities. The anatomic terminology currently in use is largely a reflection of classic Greco-Roman cultural understanding the extensive study of dead tissues.

Although modern anatomic terminology is a powerful intellectual tool, other systems of describing the human body exist and are based on cultural assumptions different from those inherited from classic Greece and Rome. For instance, in ancient China and other Asian cultures, dissection had little or no part in the understanding of human anatomy. Human anatomy was primarily a science that studied the living. The meridians of the acupuncturist exhibit little resemblance to anything that one can find in a Western anatomy text. Chi is understood to be a form of life-energy that fuels the emotions at the same time vivifing the organs, a concept that makes little allowance for the Western distinction between soma and psyche.

The efferent aspect of the autonomic nervous system (ANS) broadly consists of sympathetic and parasympathetic divisions. As seen in Table 4-1, sympathetic and parasympathetic activity generally work in opposition; what is accelerated by sympathetic stimulation will be decelerated by parasympathetic stimulation and vice versa. This oppositional relationship is similar to combining hot and cold water to produce a comfortable warm bath or shower.

For example, sympathetic stimulation accelerates heart rate, while parasympathetic stimulation slows it down.[1,2] Although special situations may require a temporary rush of scalding hot water (sympathetic dominance) and other situations need a temporary rush of ice-cold water (parasympathetic dominance), healthy cardiac function at rest is promoted by warm water (autonomic balance). In the healthy resting state, the extremes of tachycardia and bradycardia are avoided by a balance between sympathetic and parasympathetic tone. This balanced autonomic steady state is a central aspect of homeostasis.

The afferent aspect of the ANS sometimes returns information to the spinal cord with the same type of nerve that the somatic structures use. Some of the afferent autonomic tracts are tortuous and do not involve the dorsal root ganglion. However, some evidence exists that they carry pain fibers from somatic sources. Some of the nerve cell bodies of the afferent autonomics reside in the dorsal root ganglion alongside the striated afferent nerve cell bodies. They both transmit the same sensory information, proprioception or interoceptive impulses.[3] The peripheral nerves contain fibers from somatic and visceral nerve endings and some

Table 4-1 *General Effects of Autonomic Stimulation*

Sympathetic Stimulation	Parasympathetic Stimulation
Pupillary dilation	Pupillary constriction
Increased heart rate	Decreased heart rate
Increased blood pressure	Decreased blood pressure
Vasoconstriction	Vasodilation
Increased alertness	Decreased alertness
Decreased peristalsis	Increased peristalsis
Constriction of sphincters (anal and urinary)	Relaxation of sphincters
Bronchial dilation	Bronchial constriction
Orgasm and ejaculation	Sexual arousal and erection

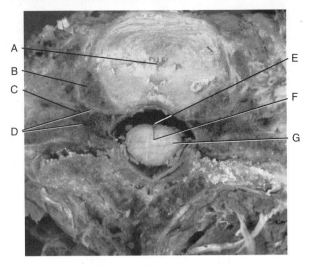

Figure 4-1 Cross section of spinal cord and vertebral column at C6-C7. In its relaxed state, the spinal cord is almost round in cross-section and lying in the posterior half of the spinal canal. **A,** Disc. **B,** Uncinate process. **C,** Dorsal root ganglion. **D,** Intervertebral foramen (IVF). **E,** Anterior spinal artery. **F,** Spinal cord. **G,** Approximate location of lateral cell column in the spinal cord.

of these nerve endings are the same. For example, Vater-Pacinian corpuscles are in striated muscle and mesentery.

Roots of the Briar Patch

The ANS is a rich network of nerve pathways with connections in both the central nervous system and the periphery. The intertwined complexity of the ANS has led some anatomists to compare it with a briar patch, with the roots of the ANS briar patch beginning within the brain and spinal cord.

Sympathetic nerve tracts originate with cell bodies in the lateral gray columns of the thoracolumbar region of the spinal cord (Figure 4-1). In most people the axons of these neurons exit the vertebral column as myelinated fibers in the ventral rami of the spinal nerve roots from T1-L2. Individuals may demonstrate a caudal or rostral shift of one to two segments in this pattern.[3] These myelinated fibers of the thoracolumbar outflow are known as *white rami communicantes* or *preganglionic fibers*.

Parasympathetic nerve tracts primarily begin with cell bodies in the brainstem and lateral gray columns of the sacral region of the spinal cord. The axons of these neurons exit at the following levels (Figure 4-2):

• Cranial nerves III (oculomotor)
• VII (facial)
• IX (glossopharyngeal) and X (vagus)
• S2, S3, S4 (and occasionally S5) spinal nerve roots

Some sensory (afferent) pathways of the ANS are served by cell bodies located in the dorsal root ganglia of the spinal nerves, which is similar to the arrangement in somatic sensory fibers.[3] The peripheral nerves are responsible for the transmission of the spinal reflex phenomenon. This is a pathway similar to that for the reflex guarding that striated muscle demonstrates with joint distress or subluxation. The experiments by Sato and others[4] show the crossover effects of the two systems. The somatoautonomic or somatovisceral reflexes show that stimuli on skin and muscle have a direct affect on visceral organ function and give an anatomic basis for acupuncture and spinal manipulation, to mention just two noninvasive or nonpharmacologic approaches to influence or change visceral organ function.

The antiquity of the physiologic systems is immense. The development of civilization is recent in this time frame. In the first week of November 1997, a tiger was killed in Nepal in the Baitadi district that had killed 100 people.[5] Concurrently, the Mir space station was having multiple problems and being labeled obsolete by critics.

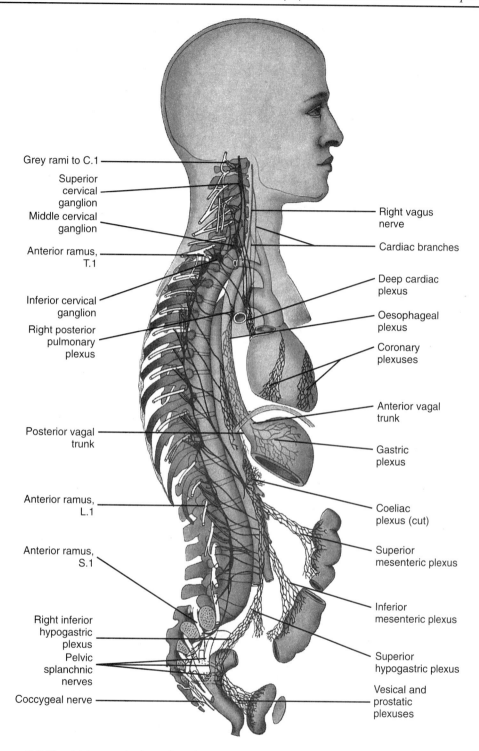

Figure 4-2 The right sympathetic trunk and its connections with the thoracic, abdominal, and pelvic plexi. Black = sympathetic trunk and branches; gray = white rami communicantes; lighter gray = parasympathetic fibres. (From William PL, editor: *Gray's Anatomy,* ed 38, New York, 1995, Churchill Livingstone.)

The human environment is changing at a phenomenal rate. As some of us live with commuter delays and computer breakdowns, others still have large carnivores in their neighborhood. The neurochemistry of the ancient needs is still with us today regardless of the current environment.

Central Vines of the Briar Patch

The sympathetic roots of the ANS briar patch converge in paired ganglia that run along the vertebral column like two vines clinging to either side of a fence. In D.D. Palmer's 1910 textbook,[6] this chain of ganglia is referred to as the "cord of sympathetics." Indeed, the paravertebral chain ganglia are reminiscent of two parallel spinal cords. The left and right paravertebral chain ganglia form a continuous body at the anterolateral aspect of the vertebral column from the upper cervical spine to the anterior aspect of the coccyx where it is joined (Figures 4-2 and 4-3).

Most of the preganglionic fibers of the thoracolumbar outflow synapse within this ganglionic chain. Other preganglionic fibers pass through and progress to more distant destinations.

Postganglionic fibers leaving the paravertebral chain are unmyelinated; many of them rejoin the spinal nerves as gray rami communicantes. Others continue on to their target organs by a number of pathways.

In the cervical region, the paravertebral chain ganglia are organized into three distinct bodies on each side of the spine (Table 4-2). The lower cervical sympathetic ganglion often fuses with the first thoracic ganglion, forming a star-shaped body, usually referred to as the *stellate ganglion* (Figures 4-3 and 4-11). Postganglionic distribution from these cervical ganglia is primarily responsible for the sympathetic innervation of the organs and vessels of the cranium, neck, thorax, and upper extremities (Figure 4-4).

Chasing a Rabbit into the Briar Patch

Beyond the paravertebral chain ganglia, the ANS briar patch thickens. Sympathetic fibers intermingle with sensory and parasympathetic fibers in increasingly complex ways. This structural combination is emblematic of a substantial degree of functional fusing. Following a neural impulse through the ANS is analogous to chasing a rabbit into a briar patch.

Some of this intermingling occurs in a series of plexi anterior to the vertebral column, following the course of the aorta and its branches. In these prevertebral plexi, postganglionic sympathetic fibers are joined by parasympathetic and sensory fibers (Table 4-3 and Figure 4-2).

The spinal nerve itself is generally comprised of somatic efferent, somatic afferent, sympathetic postganglionic, and ANS afferent fibers. This causes yet another level of joining.[3,7] Comprehending this integration of the systems is the basis for the anatomic explanation for certain aspects of chiropractic, acupuncture, and other reflex techniques.

Table 4-2 *Cervical Sympathetic Ganglia*

Ganglion	Preganglionic Origin	Location	Postganglionic Distribution
Superior	T1-T5	Occ-C2	Heart, pupils, salivary glands, pharynx, and cranial blood vessels (including those vessels serving the cranial nerves)
Middle	T1-T5	C5-C6	Heart, thyroid gland, parathyroid gland, trachea, and esophagus
Stellate	T1-T5 (in some individuals fibers destined for the stellate ganglia can originate as caudally as T10)	C7-T1 (often straddles first rib)	Heart, upper extremities, and some cranial blood vessels

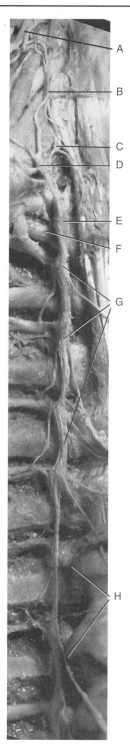

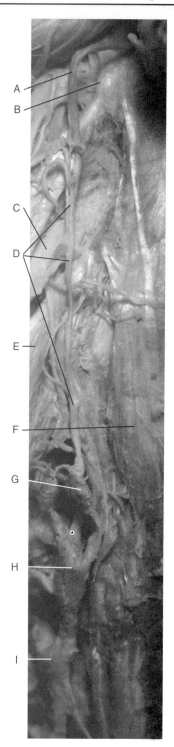

Figure 4-3 Cervical and thoracic sympathetic chain and ganglion. **A,** Superior cervical ganglion. **B,** Cervical sympathetic chain. **C,** Middle cervical ganglion. **D,** Inferior cervical ganglion (stellate ganglion). **E,** First thoracic ganglion (stellate ganglion). **F,** First rib. **G,** Sympathetic chain ganglion. **H,**Osteophytes.

Figure 4-4 Cervical and upper thoracic sympathetic ganglions and related structures. **A,** Superior cervical ganglion. **B,** C3 transverse process. **C,** Bracial plexus. **D,** Cervical sympathetic trunk. **E,** Anterior scalenes. **F,** Longus colli. **G,** Middle cervical ganglion. **H,** Inferior cervical ganglion. **I,** First thoracic ganglion.

Table 4-3 *The Prevertebral Plexi*

Plexus	Preganglionic Origin	Location	Innervation to the Following
Celiac (solar)	T5-T9	Anterior to aorta, just inferior to diaphragm	Stomach, duodenum, liver, gallbladder, pancreas, spleen, kidneys, and adrenal glands
Superior Mesenteric	T5-T11	Anterior to aorta, inferior to celiac plexus	Duodenum, small intestine, pancreas, and ascending and part of transverse colon
Inferior Mesenteric	T12-L2	Anterior to aorta, inferior to superior mesenteric	Part of transverse colon, rectum, and fibers to superior hypogastric plexus
Superior Hypogastric	T12-L2	Anterior to L4-L5 vertebral bodies	Reproductive organs, urinary bladder, rectum, and anus

Subluxation: Snaring the Rabbit

Subluxation of the spine and associated articulations can disturb the normal flow of neural impulses through the ANS in a number of ways, essentially "snaring the rabbit" as it attempts to traverse the autonomic briar patch.

Compression and Traction Snares

The intervertebral foramen (IVF) has long been a major focus of chiropractic's clinical and scientific concern. The modern vertebral subluxation complex (VSC) model continues to include consideration of the IVF.[8] If subluxation can generate enough compressive force at this level to compromise spinal nerve root function, then information flow through ANS fibers could be interrupted. Hadley[9] demonstrated that IVF constriction may be caused by displaced articular surfaces, disc bulging or herniation, and degenerative spurs projecting into the foramen. These phenomena are part of the kinesiologic and connective tissue components of the VSC model. This IVF constriction may be exacerbated in some individuals by the recently demonstrated transforaminal ligament.[10] Significant conduction block has been demonstrated with as little as 10 mmHg of compression on the spinal nerve roots.[11] This conduction block may be exacerbated by compromised vascular flow to and from the spinal nerve roots, caused by as little as 5 mmHg of compression at the IVF level.[12] Giles[13] has spotlighted the inter-

vertebral canal, which is formed by the evagination of the dura mater within which the spinal nerve roots travel to the IVF. Just before reaching the IVF, a thickening in the dorsal spinal nerve root occurs; this is the dorsal root ganglion, which contains the cell bodies of the sensory neurons, including those responsible for visceral sensation. The intervertebral foramen is barely wide enough to accommodate the dorsal root ganglion (see Figure 4-1). Buckling and hypertrophy of ligaments surrounding this part of the canal has been shown to cause compression of the dorsal root ganglion, a potential source of disturbed ANS sensory disturbance, including pain.

Although poor posture is often presumed to be entirely psychologic or simply a bad habit, postural distortion is a common consequence of subluxation, which may or may not originate in psychologic stresses. Deformation of the vertebral column, including alteration of the normal anterior-posterior curves, is a common result of this postural distortion.[14-16]

Loss of normal anterior-posterior curves causes a lengthening of the spinal canal. When the spinal canal lengthens, the dentate ligaments stretch and pull on the lateral aspect of the spinal cord. This causes an increase in the lateral diameter of the spinal cord and a reduction in the anterior-posterior diameter.[17] In some cases, the spinal cord will contact the walls of the spinal canal, causing tethering.[15,18-20] The tethered cord is a site of permanent neurologic disturbance. This process is readily seen by comparing the normal cross-

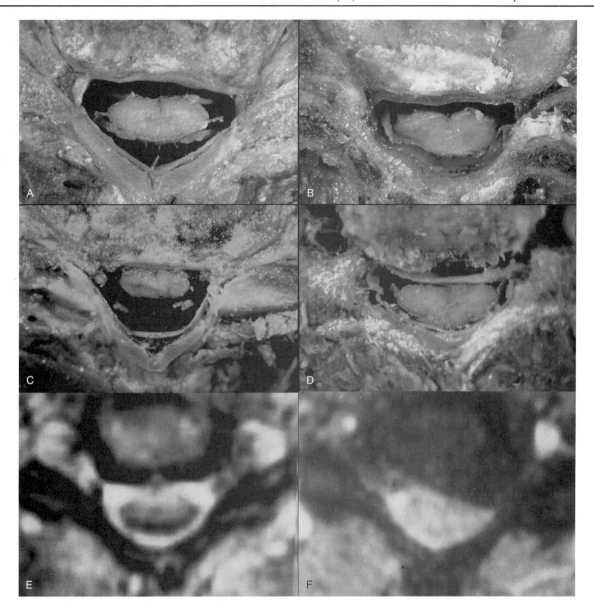

Figure 4-5 Cross sections of spinal cords in states of distress because of subluxation of the vertbral column. **A-D,** Specimens sectioned through the C7-T1 disc. **E-F,** MRIs of axial views of C5. Note changes of spinal cord shape and the position of the spinal cord in the spinal canal. The experiments on animal spinal cords that would mimic this condition show significant changes in spinal cord conductivity. In **A, C,** and **E** the increase of width and decrease of A-P diameter of the spinal cord indicates flexion deformity or increase in length of the vertebral canal. Note also, especially in **C,** the position of the spinal cord is not lying in the posterior aspect of the canal. In **B, D,** and **F** the cross-sectional shape of the canal has changed. Canal stenosis is the narrowing of the spinal canal because of various factors. In **B** and **D,** ligamentum hypertrophy has taken place; in **D** the end plate of the vertebral body has widened at the expense of the canal; and in **F** an osteophyte is compressing the spinal cord.

section of the spinal cord in Figure 4-1 with the distorted cords in the subluxated specimens in Figure 4-5. The traction or compression forces generated by altered spinal curves could also potentially distort the cauda equina or the lower brainstem, depending on the level of involvement. According to Brieg and others,[17,21] distortion of these neural structures is accompanied by distortion of their associated blood vessels, causing further neurologic insult. Animal experiments show diminishing and loss of cord conductivity.[19,20] Exacerbation of these effects would be expected when dural adhesions, posteriorly projecting osteophytes, disc bulging, or disc herniation occur. Clearly, such direct insult to the central nervous system could disturb the somatics and the sympathetic and parasympathetic portions of the ANS.[22] Typically, the onset of such problems would be gradual, insidious, and hard to explain with the usual testing and diagnostic procedures. Pharmaceutical use might mask some of the problems until the deterioration is extreme.

The jugular foramen exits the occiput in close proximity to the atlas-occiput articulation. The vagus nerve, arguably the most important single parasympathetic structure, emanates through this foramen, as do the glossopharyngeal and spinal accessory. The hypoglossal nerve is also closely related to the upper cervical area. Figure 4-6 shows that these structures are vulnerable to the altered mechanical forces of upper cervical subluxation. Upper cervical subluxation can also create cord distortion, as described earlier.

The brachial plexus transmits sympathetic and somatic fibers to the upper extremities. In Figure 4-7, the relationship of the brachial plexus to the anterior and medial scalene muscles is readily seen. Spasm of the scalene muscles is not uncommon in cervical subluxation and injury.

A number of subluxation-related processes can threaten the integrity of the paravertebral chain

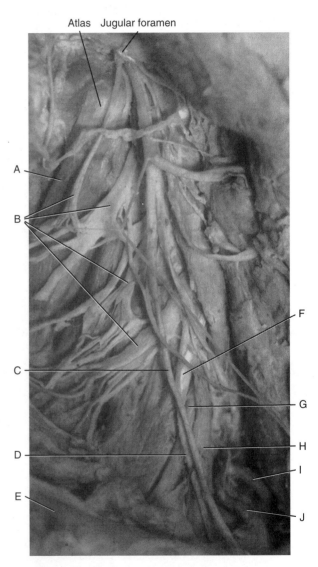

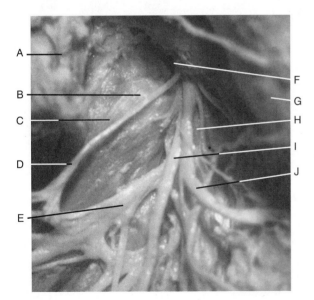

Figure 4-6 The Upper cervical neural components. Note the atlas and its proximity to the vagus nerve, superior cervical ganglion, and the C1 nerve root. Subluxation of C1 relative to the occiput can have ANS, cranial nerve, and spinal nerve consequences. **A,** Mastoid process of occiput. **B,** Atlas transverse process. **C,** Levator scapulae. **D,** C1 nerve root. **E,** C2 nerve root. **F,** Jugular foramen. **G,** Mandible. **H,** Superior cervical ganglion. **I,** Vagus nerve. **J,** Hypoglossal nerve.

Figure 4-7 The lateral aspect of the cervical spine. The structures of Figure 4-6 are in the top part of this photograph. Note the intimate relationship of the neural and muscular components. A cervical sprain and strain injury can have neurologic aspects. **A,** Levator scapulae. **B,** C1-C4 nerve roots. **C,** Vagus nerve. **D,** Phrenic nerve. **E,** Clavicle. **F,** Medial scalenes. **G,** Brachial plexus. **H,** Anterior scalenes. **I,** Vertebral artery. **J,** Sympathetic trunk.

ganglia and related sympathetic structures. Giles[23] demonstrated that degenerative spurs that project in an anterolateral direction can distort the paravertebral chain ganglia—a direct compromise of ANS tissue. Such spurs can also create traction of the sympathetic rami associated with the paravertebral chain ganglia (Figure 4-8). According to Nathan,[24] such deformation of the chain ganglia and their associated sympathetic nerves can initiate a sclerotic reaction, eventually leading to replacement of normal nervous tissue with fibrotic zones of electrical silence.

Lateral bulge or herniation of the intervertebral discs can also stretch and deform the sympathetic nerves (Figure 4-9).

The largest thickenings of the paravertebral chain, the superior cervical sympathetic ganglia, are in close proximity to the upper cervical spine (see Figure 4-6). At this important level, rotational or other types of subluxation of the C1-C2 motion segment could disturb the sympathetic chain and the other structures.

The paravertebral chain ganglia are particularly vulnerable in the thoracic spine. In Figure 4-10, the proximity of the sympathetic chain and sympathetic nerves to the costovertebral joints is readily appreciated. Costovertebral subluxation would alter the normal mechanics of the osseous

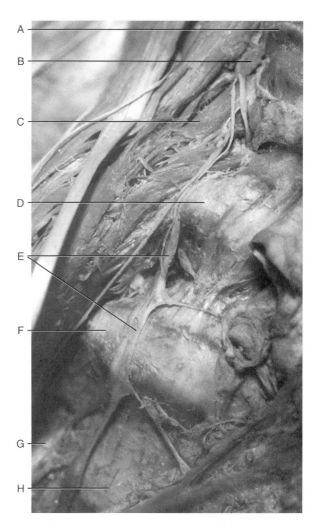

Figure 4-8 Lower thoracic vertebral osteophytes and the sympathetic chain ganglion. **A,** Sympathetic chain ganglion. **B,** Sympathetic nerves. **C,** Spinal osteophytes.

Figure 4-9 Osteophytes of the lumbar spine and sympathetic nerve deformation. **A,** Osteophyte of L3-4 disc. **B,** Third lumbar sympathetic trunk ganglion. **C,** Psoas. **D,** Bulging of L4-5 disc. **E,** Lumbar splanchnic nerve. **F,** Bulging of L5-S1 disc. **G,** L5 nerve root. **H,** Sacrum.

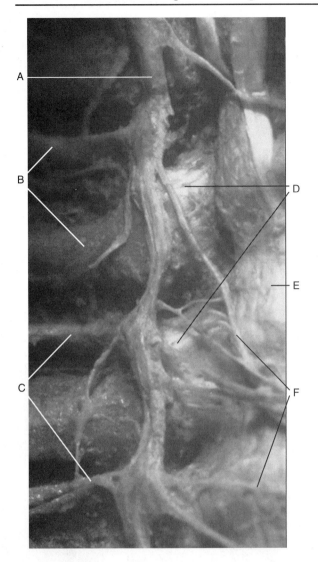

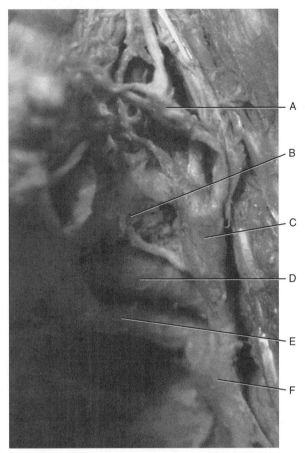

Figure 4-11 The Stellate ganglion. The stellate ganglion is also called the *cervicothoracic ganglion* and is the combination of the inferior cervical ganglion and the first thoracic sympathetic ganglion. **A,** Middle cervical ganglion. **B,** C8 nerve root. **C,** Inferior cervical ganglion. **D,** First rib. **E,** T1 nerve root. **F,** First thoracic sympathetic ganglion.

Figure 4-10 The sympathetic chain over the costovertebral joints. Note the intercostal nerves between the ribs and the rami leaving the chain and going to the vertebral column. **A,** Sympathetic chain. **B,** Ribs. **C,** Intercostal nerves. **D,** Radiate ligament of costovertebral joint. **E,** Vertebral column. **F,** Sympathetic nerves to vertebral column.

and ligamentous structures related to these joints.[25]

Costovertebral subluxation becomes particularly significant at T1. Here, a thickening or ganglion occurs in the sympathetic chain called the *stellate ganglion* (Figure 4-11). Although stellate ganglion control of the upper extremity vasculature has long been appreciated, recent studies demonstrate the existence of stellate innervation

to the blood vessels of the face and cranium, including the cochlea of the inner ear.[26-28] Intervertebral or costovertebral subluxation involving T1 or the first rib is also significant because it affects the thoracic inlet, which is bounded by the vertebral body of T1, the first ribs on each side, and the superior border of the manubrium sterni.[7] Distress of the thoracic inlet can disturb ANS function in a number of ways.[29] Mechanical stress to the muscles of the throat, including the hyoid muscles, can affect tempromandibular joint function and swallowing, functions which straddle the somatovisceral border. Also thoracic inlet distress can affect vagal innervation to the heart and other visceral structures.

Thoracic inlet distress can also alter the mechanics of the sternoclavicular joints, leading to unilateral sternocleidomastoid (SCM) spasm. This imbalance in SCM tone can contribute to upper cervical subluxation, with all of the attendant ANS involvement previously noted.

The fascia of the thoracic inlet is in close relation to the scalene muscle group. Disturbed tone in these muscles can affect the sympathetic fibers of the brachial plexus, as described previously. Subluxation of the first and second ribs will create scalene spasm and thoracic inlet distress as the ribs move away from the spine.

As significant as these mechanical snares may be, they perhaps only represent the tip of the iceberg. The rest of the iceberg involves reflex and chemical components of the VSC.

Reflex and Chemical Snares

Many of the sensory fibers of the ANS are concerned with stretch, pressure, and tonus in the walls of the visceral organs and vascular structures. In this sense, much of the ANS's sensorium can be seen as a variety of proprioception.[3] Even proprioception in the conventional (somatic) sense is crucial in the autonomic sensorium. This is because the physiologic support for posture and locomotion is organized by the sympathetic nervous system. The response of the sympathetic nervous system to the energy requirements of the locomotor system has been a central interest in the osteopathic research conducted by Korr. Korr[30] refers to this phenomenon as the *ergotropic* function of the sympathetic nervous system. Many of the components of the modern VSC model can only be properly understood in the context of this proprioceptive-sympathetic interface.

For example, the joint distress of subluxation commonly leads to a muscular guarding (sometimes referred to as *spasm*), part of the myopathology of the VSC.[31] Although some of this involuntary muscle contraction may be caused by the facilitation of simple segmental reflex arcs (much like the deep tendon reflexes elicited during physical examination), spasm has recently been proposed as an ergotropic response of the sympathetic nervous system.[32] This involuntary contraction of striated muscle coincides with similar contraction of smooth muscle or vasoconstriction. The combi-nation of striated muscle spasm and vasoconstriction would tend to promote inflammatory changes. The inflammatory process generates chemical irritants such as histamine, lactic acid, and bradykinin, which can irritate the spinal nerve roots and possibly the paravertebral chain ganglia at the molecular level. This would constitute a chemical snare for ANS signals. Chronic inflammatory conditions are part of the onset of spinal degeneration and involve permanent changes in bone, muscle, ligaments, and other structures (see Figures 4-8 and 4-9). All of this is initiated by the loss of normal architectural alignment and weight bearing. Adhesions, contracture, and eventual loss of articular components are part of this pattern of chronic subluxation. Vascular and neurologic structures are affected.

Vasoconstriction can also involve more central structures. Breig[15,17] has noted that cord elongation or flattening, such as the distortions demonstrated in Figure 4-5, are likely to reduce the lumina of the spinal arteries. The resulting ischemia and possible inflammation could contribute to myelopathy. This would certainly disturb the ANS components at the involved cord level.[33]

In the upper cervical spine, subluxation may compromise the vascular supply to the brain, either by mechanical distortion of the vertebral artery or by sympathetic reflex vasoconstriction, as suggested by Jackson[34] and more recently by Gorman.[35]

The carotid arteries and the jugular veins are closely related to the thoracic inlet. Therefore subluxations distorting the thoracic inlet may compromise the circulatory supply to the ANS structures of the brain. Hypoxia from any mechanism will produce the same loss of function.

Although much research still needs to be accomplished before the ANS implications of the subluxation will be fully understood, some of the anatomic basis of this relationship is already apparent. The subluxations or snares for the "rabbit" of ANS signals can be located in the spinal nerve roots, the brachial plexus, the paravertebral chain ganglia, the cauda equina, the cranial nerves, the spinal cord, and the brainstem. The snares can operate through compression, traction, hypoxia, chronic reflex activity, or chemical irritation.

STUDY GUIDE

1. Discuss the significance of chi in relation to soma and psyche.
2. Explain autonomic balance in relation to tone.
3. To what aspect of the ANS do parasympathetic and sympathetic refer?
4. What does the afferent aspect of a nerve do?
5. Where are the cell bodies of the sympathetic nerve tracts located and from which spinal levels do they exit?
6. Where are the cell bodies of the parasympathetic tracts located and where do they exit the spine?
7. What is the cord of the sympathetics?
8. How many ganglia exist in the cervical region? Where is the stellate ganglion?
9. What is the fiber composition of the average spinal nerve?
10. Name three causes of possible IVF constriction.
11. What is the significance of the transforaminal ligament?
12. Significant (nerve) conduction block can be caused by as little as _____ mmHg of pressure on spinal nerve roots. Significant vascular compression within the IVF can result from as little as _____ mmHg of pressure.
13. Describe the relationship of the dura mater to the intervertebral canal and to the IVF.
14. Does the loss of the normal A-P curves shorten the spinal canal? Why is this important?
15. Where does the vagus nerve exit the skull? Why is this important in relation to chiropractic and somatovisceral effects on the living body?
16. Does an upper cervical subluxation disrupt blood supply to the brain? Explain your answer.
17. How can chemical irritants promote inflammatory changes leading to subluxation?

REFERENCES

1. Mitchell JH: Neural control of the circulation during exercise, *Med Sci Sports Exerc* 2:141-154, 1990.
2. Mitchell JH, Victor RG: Neural control of the cardiovascular system: insights from muscle sympathetic nerve recordings, *Med Sci Sports Exerc Suppl* 10:S60-S69, 1996.
3. Mitchell GAG: *Anatomy of the autonomic nervous system,* 114-127, Edinburgh and London, 1953, E&S Livingstone.
4. Sato A: Physiological studies of the somatoautonomic reflexes. In Haldeman S, editor: *Modern developments in the principles and practice of chiropractic,* New York, 1979, Appleton-Century-Crofts.
5. Newman S: Earth week, a weekly diary of the planet, *San Francisco Chronicle,* November 8, 1997.
6. Palmer DD: *The science, art and philosophy of chiropractic,* Portland, Ore, 1910, Portland Printing House.
7. Williams PL, editor: *Gray's anatomy,* ed 38, New York, 1995, Churchill Livingstone.
8. Cleveland CS: Neurobiologic relations. In Redwood D, editor: *Contemporary chiropractic,* New York, 1997, Churchill Livingstone.
9. Hadley L: *Anatomico-roentgenographic studies of the spine,* Springfield, Ill, 1981, Charles C. Thomas.
10. Bakkum BW: The effects of transforaminal ligaments on the sizes of T11-L5 human interbertebral foramina, *J Manipulative Physiol Ther* 17:517, 1994.
11. Sharpless SK: Susceptibility of spinal roots to compression block, p 155. In Goldstein M, editor: *The Research status of spinal manipulative therapy,* monog no 15, Bethesda, Md, 1975, NIH/NINCDS, U.S. Department of Health, Education and Welfare.
12. Rydevik BL: The effects of compression on the physiology of nerve roots, *J Manipulative Physiol Ther* 15:62, 1992.
13. Giles LFG: A histological investigation of human lower lumbar intervertebral canal (foramen) dimensions, *J Manipulative Physiol Ther* 17:4, 1994.
14. Horwitz T: Degenerative lesions in the cervical portion of the spine, *Arch Intern Med* 1178-1191, 1942.
15. Breig A: *Adverse mechanical tension in the central nervous system,* Stockholm, 1978, Alquist and Wiksell.
16. Ruch WJ: *Atlas of common subluxations of the human spine and pelvis,* Boca Raton, Fla, 1997, CRC Press.
17. Breig A: Overstretching of and circumscribed pathological tension in the spinal cord: a basic cause of symptoms in cord disorders, *J Biomech* 3:7-9, 1970.
18. Condon BR, Hadley D: Quantification of cord deformation and dynamics during flexion and extension of the cervical spine using MR imaging, *J Comp Assist Tomog* 12:947-955, 1988.
19. Fujita Y, Yamamoto H: An experimental study on spinal cord traction effect, *Spine* 14(7):698-705, 1989.
20. Yamada S, Zinke DE, Sanders D: Pathophysiology of "tethered cord syndrome," *J Neurosurg* 54:494-503, 1981.

21. Breig A, Turnbull I, Hassler O: Effects of mechanical stresses on the spinal cord in cervical spondylosis: a study on fresh cadaver material, *J Neurosurg,* 25:45-56, 1966.

22. Hu JW, Vernon H, Tatourian I: Changes in neck electromyography associated with meningeal noxious stimulation, *J Manipulative Physiol Ther,* 9:577-581, 1995.

23. Giles LGF: Paraspinal autonomic ganglion distortion due to vertebral osteophytosis: a cause of vertebrogenic autonomic syndromes? *J Manipulative Physiol Ther* 15:551, 1992.

24. Nathan H: Compression of the sympathetic trunk by osteophytes of the vertebral column in the abdomen: an anatomical study with pathology and clinical considerations, *Surgery* 4:609-625, 1968.

25. Godwin-Austen RB: The mechanoreceptors of the costo-vertebral joints, *J Physiol* 1969, 202:737-753.

26. Drummond PD, Finch PM: Reflex control of facial flushing during body heating in man, *Brain* 112:1351-1358, 1989.

27. Lehmann LJ, Warfield CA, Bajwa ZH: Case report: migraine headache following stellate ganglion block for reflex sympathetic dystrophy, *Headache* 36:335-337, 1996.

28. Ren T et al: Effects of stellate ganglion stimulation on bilateral cochlear blood flow: annals of otology, *Rhinol Laryngol* 102:378-384, 1993.

29. Nanson EM: The anterior approach to upper dorsal sympathectomy, *Surgery, Gynecol Obstetr* 118-120, 1957.

30. Korr IM: Sustained sympatheticotonia as a factor in disease. In Korr IM, editor: *The neurobiologic mechanisms in manipulative therapy,* New York, London, 1977, Plenum Press.

31. Schafer RC, Faye LJ: *Motion palpation and chiropractic technic: principles of dynamic chiropractic,* Huntington Beach, Calif, 1989, The Motion Palpation Institute.

32. Seaman DR: A physiological explanation of subluxation and its treatment, *Calif Chiro Assoc J* 21:32, 1996.

33. Adams CBT, Logue V: Studies in cervical spondylotic myelopathy (1. Movement of the cervical roots, dura and cord, and their relation to the course of the extrathecal roots), *Brain* 94:557-658, 1971.

34. Jackson R: *The cervical syndrome,* Springfield, Ill, 1956, Charles C. Thomas.

35. Gorman RF: Monocular scotomata and spinal manipulation: the step phenomenon, *J Manipulative Physiol Ther* 19:344, 1996.

ACKNOWLEDGMENTS

I want to thank the President of Life Chiropractic College-West, Dr. Gerard Clum, for his kindness in giving me permission to use the anatomy laboratory facilities for this project. Thanks also to Dr. John Boss and Jeff Custer for their time and efforts in coordinating the use of the lab. The outstanding dissection work was done by Dr. Steve James; without his skills, these photographs could not have been taken. The outstanding assistance of the Life Chiropractic College-West Library and its staff also helped with my numerous requests for reference material.

CHAPTER 5

Referred Pain and Related Phenomena: Selected Topics

Charles S. Masarsky, DC • *Steven T. Tanaka, DC*

For the lay person, the concept of *referred pain* often seems antiintuitive. For example, when knee pain is referred from a lumbar dysfunction, one is not likely to grab the lower back and yell in pain. The patient is likely to conclude through common sense that the knee hurts; therefore something is wrong with the knee. The assumption that the locus of a pain must always be the locus of its cause is an understandable yet erroneous notion believed by many in the public. Overcoming this notion can be a challenge in patient education.

When this same assumption is acted on by a health practitioner, referred pain can lead to many expensive and dangerous blind alleys. This is especially true when a somatic dysfunction creates the impression of a serious and potentially life-threatening disease of an internal organ. Such a situation will often activate a series of hazardous diagnostic and therapeutic invasions in a futile attempt to identify and treat a visceral disease that does not exist.

This chapter was written to improve patient care by promoting a practical understanding of referred pain, referred tenderness, and related phenomena. After a general overview, we will discuss some specific referred pain syndromes of clinical importance in chiropractic.

Cross-Talk on the Spinal Switchboard

At the end of the nineteenth century, British physician Henry Head[1] began to map areas of cutaneous tenderness related to gastric disturbances. He later expanded his investigations to include such mapping in patients with various internal disorders. Many methods were used, but Head particularly favored probing with the blunt head of a pin. When he probed a tender zone on the patient's body, the patient would frequently mistake the head of the pin for the point.

Although Head was not the first physician to notice the phenomenon of referred pain and tenderness, his work took a unique turn. He correlated the zones of referred visceral tenderness with the zones of cutaneous involvement in 62 cases of herpes zoster. Because cutaneous outbreaks of herpes zoster tend to indicate distinct dermatome levels, Head was able to correlate the zones of these outbreaks with related vertebral levels. Frequently, an outbreak zone observed in a patient with herpes zoster was similar to or even identical to the zone of referred tenderness noted in patients with dysfunction of a particular internal organ. Thus visceral disorders and their related zones of tenderness were associated with vertebral levels. Head also correlated these cutaneous zones with the zones of anesthesia reported in previous descriptions of patients with traumatic spinal lesions.

Although the zones associated with herpes zoster and internal organ disorders often involved broad areas of skin, relatively small patches of maximum tenderness were usually identifiable (Table 5-1). In addition to these areas, Head also noted that organs innervated by the vagus nerve would often refer pain to cutaneous zones related to cervical spinal nerves.

Head hypothesized that sensory impulses from a distressed internal organ would create a disturbance in the segment of the cord to which such impulses are conducted. Impulses from a second

Table 5-1   *Zones of Maximum Referred Cutaneous Tenderness According to Head*

Vertebral Level	Organ Involvement	Cutaneous Zones
T1	Heart, lungs	Nape of neck over T1; third costosternal junction; inner bend of the elbow
T2	Heart, lungs	Spine of the scapula; third intercostal space, just lateral to nipple line
T3	Heart, lungs	Inferior to spine of scapula; inner border of the upper arm
T4	Heart, lungs	Medial scapular border; posterior aspect of axilla; nipple
T5	Lungs	Medial scapular border at T5 level; axilla; inferior and medial to nipple
T6	Stomach, liver, gallbladder	Angle of scapula; over fifth rib, 1 inch medial to nipple line
T7	Stomach, liver, gallbladder	Over xiphoid process; T8-9 region of midback
T8	Stomach, liver, gallbladder	Eighth intercostal space, just lateral to nipple line; 2.5 inches below angle of scapula
T9	Stomach, liver, gallbladder, upper colon	Over tip of ninth rib at costal border; T11 area of low back
T10	Liver, gall-bladder, upper colon, kidney, ureter, prostate, testes, ovaries, uterus	Over tip of twelfth rib; 1 inch inferior and 1.5 inches lateral to umbilicus
T11	Upper colon, kidney, ureter, urinary bladder, prostate, uterus, epididymis	L5-S1 area of low back; just above Poupart's ligament
T12	Same as T11	Just below crest of ilium, 4 inches lateral to midline; just below Poupart's ligament
L1	Kidney, ureter, urinary bladder, epididymis, uterus	Just superior to medial knee; over greater trochanter
L2-4	Not mapped in visceral disorders	
L5-S1	Prostate, uterus	Sole of foot, 1.5 inches anterior to heel; base of great toe
S2	Lower colon, urinary bladder, prostate, uterus	Upper calf; middle of posterior thigh
S3-4	Lower colon, urinary bladder, prostate, uterus	Lower sacral area; ischial tuberosities; glans penis

stimulus, entering the same disturbed cord segment, would create an exaggerated sensation. For instance, probing a patch of skin innervated by T1 would produce an exaggerated sensation if that segment were already disturbed by sensory impulses from a dysfunctional heart.

Head's nineteenth century explanation of referred pain and tenderness is strikingly similar to theories developed in the mid twentieth century. In 1946, Ruch[2] noted that afferent fibers carrying pain signals from somatic and visceral tissues often converged at a common synaptic site within the spinal cord. As a result, interpretation of pain by the thalamus and cerebral cortex may be projected to a larger area than the one from which the pain actually originated. Therefore visceral pain may be experienced at a segmentally related somatic region and somatic pain may be experienced at a segmentally related viscus. This convergence-projection theory of pain referral is widely considered an important mechanism of somatovisceral and viscerosomatic pain referral.

Visceral pain referred by a convergence-projection mechanism is most likely to localize in the embryonic dermatomal segment from which the visceral organ originated.[3] For instance, the heart originated in the embryonic neck and upper thorax; therefore pain signals from the heart enter

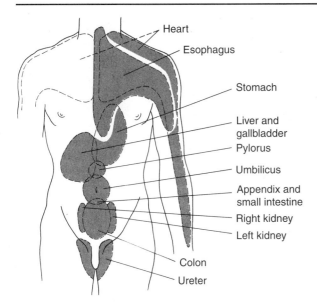

- Heart
- Esophagus
- Stomach
- Liver and gallbladder
- Pylorus
- Umbilicus
- Appendix and small intestine
- Right kidney
- Left kidney
- Colon
- Ureter

Figure 5-1 Surface areas of referred pain from different visceral organs. (From Guyton AC: *Basic neuroscience: anatomy and physiology,* p 133, Philadelphia, 1991, WB Saunders.)

between spinal segments C3 through T5, converging with pain fibers from the side of the neck, the pectoral muscles, the arm, and the substernal area of the chest. As a result, heart damage often provokes a sensation of pain in the neck, arm, and chest, generally on the left side. This same pain distribution can result from damage to spinal muscles, joint capsules, and other somatic structures whose pain signals converge at the C3 through T5 segments. Other regions of pain referral from visceral organs by this embryonic relationship appear in Figure 5-1.

Bruggemann and others[4] recently proposed that sensitization of a cord segment creates a parallel sensitization in the thalamus, which is the actual neurophysiologic site of pain referral. In any event the disturbed cord segment hypothesized by Head many years ago retains its importance as the initial field of sensory signal convergence.

Head's clinical demonstration that spinal nerve irritation via the herpes zoster virus could simulate the pain or tenderness of visceral disease was confirmed by later experimental work that involved irritating muscular or ligamentous structures innervated by various spinal levels. Lewis and Kellgren[5] simulated the referred pain of visceral disease by injecting hypertonic saline solu-

tion into the interspinous ligaments in human subjects. For example, injection into the interspinous ligament at L1 reproduced the pain usually associated with renal colic. The deep pain produced by this procedure did not always correspond to Head's zones of cutaneous tenderness and should be noted, although considerable overlap occurred.

Collectively, the findings of researchers in the past century indicate that spinal nerve irritation or disturbance of spinal musculoskeletal tissue can create perceptions of pain similar to or identical to pain experienced by patients suffering from visceral disease. Because the vertebral subluxation complex (VSC) is capable of disturbing muscular, ligamentous, and neural spinal structures, referred pain from VSC may mimic pain generated by visceral disease.

Nansel and Szlazak[6] extensively reviewed and discussed this phenomenon of visceral disease mimicry by somatic dysfunction in general and the VSC in particular. In their review, the authors cited 351 papers and textbook chapters, originating primarily from the biomedical literature. They concluded that visceral disease mimicry by somatic dysfunction was a relatively frequent phenomenon and suggested that health interventions that correct somatic dysfunction (chiropractic, acupuncture, Rolfing, Qi Gong, and others) would be expected to reduce symptoms of apparent visceral disorders. Based on these observations, the authors urged chiropractic clinicians to be cautious in interpreting their patients' often dramatic relief from apparent internal organ pain and other visceral symptoms. Basing claims of visceral disease cure or treatment on such experiences was viewed as irresponsible, especially with the current knowledge of somatovisceral pain referral.

Nansel's and Szlazak's conclusions were not as reasonable as their previous argument. They stated that they were unable to find any scientifically sound support for a somatovisceral disease mechanism and have voiced the following opinion[6]:

Nor does there seem to be any clinical evidence, even of a purely correlative nature, that would support the notion of a regional or segmentally induced 'somatovisceral disease' connection.

Admittedly, the evidence demonstrating frank visceral tissue pathology related to somatic dys-

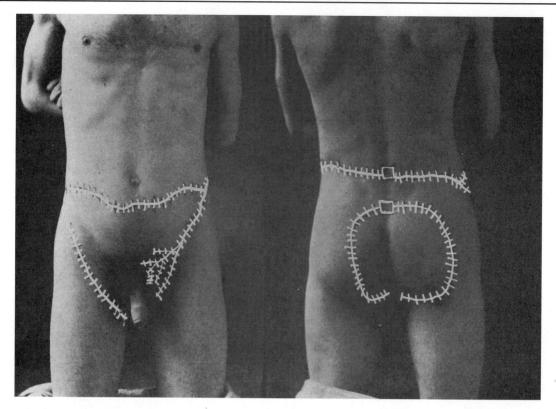

Figure 5-2 Nerve trace of a patient with a history of inguinal hernia. The results of the nerve trace indicated an apparent relationship between the inguinal and scrotal areas and a lumbar and lumbosacral subluxation. (Courtesy Palmer College of Chiropractic.)

function is not yet voluminous and is certainly not incontrovertible. Much remains to be done. However, this is a far cry from the contention that no evidence exists, experimental or clinical, supporting the existence of this phenomenon. Seminal work in this area by medical scientist Henry K. Winsor,[7] osteopathic researcher Louisa Burns,[8-10] and chiropractic investigator Carl S. Cleveland, Jr.[11] represent only the beginnings of this work. These references, and many others that

are discussed in this textbook, are not cited in Nansel's and Szlazak's paper.[6]

Visceral dysfunction, even in the absence of frank tissue pathology, is not a condition of optimal health. Dyspnea without alveolar destruction; cardiac arrhythmia without infarct; vomiting without gastric ulceration; and urinary incontinence without bladder lesions are in a separate category than referred pain or tenderness. They represent disturbances in the actual physiology of

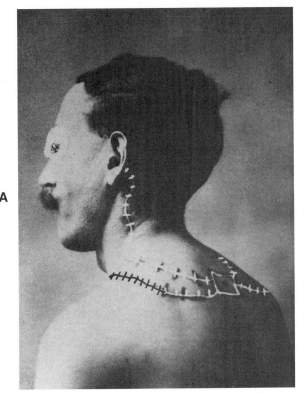 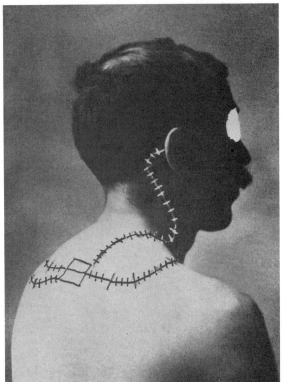

Figure 5-3 Nerve trace of a patient with a history of deafness in both ears. The results of the nerve trace indicated an apparent relationship between the dysfunctional ears and a subluxation at T2-3. (Courtesy Palmer College of Chiropractic.)

the involved organs. Whether such pathophysiology leads to histopathology in every case is irrelevant. Patients with persistent syndromes of such pathophysiology are sick in a manifestly visceral way, and considerable literature, much of which was, in fact, cited by Nansel and Szlazak, exists indicating that somatic dysfunction can lead to such pathophysiology.

Chiropractic Approaches to the Assessment of Referred Visceral Pain and Tenderness

The original chiropractic method of analysis took advantage of the phenomenon of referred tenderness. D.D. Palmer[12] was able to use digital pressure to probe for a line of tenderness from a painful peripheral area to the spine or vice versa. This technique was called *nerve tracing*. A nerve trace to a particular spinal segment was believed to

represent disturbed tone in the indicated spinal nerve. The chiropractor would suspect disturbed neurologic tone as a potential cause of dysfunction in all tissues—somatic or visceral—innervated by the indicated nerve. Originating a nerve trace from a patient with a nauseated stomach or a painful kidney was thought to be as legitimate as tracing from a patient's sore shoulder or painful hip.

D.D. Palmer's son B.J. Palmer[13] published photographs of many such nerve traces in a book written in 1911. Two such photographic records are reproduced in Figures 5-2 and 5-3.

Although nerve tracing in the traditional sense has been largely supplanted by newer methods of analysis, tenderness and digital pain provocation linking the VSC to visceral regions continue to be essential in contemporary chiropractic clinical assessment (see Chapter 8).

Two contemporary chiropractic techniques, Sacrooccipital Technique and Applied Kinesiology, employ points of referred tenderness at the lateral aspects of the head, along what is known as the *temporal sphenoidal line (TS line)*.[14] The points of the TS line have been correlated with skeletal muscle dysfunction, internal organ dysfunction, and vertebral subluxation (Figure 5-4).

Diagnostic points called *alarm points* have existed in classic acupuncture for centuries (Figure 5-5). Pain or tenderness at an alarm point indicates a disturbance in a pathway known as a *meridian.* Meridians are traditionally believed to be pathways of biologic energy called *chi.* Because most meridians have a close association with one or more internal organs, the alarm points may represent the first formally described instance of visceral pain or tenderness referred to somatic structures. Most meridians also have an *associated point* along the spine (Figure 5-6). Some chiropractic authors maintain that disturbance in a particular meridian, as indicated by assessment of the alarm points and other techniques (including pulse analysis and other methods associated with classic accupuncture), is likely to be corre-

lated with a subluxation at the level of the relevant associated point.[15] For this reason, assessment of the alarm points has been included in the analysis procedures of some doctors of chiropractic.

In the 1930s, fascial zones of palpable swelling and tenderness were reported by doctor of osteopathy Frank Chapman to correspond with dysfunctional lymphatic circulation in the internal organs.[16] Stimulation of these *Chapman's reflexes* or *neurolymphatic reflexes* is purported to normalize this dysfunctional lymphatic circulation. Some DCs assess these neurolymphatic reflexes to gain insight into their patients' somatovisceral health status. (Figures 5-7 to 5-12 and Table 5-2).

For chiropractic clinicians of all technique schools, the presence of referred pain or tenderness patterns associated with visceral involvement should be correlated with the patient's history and other current signs and symptoms. When this depiction suggests a potentially serious visceral disease or dysfunction, referral for a medical opinion and possible comanagement is indicated.

Text continued on p. 65

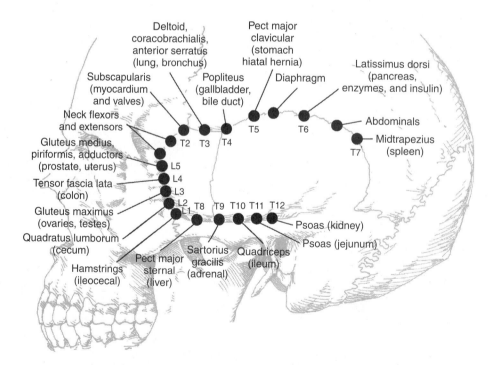

Figure 5-4 Tender points along the temporal sphenoidal line have been correlated with skeletal muscle dysfunction, visceral organ dysfunction, and subluxation at vertebral levels. (Courtesy Walther DS: *Applied kinesiology, synopsis,* ed. 2, Pueblo, Colo, 1999, Systems DC.)

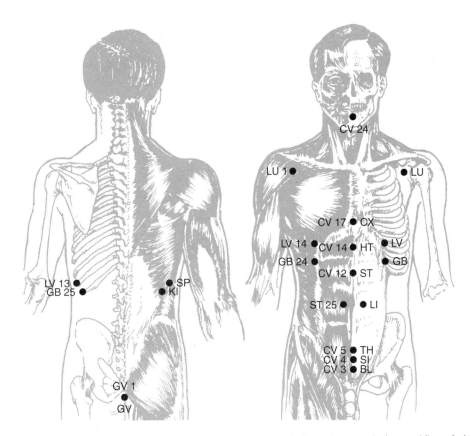

Figure 5-5 Pain or tenderness at the alarm points indicate imbalance in a particular meridian of classic acupuncture. The following meridians are indicated by the following designations: gallbladder *(GB)*, liver *(LV)*, kidney *(KI)*, spleen *(SP)*, governing vessel *(GV)*, conception vessel *(CV)*, lung *(LU)*, circulation sex *(CX)*, heart *(HT)*, stomach *(ST)*, triple heater *(TH)*, large intestine *(LI)*, small intestine *(SI)*, bladder *(BL)*. (Courtesy Walther DS: *Applied kinesiology, synopsis,* ed. 2, Pueblo, Colo, 1999, Systems DC.)

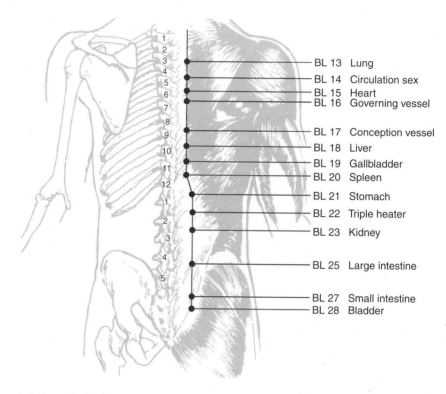

Figure 5-6 Along the bladder meridian of classic acupuncture are associated points correlating each meridian with a vertebral level. This association is used in some forms of chiropractic analysis. (Courtesy Walther DS: *Applied kinesiology, synopsis,* ed. 2, Pueblo, Colo, 1999, Systems DC.)

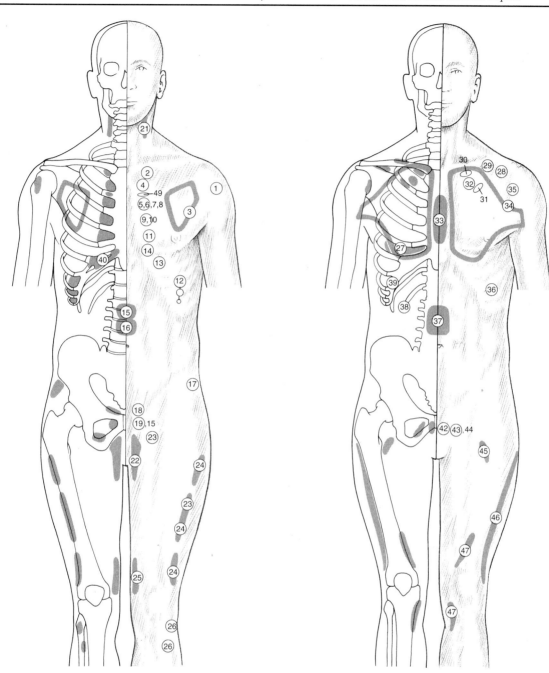

Figure 5-7 Chapman's neurolymphatic reflexes. Refer to Table 5-2 for visceral correlation of Chapman's reflexes illustrated here. (From Chaitow L: *Palpation skills: assessment and diagnosis through touch,* 89, New York, 1997, Churchill Livingstone.)

Figure 5-8 Chapman's neurolymphatic reflexes. Refer to Table 5-2 for visceral correlation of Chapman's reflexes illustrated here. (From Chaitow L: *Palpation skills: assessment and diagnosis through touch,* 89, New York, 1997, Churchill Livingstone.)

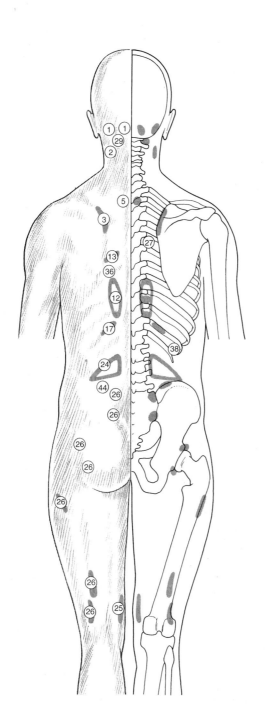

Figure 5-9 Chapman's neurolymphatic reflexes. Refer to Table 5-2 for visceral correlation of Chapman's reflexes illustrated here. (From Chaitow L: *Palpation skills: assessment and diagnosis through touch,* 90, New York, 1997, Churchill Livingstone.)

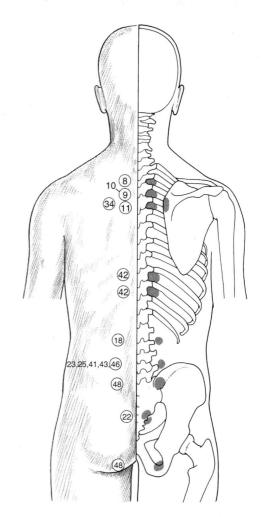

Figure 5-10 Chapman's neurolymphatic reflexes. Refer to Table 5-2 for visceral correlation of Chapman's reflexes illustrated here. (From Chaitow L: *Palpation skills: assessment and diagnosis through touch,* 90, New York, 1997, Churchill Livingstone.)

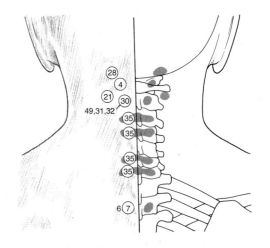

Figure 5-11 Chapman's neurolymphatic reflexes. Refer to Table 5-2 for visceral correlation of Chapman's reflexes illustrated here. (From Chaitow L: *Palpation skills: assessment and diagnosis through touch,* 90, New York, 1997, Churchill Livingstone.)

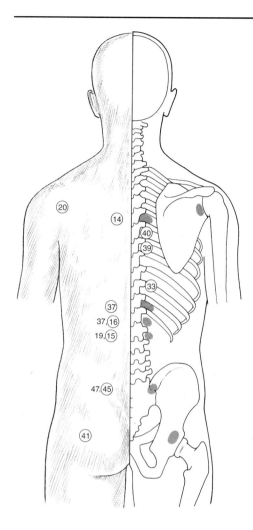

Figure 5-12 Chapman's neurolymphatic reflexes. Refer to Table 5-2 for visceral correlation of Chapman's reflexes illustrated here. (From Chaitow L: *Palpation skills: assessment and diagnosis through touch,* 91, New York, 1997, Churchill Livingstone.)

Table 5-2   *Location of Chapman's Neurolymphatic Reflexes*

No. Symptoms/Area	Anterior	Fig.	Posterior	Fig.
1. Conjunctivitis and retinitis	Upper humerus	5-7	Occipital area	5-9
2. Nasal problems	Anterior aspect of first rib close to sternum	5-7	Posterior the angle of the jaw on the tip of the transverse process of the first cervical vertebra	5-9
3. Arms (circulation)	Muscular attachments pectoralis minor to third, fourth, and fifth ribs	5-7	Superior angle of scapula and superior third of the medial margin of the scapula	5-9
4. Tonsillitis	Between first and second ribs close to sternum	5-7	Midway between spinous process and tip of transverse process of first cervical vertebra	5-11
5. Thyroid	Second intercostal space close to sternum	5-7	Midway between spinous process and tip of transverse process of second thoracic vertebra	5-9

From Chaitow L: *Palpation skills: assessment and diagnosis through touch,* p 273, New York, 1997, Churchill Livingstone.

Continued

Table 5-2   *Location of Chapman's Neurolymphatic Reflexes—cont'd*

No. Symptoms/Area	Anterior	Fig.	Posterior	Fig.
6. Bronchitis	Second intercostal space close to sternum	5-7	Midway between spinous process and tip of transverse process of second thoracic vertebra	5-11
7. Oesophagus	As no. 6	5-7	As no. 6	5-11
8. Myocarditis	As no. 6	5-7	Between the second and third thoracic transverse processes. Midway between the spinous process and the tip of the transverse process	5-10
9. Upper lung	Third intercostal space close to the sternum	5-7	As no. 8	5-10
10. Neuritis of upper limb	As no. 9	5-7	Between the third and fourth transverse processes, midway between the spinous process and the tip of the transverse process	5-10
11. Lower lung	Fourth intercostal space, close to sternum	5-7	Between fourth and fifth transverse processes, midway between the spinous process and the tip of the transverse process	5-10
12. Small intestines	Eighth, ninth, and tenth intercostal spaces close to cartilage	5-7	Eighth, ninth, and tenth thoracic intertransverse spaces	5-9
13. Gastric hypercongestion	Sixth intercostal space to the left of the sternum	5-7	Sixth thoracic intertransverse space, left side	5-9
14. Gastric hyperacidity	Fifth intercostal space to the left of the sternum	5-7	Fifth thoracic intertransverse space, left side	5-12
15. Cystitis	Around the umbilicus and on the pubic symphysis close to the midline	5-7	Upper edge of the transverse processes of the second lumbar vertebra	5-12
16. Kidneys	Slightly superior to and lateral to the umbilicus	5-7	In the intertransverse space between the twelfth thoracic and the first lumbar vertebrae	5-12
17. Atonic constipation	Between the anterior superior spine of the ilium and the trochanter	5-7	Eleventh costal vertebral junction	5-9
18. Abdominal tension	Superior border of the pubic bone	5-7	Tip of the transverse process of the second lumbar vertebra	5-10
19. Urethra	Inner edge of pubic ramus near superior aspect of symphysis	5-7	Superior aspect of transverse process of second lumbar vertebra	5-12
20. Dupuytren's contracture and arm and shoulder pain	None		Anterior aspect of lateral margin of scapulae, inferior to the head of humerus	5-12
21. Cerebral congestion (related to paralysis or paresis)	(On the posterior aspect of the body) lateral from the spines of the third, fourth, and fifth cervical vertebrae	5-7	Between the transverse processes of the first and second cervical vertebrae	5-11

From Chaitow L: *Palpation skills: assessment and diagnosis through touch*, p 273, New York, 1997, Churchill Livingstone.

Table 5-2   *Location of Chapman's Neurolymphatic Reflexes—cont'd*

No. Symptoms/Area	Anterior	Fig.	Posterior	Fig.
22. Clitoral irritation and vaginismus	Upper medial aspect of the thigh	5-7	Lateral to the junction of the sacrum and the coccyx	5-10
23. Prostate	Lateral aspect of the thigh from the trochanter to just above the knee. Also lateral to symphysis pubis as in uterine conditions (see no. 43)	5-7	Between the posterior superior spine of the ilium and the spinous process of the fifth lumbar vertebra	5-10
24. Spastic constipation or colitis	Within an area of 1-2 inches wide extending from the trochanter to within 1 inch of the patella	5-7	From the transverse processes of the second, third, and fourth lumbar vertebrae to the crest of the ilium	5-9
25. Leucorrhoea	Lower medial aspect of thigh, slightly posteriorly (on the posterior aspect of the body)	5-7 & 5-9	Between the posterior and superior spine of the ilium and the spinous process of the fifth lumbar vertebra	5-10
26. Sciatic neuritis	Anterior and posterior to the tibiofibular junction	5-7	1. On the sacroiliac synchondrosis 2. Between the ischial tuberosity and the acetabulum 3. Lateral and posterior aspects of the thigh	5-9
27. Torpid liver (nausea, fullness, malaise)	Fifth intercostal space, from the midmammillary line to the sternum	5-8	Fifth thoracic intertransverse space on the right side	5-9
28. Cerebellar congestion (memory and concentration lapses)	Tip of coracoid process of scapula	5-8	Just inferior to the base of the skull on the first cervical vertebra	5-11
29. Otitis media	Upper edge of clavicle where it crosses the first rib	5-8	Superior aspect of first cervical transverse process (tip)	5-9
30. Pharyngitis	Anterior aspect of the first rib close to the sternum	5-8	Midway between the spinous process and the tip of the transverse process of the second cervical vertebra	5-11
31. Laryngitis	Upper surface of the second rib, 2 or 3 inches (5-8 cm) from the sternum	5-8	Midway between the spinous process and the tip of the second cervical vertebra	5-11
32. Sinusitis	Lateral to the sternum on the superior edge of the second rib in the first intercostal space	5-8	As no. 31	5-11
33. Pyloric stenosis	On the sternum	5-8	Tenth costovertebral junction on the right side	5-12

Continued

Table 5-2 *Location of Chapman's Neurolymphatic Reflexes—cont'd*

No. Symptoms/Area	Anterior	Fig.	Posterior	Fig.
34. Neurasthenia (chronic fatigue)	All the muscular attachments of pectoralis major on the humerus, clavicle, sternum, and ribs (especially fourth rib)	5-8	Below the superior medial edge of the scapula on the face of the fourth rib	5-10
35. Wry neck (torticollis)	Medial aspect of upper edge of the humerus	5-8	Transverse processes of the third, fourth, sixth, and seventh cervical vertebrae	5-11
36. Splenitis	Seventh intercostal space close to the cartilaginous junction, on the left	5-8	Seventh intertransverse space on the left	5-9
37. Adrenals (allergies, exhaustion)	Superior and lateral to umbilicus	5-8	In the intertransverse space between the eleventh and twelfth thoracic vertebrae	5-12
38. Mesoappendix	Superior aspect of the twelfth rib, close to the tip, on right	5-8	Lateral aspect of the eleventh intercostal space on the right	5-9
39. Pancreas	Seventh intercostal space on the right, close to the cartilage	5-8	Seventh thoracic intertransverse space on the right	5-12
40. Liver and gallbladder congestion	Sixth intercostal space, from the midmammillary line to the sternum (right side)	5-7	Sixth thoracic intertransverse space, right side	5-12
41. Salpingitis or vesiculitis	Midway between the acetabulum and the sciatic notch (this is on the posterior aspect of the body)	5-12	Between the posterior, superior spine of the ilium and the spinous process of the fifth lumbar vertebra	5-10
42. Ovaries	The round ligaments from the superior border of the pubic bone, inferiorly	5-8	Between the ninth and tenth intertransverse space and the tenth and eleventh intertransverse space	5-10
43. Uterus	Anterior aspect of the junction of the ramus of the pubis and the ischium	5-8	Between the posterior, superior spine of the ilium and the fifth lumbar spinous process	5-10
44. Uterine fibroma	Lateral to the symphysis, extending diagonally inferiorly	5-8	Between the tip of the transverse process of the fifth lumbar vertebra and the crest of the ilium	5-9
45. Rectum	Just inferior to the lesser trochanter	5-8	On the sacrum close to the ilium at the lower end of the iliosacral synchondrosis	5-12
46. Broad ligament (uterine involvement usual)	Lateral aspect of the thigh from the trochanter to just above the knee	5-8	Between the posterior, superior spine of the ilium and the fifth lumbar spinous process	5-10

From Chaitow L: *Palpation skills: assessment and diagnosis through touch,* p 273, New York, 1997, Churchill Livingstone.

Table 5-2 *Location of Chapman's Neurolymphatic Reflexes—cont'd*

No. Symptoms/Area	Anterior	Fig.	Posterior	Fig.
47. Groin glands (circulation and drainage of legs and pelvic organs)	Lower quarter of the sartorius muscle and its attachment to the tibia	5-8	On the sacrum close to the ilium at the lower end of iliosacral synchondrosis	5-12
48. Hemorrhoids	Just superior to the ischial tuberosity (these areas are on the posterior surface of the body)	5-10	On the sacrum close to the ilium, at the lower end of the iliosacral synchondrosis	5-10
49. Tongue	Anterior aspect of second rib at the cartilaginous junction with the sternum	5-7	Midway between the spinous process and the tip of the transverse process of the second cervical vertebra	5-11

Selected Clinical Syndromes

Pseudoangina

The phenomenon of precordial pain originating in the cervical area simulating coronary ischemic disease was described in the biomedical literature at least as early as 1927.[17] This occurence is called *cervical angina.*

Booth and Rothman[18] described a series of seven cases of cervical angina. In each case, the primary complaint from the patient was precordial pain, often accompanied by nausea, dyspnea, and diaphoresis. Although cardiovascular findings such as murmurs and blood pressure variations were notably absent on physical examination, reduced cervical range of motion was present in all cases. In two patients, the precordial pain could be reproduced with digital pressure at paracervical trigger points. Roentgenographic evidence of cervical spondylosis was found in all seven patients, with findings clustering at the C5-6 motion segment. Two patients received substantial relief of the angina symptoms by using soft cervical collars. Three additional patients underwent surgical disc excision and fusion at the involved cervical level and displayed full recovery from angina symptoms at 1 year of follow-up.

Jacobs[19] presented 164 cases of cervical angina treated over 22 years. Each of these patients had experienced precordial pain for 10 months or more and most of the patients had consulted at least two cardiologists before diagnosis. Neck pain, occipital headache, and arm pain indicated probable cervical involvement, which was then confirmed by x-ray examination. Although surgical intervention was required in 38 cases, the majority of problems were successfully managed by 3 months or more of conservative medical management such as the patient receiving intermittent traction, wearing a hard collar, engaging in isometric exercise, and taking antiinflammatories and muscle relaxants.

Wells[20] reported the case of a 48-year-old woman who went to her cardiologist because she had symptoms of chest pain, nausea, and shortness of breath for 2 weeks. A cardiologic work-up including electrocardiogram, echocardiogram, treadmill test, and blood chemistry was unremarkable. Wells noted a reduced triceps reflex on the patient's left side and reproduction of the patient's chest pain on left lateral head tilt. A C6-7 left-sided disc herniation was noted on magnetic resonance imaging (MRI). The patient's pain was reduced by 70% to 80% after 2 months of conservative medical management, including wearing a cervical collar, receiving cervical traction, performing isometric exercises, and taking nonsteroidal antiinflammatory medication.

Successful management of cervical angina by conservative medical methods suggests the possibility that a more direct approach by manual spinal methods would work. Indeed, manual medicine advocate Mennell[21] frequently found manipulation to resolve cervical angina.

Homewood[22] noted that the VSC at the C3-6 levels could irritate the roots of the phrenic nerve, causing diaphragm spasm. If this occurred in the left hemidiaphragm, chest pain, dyspnea, and nausea could easily result. The anxiety related to such symptoms could provoke tachycardia and diaphoresis in the patient. If the roots of the brachial plexus were also involved, left arm pain could complete the classic clinical description of a patient suffering a coronary ischemic episode. Homewood stated that many such cases were resolved by chiropractic adjustment of the involved cervical level, often with one visit.

Pseudoangina unrelated to cervical dysfunction has also been widely reported in the biomedical literature. Kellgren[23] reported four cases in which pressure over tender spots in the thoracic spine or shoulder girdle reproduced the precordial pain of apparent angina. Novocaine injection into these tender spots resolved the pain in all but one patient, who proved to have genuine coronary disease. Kellgren noted that spontaneous movement rarely provoked the angina-like pain and that each segment of the spine must be examined to find the connection. Precordial pain that continued day and night for long periods was seen as more likely to be somatic in origin, and true coronary pain tends to manifest in attacks. Kellgren also noted that areas of locally increased thoracic kyphosis were most likely to harbor trigger areas for pseudoangina pain.

Six cases of thoracic pseudoangina were presented by Hamberg and Lindahl.[24] The major examination finding was spinous process tenderness, demonstrated by a jump reaction by the patient as the examiner's finger pressed on the spinous process. The spinal manipulation technique described resembles chiropractic techniques for adjusting thoracic anteriorities. This manipulative intervention resulted in relief for all six patients, sometimes in as little as one visit, with follow-up periods as long as 10 years. A study by Bechgaard[25] in the same volume and journal as Hamberg's and Lindahl's study found that thoracic pseudoangina was the third most common diagnosis after coronary thrombosis and true angina pectoris in a series of 1,097 patients admitted to a hospital coronary unit.

Pellegrino[26] described four cases of pseudoangina related to myofascial trigger points. These trigger points were located in a variety of muscles, including the pectorals, trapezii, brachioradialis, and supraspinatous. All of the patients in this group had chest pain; three patients had tachycardia or palpitations; and two patients were experiencing dyspnea. Before referral to Pellegrino's department, all of these patients underwent extensive and inconclusive cardiologic work-ups, including cardiac catheterization in two cases. In addition to trigger point injection with Lidocaine, more general physical medicine interventions were used, including hot packs, ice packs, massage, whirlpool baths, therapeutic exercise, and antidepressant drugs. These treatments produced favorable results for all four patients.

Benhamou and others[27] reported several cases of pseudoangina in a group of patients with pseudovisceral pain from costovertebral dysfunction. Provocation of the angina-like pain during paravertebral palpation, mobilization of a rib in the horizontal or vertical plane, or "vigorous thoracic compression between the hands of the physician" were helpful in physical examination.[27] Special studies included provocation of the pain by contrast medium injection into the related costovertebral joint and elimination of the pain by anesthetic injection into the same joint. Treatment by corticosteroid injections and oral nonsteroidal antiinflammatory drugs was generally successful.

T4 syndrome is a catch-all term for a constellation of symptoms related to the VSC of the upper thoracic vertebrae in general and T4 in particular. Prominent among these symptoms is pain, tingling, or a tight band feeling around one or both arms or hands. In a recent literature review, Evans[28] stated that patients with T4 syndrome often go to hospital emergency rooms because of their frequent angina-like pain accompanied by left upper extremity paresthesia. Chiropractors DeFranca and Levine[29] presented two patients with T4 syndrome who responded well to thoracic anteriority adjusting. However, their cases did not involve pseudoangina as such.

For some reason the chiropractic literature on pseudoangina is sparse. Perhaps this is because chiropractic clinicians often find out about relief of angina-like pain long after the fact from patients reluctant to discuss their fears, making proper documentation and follow-up difficult.

Conversely, relief of pseudoangina is perhaps a frequent event in chiropractic practice and the commonplace diagnosis is likely to be ignored. Nansel and Szlazak begin their previously cited paper with the following statement[6]:

> One need not be in residence at a chiropractic college for very long before one hears of a patient exhibiting deep radiating pain involving their upper back, chest and arm (symptoms most often associated with cardiac angina) who has experienced significant amelioration of their symptoms immediately following a single upper thoracic or lower cervical spinal adjustment.

We have indeed had similar experiences in our practices, and anecdotal descriptions of such occurrences by our colleagues are not at all rare.

Pseudoangina may not always be entirely "psuedo." Obviously, referred cervical or thoracic pain can coexist with genuine coronary disease. A medical opinion to rule this out is always wise, although in acute situations, the patient often has already taken this step before visiting the chiropractor. The presence of frank cardiovascular disease is not a contraindication to chiropractic care, provided that appropriate precautions are observed (see Chapter 10).

Apparent pseudoangina may sometimes represent a disturbance in cardiac physiology that has not yet progressed to the point of full-blown disease. One of the cases of cervical angina reported by Booth and Rothman demonstrated electrocardiographic abnormalities.[18] These abnormalities reverted to normal after cervical spine surgery. The results of stress tests were abnormal in 10 out of 164 of Jacobs' cervical angina patients.[19] Electrocardiographic abnormalities were also found in one of Kellgren's pseudoangina patients,[23] and a history of fainting spells was discovered in another. A history of fainting in connection with precordial pain was also reported in two of Hamberg's and Lindahl's pseudoangina patients.[24]

The possibility that the same vertebral dysfunctions leading to pseudoangina may also be associated with cardiac pathophysiology should be seriously considered. Pseudoangina may lie on a continuum, somewhere between optimal cardiovascular health and frank cardiovascular disease.

Other Syndromes Involving the Chest

The previously cited paper by Benhamou and others[27] involved at least one case of costovertebral arthropathy mimicking the pain of pulmonary embolism. Relief was obtained by corticosteroid injection and nonsteroidal antiinflammatory drugs.

LaBan and others[30] described 18 cases of breast pain from cervical dysfunction. All of these patients had extensive but noninformative breast evaluations, including 10 mammograms and 4 biopsies. When they were evaluated by the physical medicine department, no masses were palpated in their breasts, but the underlying pectoral musculature was invariably the site of multiple myofascial trigger points. Physical examination, x-ray, and electromyography revealed cervical spondylosis in every instance, with findings clustering at C6-7. Cervical traction resolved this referred breast pain in all cases.

Pain and Tenderness Referral Involving the Upper Abdomen

Kellgren's previously cited paper[23] involved two cases of upper abdominal pain. One patient was a 48-year-old woman with a history suggestive of gastric ulcer, which included 1 year of epigastric pain associated with nausea. A barium study revealed no sign of ulcer. Forced extension of the midthoracic spine reproduced the epigastric pain. Novocaine injection at the T8-9 level abolished this patient's symptoms.

The second patient had a history suggestive of cholecystitis, including pain at the right costal margin and right scapula associated with nausea and flatulence. A cholecystogram failed to show any abnormality of the gallbladder. Marked tenderness was noted at the T6-7 interspinous ligament. Novocaine injection at that site resolved the abdominal symptoms.

Ashby[31] presented a number of cases of abdominal pain originating in the spine. One case involved a 41-year-old man whose 12-year history of right subcostal pain suggested cholecystitis. Two cholecystograms showed no abnormality. However, spinal examination revealed dysfunction at the right T8 costovertebral joint. After a right T8 intercostal block by injection of Lignocaine was administered, the right subcostal pain was abolished and did not recur.

Jorgensen and Fossgreen[32] compared spinal history and examination findings of 39 patients with upper abdominal pain with 28 controls. After extensive work-ups as hospital inpatients, the patients with abdominal pain were not found to have any demonstrable visceral pathology. Approximately 72% of the patients versus 17% of the controls reported back pain as a current complaint. Palpation for tenderness revealed spinal dysfunction in 75% of the patients with reported back pain, with abnormalities gathered in the lower thoracic segments.

In Benhamou's study,[27] what was previously said about pseudoangina and false pulmonary embolism also applies to upper abdominal pain, including symptoms suggestive of duodenal ulcer and pancreatitis. These upper abdominal pains were found to be related to costovertebral dysfunction, and were resolved with injected and oral antiinflammatory medications.

In a mechanism similar to the one he proposed for cervical angina, Homewood[22] suggested that right hemidiaphragm spasm from cervical subluxation could refer pain to the right flank and shoulder. This could give the impression of gallbladder or liver disease. Favorable results were often obtained by chiropractic adjustment of the involved levels, usually between C3 and C6.

Schafer[33] suggested that pain referable to upper cervical subluxation can originate in upper gastrointestinal tract disorders. In such cases, cervicogenic headache could actually be a viscerosomatic disorder.

Pain and Tenderness Involving the Lower Abdomen

Kellgren's paper[23] included three cases involving lower abdominal pain. One patient was a 42-year-old woman presumed to be suffering from acute appendicitis. She went to the hospital because she was suffering from severe pain in the right iliac fossa. She was also nauseated and vomiting. After appendicitis was ruled out, a musculoskeletal examination revealed loss of thoracolumbar range of motion in all planes. A trigger point in the patient's erector spinae muscles to the right of T12 was injected with Novocaine. This resulted in prompt relief of the abdominal pain and the spinal stiffness.

The other two patients were men complaining of testicular pain. In each case, a full urologic work-up was noninformative. Both patients also had a recent history of low back pain. Spinal examination revealed trigger areas in the paravertebral region around L1; Novocaine injected into the region resolved the testicular pain in both instances.

Ashby[31] reported four cases of lower abdominal pain. Three of the patients were women with right iliac pain suggestive of appendicitis. Physical examination, barium studies, and other tests ruled out this diagnosis in all three cases. In one patient, a right T10 intercostal block with Lignocaine produced immediate and complete resolution. In another case, a single intercostal block (level not noted) did bring complete ease but only after a week. In the third case, intercostal block only generated temporary relief, and multiple visits were required until the condition finally subsided 18 months after examination.

Ashby's fourth case was a 75-year-old man with a 3 month history of left groin pain with intermittent hematuria. An intravenous pyelogram did demonstrate bladder outlet obstruction, possibly caused by the passage of a renal stone. A T12 intercostal block relieved this pain. This may have been an instance in which referred pain exacerbated a genuine underlying pathology.

Rubenstein[34] reported the case of a 39-year-old man who endured several months of severe right lower abdominal pain. During physical examination, gastrointestinal and genitourinary pathology were dismissed by sigmoidoscopy, barium enema, and intravenous urography. At a subsequent visit, tenderness to digital pressure was noted just superior to the right pubic bone. Lidocaine injection at this site relieved the abdominal pain for several hours. At a follow-up visit, corticosteroid injection at the same site resulted in lasting relief.

Twelve additional cases of this syndrome called *periostitis pubis* were described by Rubenstein over the next 5 years. Right- and left-sided involvement were equally frequent. Duration of symptoms before the physical examination ranged from several weeks to 2 years. Ipsilateral suprapubic tenderness was invariably found, and response to tender point corticosteroid injection was favorable in all cases except one.

Rubenstein does not offer a detailed mechanism for periostitis pubis, except to hypothesize that it may be of mechanical origin. In this connection, subluxation at the pubic symphysis being a frequent radiographic finding in the sacroiliac subluxation syndrome is interesting to note.[35] Sacroiliac subluxation often being the "mechanical origin" referred to by Rubenstein would not be a surprising discovery, although specific chiropractic clinical research documenting this has not been discovered.

Jamelick and others[36] reported 10 cases of testalgia. After urogenital disease was ruled out, a musculoskeletal examination revealed ipsilateral thoracolumbar dysfunction in every case. Nine of the patients also exhibited psoas muscle spasm, and five had ipsilateral dysfunction of the sacroiliac joint. The testicular pain completely disappeared after spinal manipulation, often with one visit. Interestingly, every one of these patients denied a history of back pain; testalgia was the only presenting symptom.

The previously cited paper by Benhamou and others[27] mentions one case of costovertebral arthropathy causing referred pain suggestive of renal colic. This pain was resolved by giving the patient injected and oral antiinflammatory medication.

Lower sacral nerve root irritation has been found to be associated with a myriad of lower abdominal pain syndromes and actual pathophysiology of the lower abdominal organs. Chiropractic care often resolves this lower sacral nerve root involvement and the related symptoms, even in the face of considerable chronicity (see Chapter 8).

STUDY GUIDE

1. Where is visceral pain referred by a convergence-projection mechanism most likely to localize? Define a convergence-projection mechanism.
2. What organ is currently assumed to be the actual neurophysiologic site of pain referral? Is this considered an endocrine organ?
3. Can referred pain from the VSC mimic visceral disease? Why?
4. What is the significance of the work of Henry Winsor?
5. At what stage of dis-ease can the patient be said to be exhibiting frank visceral dysfunction?
6. How would somatic dysfunction lead to pathophysiology?
7. Name an early means of analysis that used the phenomenon of referred pain.
8. Describe the use of the temporosphenoidal line.
9. What is an alarm point? Relate this to the concept of tone.
10. What is the concept behind Chapman's reflexes?
11. Describe the symptoms of cervical angina. Describe at least one mechanism by which the VSC could cause this problem.
12. What is T4 syndrome?
13. Considering the source of pseudoangina, why does so little chiropractic research exist on the problem, despite a national emphasis on detecting heart disease?
14. At what point would you refer a patient with signs of possible visceral disease for medical comanagement?
15. Name three organs that might be directly affected by the VSC at T12.

REFERENCES

1. Head H: On disturbances of sensation with especial reference to the pain of visceral disease, *Brain* 16:1, 1893.
2. Ruch TC: Visceral sensation and referred pain. In Fulton JF, editor: *Howell's textbook of physiology,* vol 15, Philadelphia, 1946, WB Saunders.
3. Guyton AC: *Basic neuroscience: anatomy and physiology,* p 133, Philadelphia, 1991, WB Saunders.
4. Bruggemann J, Shi T, Apkarian V: Squirrel monkey lateral thalamus, II, viscerosomatic convergent representation of urinary bladder, colon, and esophagus, *J Neurosci* 14:6796, 1994.
5. Lewis T, Kellgren JH: Observations relating to referred pain, visceromotor reflexes and other associated phenomena, *Clin Sci* 4:47, 1939.
6. Nansel D, Szlazak M: Somatic dysfunction and the phenomenon of visceral disease simulation: a probable explanation for the apparent effectiveness of somatic therapy in patients presumed to be suffering from true visceral disease, *J Manipulative Physiol Ther* 18:379, 1995.

7. Winsor HK: Sympathetic segmental disturbances, II, *Med Times* 49:267, 1922.

8. Burns L, Steudenberg G, Vollbrecht WJ: Family of rabbits with second thoracic and other lesions, *J Am Osteopath Assoc* 42:3, 1937.

9. Burns L: Preliminary report of cardiac changes following the correction of third thoracic lesions, *J Am Osteopath Assoc* 42:3, 1943.

10. Burns L, Candler L, Rice R: *Pathogenesis of visceral diseases following vertebral lesions,* Chicago, 1948, American Osteopathic Association.

11. Cleveland CS Jr: Researching the subluxation on the domestic rabbit, *Sci Rev Chiro* 1(4):5, 1965.

12. Palmer DD: *The science, art and philosophy of chiropractic,* Portland, Ore, 1910, Portland Printing House.

13. Palmer BJ: *The Philosophy, science, and art of chiropractic nerve tracing,* Davenport, Iowa, 1911, Palmer School of Chiropractic.

14. Walther DS: *Applied kinesiology,* vol I, p 39, Pueblo, Colo, 1981, Systems DC.

15. Walther DS: *Applied kinesiology: synopsis,* p 247, Pueblo, Colo, 1988, Systems DC.

16. Chaitow L: *Palpation skills: assessment and diagnosis through touch,* p 86, New York, 1997, Churchill Livingstone.

17. Phillips J: The importance of examination of the spine in the presence of intrathoracic or abdominal pain, *Proc Interst Postgrad MA North America* 3:70, 1927.

18. Booth RE, Rothman RH: Cervical angina, *Spine* 1:28, 1976.

19. Jacobs B: Cervical angina, *NY State J Med* 90:8, 1990.

20. Wells P: Cervical angina, *Am Fam Physician* 55:2262, 1997.

21. Mennell JMCM: The validation of the diagnosis "joint dysfunction" in the synovial joints of the cervical spine, *J Manipulative Physiol Ther* 13:7, 1990.

22. Homewood AE: *The neurodynamics of the vertebral subluxation,* p 193, St. Petersburg, Fla, 1977, Valkyrie Press.

23. Kellgren JH: Somatic simulating visceral pain, *Clin Sci* 4:303, 1940.

24. Hamberg J, Lindahl O: Angina pectoris symptoms caused by thoracic spine disorders: clinical examination and treatment, *Acta Med Scand* 644(suppl):34, 1981.

25. Bechgaard P: Segmental thoracic pain in patients admitted to a medical department and a coronary unit, *Acta Med Scand* 644(suppl):87, 1981.

26. Pellegrino MJ: Atypical chest pain as an initial presentation of primary fibromyalgia. *Arch Phys Med Rehabil* 71:526, 1990.

27. Benhamou CL et al: Pseudovisceral pain referred from costovertebral arthropathies, *Spine* 18:790, 1993.

28. Evans P: The T4 syndrome: some basic science aspects, *Physiother* 83:186, 1997.

29. DeFranca GG, Levine LJ: The T4 syndrome, *J Manipulative Physiol Ther* 18:34, 1995.

30. LaBan MM, Meerschaert JR, Taylor RS: Breast pain: a symptom of cervical radiculopathy, *Arch Phys Med Rehabil* 60:315, 1979.

31. Ashby EC: Abdominal pain of spinal origin: value of intercostal block, *Ann R Coll Surg Engl* 59:242, 1977.

32. Jorgensen LS, Fossgreen J: Back pain and spinal pathology in patients with functional upper abdominal pain, *Scand J Gastroenterol* 25:1235, 1990.

33. Schafer RC: *Symptomatology and differential diagnosis: a conspectus of clinical semeiographies,* p 737, Arlington, Va, 1986, American Chiropractic Association.

34. Rubenstein NH: Chronic abdominal pain due to periostitis pubis, *Postgrad Med* 91:147, 1992.

35. Panzer DM, Gatterman MI: Sacroiliac subluxation syndrome. In Gatterman MI, editor: *Foundations of chiropractic: subluxation,* p 452, St Louis, 1995, Mosby.

36. Jamelick R, Penickova V, Vyborny K: Testalgia caused by dysfunction at the throaco-lumbar junction, *J Man Med* 6:189, 1992.

CHAPTER 6

Patient-Based Outcomes Assessment: "Pencil-and-Paper" Instruments

Cheryl Hawk, DC, PhD

What Are "Patient-Based" Outcomes Assessments?

Chiropractic's patient-centered and health-oriented approach to care has always been a strong feature with the public. Chiropractors give understandable explanations of health problems, communicate, and treat their patients through physical touch.[1,2] They emphasize *health* rather than *disease* and treat the person rather than the symptoms.[1] However, for purposes of assessing the outcomes of care, chiropractors have generally imitated the medical physician's reliance on mechanistic, practitioner-based methods.[3-5] These methods are perceived as objective. If a doctor uses mechanical or electronic instrumentation, this proves that the measurement is objective, but if a patient reports a perception, this is viewed as subjective and devalued as a valid measure.[6]

However, in the evolving health care system, self-assessed, or subjective measures are gaining credibility.[4,7,8] Consumer satisfaction with care and perception of improvement are not marginal but primary considerations.[9] Once devalued as subjective, patient-based measures of pain and disability are now becoming the standard for outcome measures in clinical trials and practice-based research.[10,11] Clinicians and health policymakers are recognizing the importance of positive measures of quality of life and general health status.[4] Even pharmaceutical trials are now including quality of life outcomes assessments.[12] For example, a trial of hypertension drugs included a subject-reported psychometric test to assess patients' psychologic well-being.[12] Furthermore, patient-based measures have been demonstrated to be *more* predictive of outcomes than physiologic measures.[13] For example, patient-reported symptoms of disability have been found to be more predictive of outcomes such as returning to work than diagnostic tests or signs such as x-rays or orthopedic examinations of physical abnormalities.[13]

Why Should Clinicians use "Pencil-and-Paper" Instruments?

To substantiate the effects of chiropractic care, outcome measures must be available to determine those effects as follows[14]:

> The failure to develop consistent outcome measures that reflect clinically meaningful changes in the patient's status is the most serious flaw in clinical studies. The unreliability of physical measurements in defining outcomes has led to a shift toward using patient-reported perceptions as outcome measures.

Evidence-based decision-making in clinical practice requires, first of all, *evidence*. Evidence of the effect of chiropractic care on patients' functional status such as patients' ability to function effectively in their daily lives requires input not only from the doctor but also from the patient. Evidence of the effect of chiropractic on states of positive health and well-being that are even more elusive to identify through traditional instrumentation requires the collection of attitudinal data from the patient. Positive health is difficult to detect solely through currently existing physiologic measures. Collecting information on how the patient feels facilitates interpretation of other data and adds an important dimension to the available evidence.

Patient-based measures are an important component of evidence-based practice for the following reasons:

- They can measure factors important to the patient.
- They can predict clinical outcomes.
- They can measure quality of life and other global concepts that interest chiropractors such as correcting causes of dis-ease.
- They can assess positive characteristics such as well-being and negative traits such as pain.
- They can provide indirect information on physiologic functions that cannot be directly monitored in a noninvasive, cost-effective way.

However, like any other instruments used in clinical practice, patient-based measures must be used correctly or their results are meaningless or even misleading. Therefore in this chapter, information will be presented about how to use patient-based instruments in general and specific descriptions and instructions for use of several of the most useful instruments for chiropractic clinicians interested in assessing states of health not exclusively related to the musculoskeletal system.

How to Use Patient-Based Instruments

The purpose of this chapter is not simply to provide instruments for clinicians to use in practice. It is to provide the necessary background on patient-based instruments to allow a clinician to make informed decisions about when such instruments are appropriate, how to select the best one, and how to interpret it in a meaningful manner.

So-called *soft* assessment instruments, although administered by pencil and paper, share the same requirements for effective use with *hard* instruments made of chrome and electronic circuitry: demonstration of reliability, validity, and clinical responsiveness.[15] A real distinction exists between outcome measures that are objective and those that are subjective. Any measurement cannot be called *objective* unless it yields the same measure regardless of who administers it. This type of re-

producibility is actually easier to achieve with a standardized questionnaire than with a goniometer or an x-ray line drawing. In the case of patient-assessed measures, objectivity and minimization of bias are maintained through appropriate procedures of instrument selection, data collection, and interpretation.[12]

Instrument Selection

Selection of the most appropriate pencil-and-paper instrument is made by the clinician doing the following:

1. Considering the reliability, validity, and clinical responsiveness of the instrument.
2. Determining that the instrument measures the characteristic of interest.

Reliability, Validity, and Clinical Responsiveness For a given instrument, formal tests of reliability, validity, and clinical responsiveness should be published in the literature and available for review. This does not mean chiropractors cannot develop new instruments; the Neck Disability Index and the Global Well-Being Scale are proof of this.[16,17] Clinicians should be aware of the importance of these properties and make some assessment of whether they have been demonstrated, and new instruments should be formally tested before they are made available for general use. Although many doctors of chiropractic (DC) have developed ingenious and intuitive questionnaires to assess various aspects of health, few have had the resources to perform tests for reliability and validity; tests for clinical responsiveness are even less likely to have occurred in any arena.

Measuring the Characteristic of Interest Measuring the characteristic expected to be affected may obviously be necessary, however, clinicians often simply measure what they are capable of measuring rather than what they are actually affecting. If the patient's improvement in physical function—the ability to perform necessary activities—is the characteristic of interest and the clinician measures only the patient's range of motion (ROM), no meaningful outcomes data will be available because ROM does not have a close correlation with function.[18] A questionnaire that directly asks patients about their ability to perform daily activities is more appropriate. Consider an example relevant to chiropractic wellness and health promotion practice: for a patient who is not in pain and has no disability but feels depressed and low in energy, any clinical change that occurs postintervention will not be detected if the clinician only measures ROM, pain, and disability. Instead, evidence of *no change* will be present when the clinician and patient know a significant change has occurred. In this case, the appropriate instruments should measure mental state, mood, energy, or fatigue. These conditions would then reflect the real improvement that took place.

Data Collection

Clinicians can use outcomes assessment instruments in the following two ways:

1. To assess individual patients' progress for the purpose of monitoring clinical improvement and reporting to third-party payors or for writing case reports or case series.
2. To collect aggregate data, most often as part of a large, multipractice study such as those conducted through practice-based research programs.

Each of these circumstances requires different methods to administer forms and collect and interpret results.

Collecting Data on Individual Patients Collecting data should be the most common use of patient-based outcomes instruments. It is as integral to patient management as taking a history and performing a physical examination. However, most students in the health professions did not learn about these instruments; therefore most practitioners are still unfamiliar with their use. As practitioners are increasingly expected to demonstrate accountability by showing evidence of efficacy, health professions institutions, including chiropractic colleges, will begin to incorporate use of such instruments into their curriculum. Until then, progressive practitioners will need to learn the functions on their own through professional textbooks such as this one or journals such as *Topics in Clinical Chiropractic,* which provided instruction on the SF-36 health survey (RAND version 1.0) in 1994.[4]

Using patient-based instruments to document both baseline, or preintervention, patient status and outcomes, or postintervention effects is simple. However, the clinician should observe the following basic rules to achieve meaningful results:

1. *Administer the instruments before any intervention.* My experience in directing a practice-based research program has shown that clinicians frequently violate this rule because of scheduling problems. Often, new patients have many forms to complete therefore finishing the outcomes assessment forms is delayed until the second visit. This is a problem if the patient has already interacted with the doctor on the first visit and completed the history and examination, at which point an intervention has already occurred; therefore doctor-patient interaction has an effect on the patient's health status.[19] Thus the patient's baseline will not accurately reflect preintervention status and the chances are good that the patient will have already made some improvement before even receiving the form to complete. As a result, the outcomes data will not reflect as large an improvement as it would have if the patient had completed the form before any interaction. Ideally, office staff administers all questionnaires either in the reception area or in the room where histories are taken, before any sustained interaction with the doctor. Although administering a baseline (preintervention) instrument may seem obvious, it is not always recognized by clinicians and should be done. Even well-respected researchers have designed studies in which patients were asked to try to estimate how much improvement they had made because no baseline information was collected to actually document it. This will not provide useful information for the clinician or patient.
2. *Administer the follow-up instruments at a predetermined interval.* The follow-up instruments should be given when the patient is discharged or at a regularly scheduled reevaluation interval. It could also be mailed to the patient at home. Appropriate intervals vary according to the requirements of specific instruments. Again, although the forms should obviously be administered postintervention and at baseline to assess progress, patients and some doctors do

not immediately understand this principle. The staff should explain to patients at the beginning of treatment that they will be completing the *same form* later to evaluate any changes in their health; otherwise they often wonder why they are filling out an exact duplicate of the instrument they completed when care began.[19]

3. *Assure patients that the forms are used only to improve the care plan and allow them to complete the forms in private if possible.* Patients want to please their doctor and may not be forthcoming with their perceptions, especially if the doctor is observing them while they complete forms such as a Visual Analog Scale. For aggregate data, patients should be fully informed that the results will be reported in group form only and that their responses are confidential, even from the doctor. This is not the case for individual patient management, but the doctor still needs to make patients feel comfortable about reporting their perceptions by assuring them that finding out how to deliver the best possible care is the primary interest.

Collecting Aggregate Data Collecting aggregate data has more stringent requirements because including many different patients in the research increases the variability of the results and the number of extraneous factors that must be considered. For most full-time clinicians, collecting data is probably not feasible unless it is part of a practice-based research program in which an academic institution supplies the requisite infrastructure. Many practice-based research networks exist in family practice medicine, where the field has been developing for over 20 years. In chiropractic, at least three well-established networks are operating: one between chiropractors and family practice medical doctors in Oregon through the Center for Outcomes Studies at Western States College of Chiropractic[10]; one in the United States and Canada through the Practice-Based Research Program of the Palmer Center for Chiropractic Research[20]; and one through Life College of Chiropractic.[21]

Because most clinicians will not have the problems of aggregate data collection and interpretation, I will only describe how they relate to individual patient data concerns. The major problems in aggregate data are generalizability and compa-

rability of results and bias or systematic error. The two main remedies of these problems are standardization of data collection and appropriate interpretation of data.[12]

Standardization of Data Collection Standardizing data collection is a much more critical concern for collection of aggregate data than for individual data. Even when clinicians use the best instruments, results will not be comparable with other populations and will be subject to bias if they do not reflect baseline and outcomes data on *all* eligible subjects and possible extraneous or confounding information on variables. When professionals collect data from private practice in an ambulatory setting, bias is particularly likely because the conditions are nonrandom and difficult to control. For example, patients who discontinue care without completing follow-up questionnaires may do so because they have improved greatly; therefore their lack of follow-up makes the results less positive. Conversely, patients may discontinue care because it is not helping them, and their lack of follow-up may make the results appear more positive. Assessing results when data have not been collected completely and in a standardized manner is impossible.

In addition to thoroughly gathering data, carefully labeling instruments is another important part of standardization for individual and aggregate data collection. To facilitate record-keeping, the clinician should always place each instrument on a form that specifies "pre" or "post," the date, and patient identifier. Similar to many of the other simple procedures important to effective data management, this may seem obvious but is often neglected, resulting in wasted time in correctly differentiating "pre" from "post" at best, and unusable data at worst.

Data Interpretation

Appropriate interpretation of results is crucial for the clinician to avoid bias when compiling data. This becomes even more important when characteristics are difficult to quantify such as those particularly positive quantifiers such as well-being and quality of life assessed by patient-based measures.[12,22] The clinician should use instruments that have a track record of wide use and thorough testing on large populations and explicit instructions for scoring and analysis.[17,19] However, because patient-based instruments as outcome measures are still being developed, no one yet knows exactly how to interpret changes in scores in many cases, especially aggregate scores; for this reason, caution should be used in grouping patient data.[19] Another important concern in data interpretation is nonresponse. Collecting data on some patients only and missing patients in the follow-up questioning present real problems in interpretation. For individual patient management, interpretation is less problematic because the doctor can take individual factors into consideration.

If several cases are being considered together, viewing each patient's case individually is more informative than combining a few scores and taking averages. For example, if a doctor has collected SF-36 Health Survey (discussed next) scores for five patients, the clinician should look at each patient's scores within the context of that patient's total case work-up rather than aggregating such a small amount of data. However, if the clinician collects SF-36 scores for all patients in a given time and also collects follow-up data on all patients, aggregating and averaging scores for 20 or more patients may be helpful in assessing a patient profile for the practice. However, the collector should always provide descriptive background information along with any set of outcomes scores. Scores alone are meaningless unless some information on the gender, age, major and concurrent complaints, and other characteristics that might affect outcomes is available to help interpretation.[18]

Another essential component of interpretation of data, particularly for determining quality of life and other constructs that measure characteristics other than pain and disability, is knowledge of population norms. A patient already scoring in the high-functioning range of the SF-36 for the normal population will be unlikely to show much improvement on this instrument with chiropractic or other types of care. For almost all measures, change is most likely and most dramatic with patients who are sick or functioning lower than normal. Knowing the normal range for the general, nonpatient population is also helpful to illustrate in solid descriptions that a patient has regained normal function and improved or returned to health.

Instruments

Pencil-and-paper instruments that have been useful in maintaining data on pain and physical function and general health status and well-being will be described. These instruments should be considered part of the chiropractic clinician's general collection of assessment tools. The instruments that are proven to be the most effective and have the widest application for chiropractors interested in visceral and nonmusculoskeletal conditions will be discussed in detail. The following two issues regarding each instrument will be addressed: (1) its documented reliability and validity; and (2) its usefulness for assessing outcomes of care. Appropriate application, administration, and interpretation of each instrument will also be discussed. The instruments provided in this chapter are in the public domain and may be used by clinicians without obtaining permission. In addition, a brief discussion of other patient-based instruments that may be used to monitor specific conditions will be provided, including sources for obtaining them.

Pain and Physical Function

The majority of chiropractic patients seek treatment for pain-related complaints, mainly but not exclusively in the musculoskeletal system. Instruments for measuring pain are neither condition-specific nor system-specific; they can be used to assess back pain, ulcer pain, cancer-related pain, or pain of any other origin. Because pain is a subjective interpretation of sensation, its assessment is best accomplished through patient-based measures.[13] The most important distinction clinicians should make when selecting an instrument to assess pain is whether the pain is chronic or acute. Chronic pain is often less intense at any given time, may be intermittent, is associated with a higher degree of disability, and is accompanied by a strong psychologic component. All these factors must be considered to select an instrument that will encompass the patients' perception of their pain accurately and be sensitive to treatment effects.

Physical function, like pain, is unrelated to any specific condition, although musculoskeletal conditions are particularly debilitating in terms of physical function. Actual physical ability or activity can be assessed through physiologic and biomechanical tests. However, an important distinction to make in the assessment of physical function is between physical function, which is the ability to perform physical activities, and disability, which is *perception* of their ability to perform these activities. Disability, a subjective phenomenon, is best assessed through patient-based measures.[13] Furthermore, clinicians should make these assessments because patient-assessed disability has been proven to be more predictive of objective outcomes such as return to work than physiologic measures.[13,18] However, physical function descriptions are completely distinct from legal definitions of disability and classification of compensation claims concerning disability or impairment. Thus the role of the patient-based instruments must be considered by the clinician making the assessment.

The Visual Analog Scale (VAS) for Pain The visual analog scale (VAS) for pain assesses the subject's perception of current pain intensity (Figure 6-1).[23,24] Visual analog scales are widely used for pain measurement.[25] The VAS is a 10 cm line that may be horizontal or vertical; however, the horizontal scale has resulted in a more uniform score distribution.[24,26] The VAS has been shown to be reliable, valid, and sensitive to clinical change.[27,28] Furthermore, the VASs are often used in drug analgesic trials where they are considered a standard and have been used successfully as outcome measures in studies of the effect of chiropractic on spinal pain and chronic pelvic pain.[27,29,30]

Application and Administration The VAS is a useful instrument for assessing current intensity of pain. Using it to recall average pain or previous pain is not as beneficial. Pain is difficult to remember, and the perception measured on recollection may have little to do with the actual pain; it's more of a reflection on how patients currently feel about the health care being provided or their confidence in the practitioner. The VAS may be used preadjustment and postadjustment to reflect immediate changes in level of pain, or it may be used routinely as part of each clinician's assessment per office visit. The VAS is not helpful as a measure of long-term outcomes for conditions that occur intermittently such as migraines unless the findings are recorded daily by patients in a diary and averaged over time. It is most practical for relatively consistent or very acute pain or for short-term assessments in which a decrease in pain is rapid. The VAS form should specify the pain to be described; for example, the clinician could ask the patient, "please indicate your level of migraine headache pain." Patients with multiple pain sites may be given a separate VAS for each site; characterizing several sites together is difficult for patients unless they are closely related such as the multiple joint pain of arthritis. A pain drawing combined with a VAS might produce helpful information for tracking patients with multiple pain sites.

Interpretation The same person should always measure the VAS to reduce variability in measurement. Another often unrecognized factor in VAS inconsistencies is photocopying, which increases the length of a VAS line. After several successive photocopies have been made, the line may in-

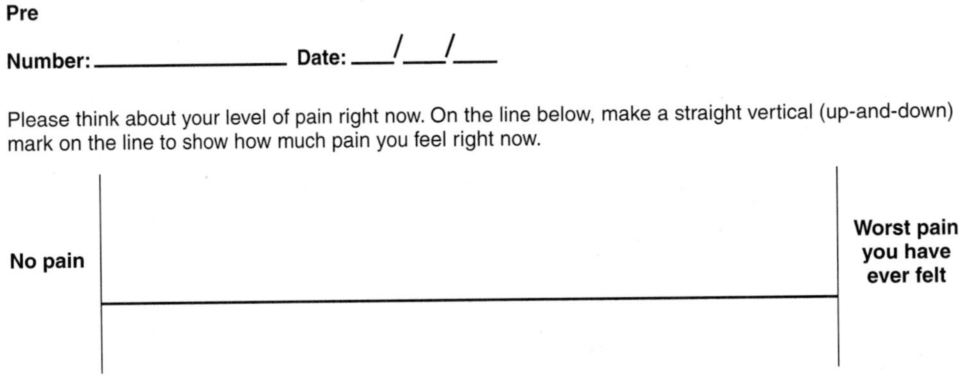

Pre

Number: _____ **Date:** ___/___/___

Please think about your level of pain right now. On the line below, make a straight vertical (up-and-down) mark on the line to show how much pain you feel right now.

No pain   **Worst pain you have ever felt**

Figure 6-1 The visual analog scale for pain (VAS).

crease by several millimeters, making precise comparisons impossible. Usually, however, these are major concerns only in controlled research settings. For purposes of case management, changes postintervention are usually marked and easy for patients and payors to appreciate. Slide algometers, which are plastic rulers printed with the same measurement scale as a paper VAS, are also useful clinical tools and not subject to the distortion problems created by photocopying.

The Pain Disability Index (PDI) The pain disability index (PDI) evaluates subjects' perception of their disability associated with pain. Interpretation of pain sensations from patients with chronic pain is influenced by their mental state and other psychosocial factors.[29] An instrument measuring only pain will not capture the effect of that pain on patients' ability to function. Consequently, clinicians should not only assess pain but also its effect on daily activities.[28] The PDI is designed specifically for use with chronic pain patients.[31,32] Originally developed by Pollard, the PDI is a seven-item self-report instrument for patients that provides general and specific indices of disability related to chronic pain (Figure 6-2).[33-35] Normative data were collected from patients with chronic pain, referred from a hospital; therefore its generalizability is best ascertained for patient populations with relatively severe pain.[32] Several studies have documented that the PDI is reliable and valid in assessing chronic pain.[32-38] In a feasibility study on the effect of chiropractic care on women with chronic pelvic pain, the PDI was used as an outcome measure and demonstrated sensitivity to clinical change after 6 weeks of chiropractic care.[30]

Application and Administration The PDI is not appropriate for patients with acute pain. It is not as useful for patients with chronic intermittent pain such as migraines as it is for patients with chronic unrelenting pain such as back pain or peripheral neuropathies.[36] Although the PDI was developed for use by patients with relatively severe and extended disability, it is also valuable for ambulatory patients with chronic pain who are not restricted from working or performing everyday activities but are somewhat impaired in normal function. These patients commonly suffer from musculoskeletal pain, but the PDI is sensitive to chronic pain of any origin. For example, it was used as the primary outcome measure in a large random experiment of chiropractic care for women with chronic pelvic pain.[30]

Interpretation The PDI has seven questions with categoric scaling ranging from 0 (no disability) to 10 (total disability). The average PDI score for inpatients with chronic pain was 32, and the average total for outpatients with chronic pain was 19.[36] Patients with chronic pain on sick leave from work have shown average scores of 32, and those who were still working had average totals of 20.[36-38] High disability should be assumed for scores over 55.[13] Because its use as an outcome measure is still exploratory, identifying a changed number that indicates clinically significant improvement is difficult. In the only chiropractic study published using the PDI as an outcome measure, a change of 13 points was found in the baseline PDI score (19 to 6) after 6 weeks of chiropractic care for women with chronic pelvic pain. This change definitely reflected clinical improvement in symptoms.[30]

General Health Status

Many patient-based-instruments that rely on the patient's perceptions rather than pathophysiology still tend to emphasize the negative side of health rather than to measure positive aspects of health, "consistent with a disease orientation."[39] However, several pencil-and-paper instruments are available for measuring quality of life, well-being, or positive health, all terms consistent with the World Health Organization's (WHO) definition of health as a "state of complete physical, mental, and social well-being and not merely the absence of disease or infirmity.[39,40] Collectively, the two instruments discussed earlier can readily provide information on immediate changes in positive health and long-term improvements in multiple aspects of health and well-being.

The Global Well-Being Scale (GWBS) The global well-being scale (GWBS) is a visual analogue scale assessing the patient's perception of general positive well-being.[17] Initial investigation suggested that it measures a perception distinct from pain and positively correlated with subscales on the SF-36 determining vitality and mental health and has high test-retest reliability.[17,41] It has been used in chiropractic clinical settings as a method to assess

The rating scales below measure the effect of chronic pain in your everyday life. We want to know how much your pain is preventing you from doing your normal activities.

For each of the seven categories of life activity listed, fill in the **one circle** above the number that best reflects the level of disability you typically experience. A score of 0 means no disability at all. A score of 10 means that all the activities that you would normally do have been disrupted or prevented by your pain.

Your rating should reflect the **overall** effect of pain in your life not just when the pain is at its worst. Fill in one circle for **every** category. If you think a category **does not** apply to you, **fill in the "0" circle**.

1. **Family and home responsibilities**. This category refers to activities related to the home or family. It includes chores and duties performed around the house (e.g., yard work) and errands or favors for other family members (e.g., driving the children to school).

⓪ ① ② ③ ④ ⑤ ⑥ ⑦ ⑧ ⑨ ⑩
No disability   Mild   Moderate   Severe   Total disability

2. **Recreation**. This category includes hobbies, sports, and other leisure-time activities.

⓪ ① ② ③ ④ ⑤ ⑥ ⑦ ⑧ ⑨ ⑩
No disability   Mild   Moderate   Severe   Total disability

3. **Social activity**. This category includes parties, theater, concerts, dining out, and other social activities that are attended with family or friends.

⓪ ① ② ③ ④ ⑤ ⑥ ⑦ ⑧ ⑨ ⑩
No disability   Mild   Moderate   Severe   Total disability

4. **Occupation**. This category refers to activities that are directly related to one's job. This also includes nonpaying jobs, such as homemaker or volunteer.

⓪ ① ② ③ ④ ⑤ ⑥ ⑦ ⑧ ⑨ ⑩
No disability   Mild   Moderate   Severe   Total disability

5. **Sexual behavior**. This category refers to the frequency and quality of one's sex life.

⓪ ① ② ③ ④ ⑤ ⑥ ⑦ ⑧ ⑨ ⑩
No disability   Mild   Moderate   Severe   Total disability

6. **Self care**. This category includes personal maintenance and independent daily living activities (e.g., taking a shower, driving, getting dressed, etc.).

⓪ ① ② ③ ④ ⑤ ⑥ ⑦ ⑧ ⑨ ⑩
No disability   Mild   Moderate   Severe   Total disability

7. **Life-support activity**. This category refers to basic life-supporting behaviors such as eating, sleeping, and breathing.

⓪ ① ② ③ ④ ⑤ ⑥ ⑦ ⑧ ⑨ ⑩
No disability   Mild   Moderate   Severe   Total disability

PLEASE DO NOT WRITE IN THIS AREA   SERIAL #

Figure 6-2 The pain disability index (PDI). (From Tait RC, Chibnall JT, Krause S: The pain disability index: psychometric properties, *Pain* 40:171-182, 1990. Format of PDI shown in Figure 6-1 is that used in the Palmer Practice-Based Research Program.)

immediate postadjustment changes and also showed sensitivity to longer-range (6 to 8 weeks) outcomes.[17,30,41]

The GWBS is basically a VAS in form but with a different function. It consists of a horizontal line 10 cm long, representing a continuum of well-being; the left end represents "the worst you could possibly feel" and the right represents "the best you could possibly feel" (Figure 6-3).

Application and Administration The GWBS should be administered with the same procedures as the VAS for pain. The clinician should separate the two scales to be sure patients do not confuse them or verbally note the difference in the two scales when the patient completes the forms. The GWBS was designed specifically to identify changes in positive perceptions rather than negative ones such as pain; therefore all patients, even those under maintenance care can use it. However, young, healthy patients who have an acute injury or other relatively straightforward complaint will likely show little improvement in well-being after an adjustment because they already have a positive sense of well-being.

The GWBS is especially useful for identifying nonspecific treatment effects that are sometimes referred to as *placebo,* which are actually real effects with poorly understood mechanisms of action. For example, anecdotal evidence repeatedly indicates that chiropractic adjustments give many patients a rush of energy unrelated to their specific symptoms or the local spinal segment adjusted. The exact mechanism of this effect is unknown, although endorphin release may be involved, triggered by a complex psychophysiologic interaction between the doctor and patient, which results in the sudden improvement in energy and well-being. The GWBS was developed precisely to measure this effect and to investigate whether that effect is short-term or long-term. Thus it has particular benefits for clinicians to record which of their adjustments and interactions produced this effect most strongly and to track the patient's progress related to it.

Interpretation The same scoring procedures apply to the GWBS as to the VAS. Young, healthy patients with uncomplicated conditions may be expected to show little change postintervention because their initial score was so high. In pilot studies including such subjects and in studies in which otherwise asymptomatic young migraine sufferers who were also chiropractic students received the GWBS, baseline scores were already so high (8 to 9 cm) that postintervention scores, although higher, were not significantly so. However, for patients in poor health with chronic conditions or elderly patients with low physical function whose baseline scores were 3 to 4 cm, both immediate postadjustment scores and long-range follow-up scores were 3 to 4 cm higher.[41]

SF-36 Health Survey The SF-36 health survey evolved from longer and more difficult-to-score psychometric instruments associated with the medical outcomes study.[19] The SF-36 has been documented to be reliable, valid, and sensitive to

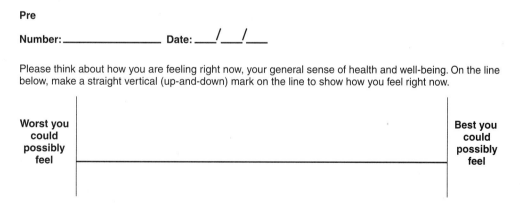

Figure 6-3 The global well-being scale (GWBS). (From Hawk C et al: A study of the reliability, validity, and responsiveness of a self-administered instrument to measure global well-being, *Palmer J Res* 2(1):15-22, 1995.)

clinical change. It is also capable of providing normative data on the general population and is used for patients with specific chronic conditions.[19] The SF-36 is currently being employed routinely in many chiropractic settings, providing baseline characteristics of patients and assessing outcomes of care.[20]

The SF-36 assesses eight different elements of health (Figure 6-4 on pp 82-83): pain, physical function, role limitation because of physical and emotional problems, social function, mental health and well-being, energy and fatigue, and general health (Table 6-1).

Application and Administration The SF-36 takes 5 to 10 minutes to complete. It was developed for adults and therefore should not be administered to children (although children's versions are available). Urge patients to complete the form entirely, answering all questions to the best of their ability.[19] For outcomes assessment, some have recommended that the SF-36 be used to assess long-term outcomes, at least 4 to 6 weeks from the baseline administration.

Interpretation The RAND version 1.0 of the SF-36 differs primarily in its scoring method; it is the version provided in this chapter because it is relatively easy to score by hand.[42] Negligible differences occur in scores computed for the SF-36 versus the RAND-36; therefore for most purposes they may be considered interchangeable. However, for accuracy, the form included in this chapter should be called the *RAND-36 (version 1.0).*[42] The scoring instructions are provided in Tables 6-2 and 6-3. A total score is not compiled; the eight subscales are reported as separate figures. Generally, chiropractic patients tend to be healthier than other patient populations, coming close to the general nonpatient population on most of the subscales, with the exception of pain, physical function, and role limitation because of physical problems. Chiropractors who treat higher proportions of patients with visceral and other problems not related to the musculoskeletal system may expect their patient profiles to be different.

To provide some perspective, Figure 6-5 compares, in graphic form, SF-36 profiles of the following:

Table 6-1   *Subscales of the SF-36*

Subscale	Abbreviation	Description	Number of Questions
Physical functioning	PF	Limitation on physical abilities	10
Role—physical	RP	Limitations on ability to perform normal activities because of physical problems	4
Bodily pain	BP	Pain severity and degree to which it impairs normal function	2
General health	GH	Physical health status; has been found to be predictive of health outcomes	5
Vitality	VT	Energy level and fatigue; sense of well-being distinct from disease symptomatology	4
Social functioning	SF	Quality and quantity of interpersonal interactions, an important aspect of multifactorial health assessment	2
Role—emotional	RE	Limitations on ability to perform normal activities because of emotional problems	4
Mental health	MH	Sense of emotional well-being reflected by the four major mental health dimensions: anxiety, depression, loss of behavioral control, and psychologic well-being	5

From RAND Health Sciences Program: *RAND 36-Item Health Survey 1.0, Santa Monica, Calif,* 1992, RAND.

Table 6-2 *Scoring the RAND-36 version 1.0 of the SF-36*

Item	Original Response Value	Recode Value
1, 2, 20, 22, 34, 36	1	100
	2	75
	3	50
	4	25
	5	0
3-12	1	0
	2	50
	3	100
13-19	1	0
	2	100
21, 23, 26, 27, 30	1	100
	2	80
	3	60
	4	40
	5	20
	6	0
24, 25, 28, 29, 31	1	0
	2	20
	3	40
	4	60
	5	80
	6	100
32, 33, 35	1	0
	2	25
	3	50
	4	75
	5	100

From RAND Health Sciences Program: *RAND 36-Item Health Survey 1.0*, Santa Monica, Calif, 1992, RAND.

1. General, nonpatient population[19]
2. Outpatients with a diagnosis of clinical depression[19]
3. Patients in a tertiary chiropractic practice that cares for patients only after their regular chiropractor could not help them further. About 38% of the chief complaints were nonmusculoskeletal symptoms that lasted longer than 1 year[41] (over 90% of the main complaints in chiropractic in the United States involve the musculoskeletal system)
4. Chiropractic patients in a practice-based research program with primarily (>90%) musculoskeletal chief complaints[20]

Table 6-3 *Subscale Formation for RAND-36 version 1.0 of the SF-36*

Scale	Average these Items	Total Number of Items in Subscale
Physical function	3-12	10
Role—physical	13-16	4
Bodily pain	21, 22	2
General health	1, 2, 33-36	6
Vitality	23, 27, 29, 31	4
Social function	20, 32	2
Role—emotional	17-19	3
Mental health	24-26, 28, 30	5

From RAND Health Sciences Program: *RAND 36-Item Health Survey 1.0*, Santa Monica, Calif, 1992, RAND.

As with other measures, those patients with the lowest scores are expected to show the greatest improvement. For patient management, graphically illustrating prescores and postscores is useful. Two options exist for viewing SF-36 scores to track patient progress. One is to graph baseline and postintervention and progress report scores in the manner shown in Figure 6-3. Figure 6-6 illustrates this method, displaying results of a feasibility study of chiropractic care for women with chronic pelvic pain. Although these are aggregate data for a controlled clinical study, individual patient scores can be displayed in the same way. Graphing the population norm and a point of comparison are helpful for the clinician. The other option for tracking patient progress over an extended period is to graph the subscales of greatest concern separately with a horizontal line displaying the population norm: The patient's scores over time can be graphed under (or hopefully, eventually, above) it (Figure 6-7).

Although the illustrations presented in this chapter use overall population norms for purposes of example, for individual patient management, using population norms for the patient's gender and age because these differ considerably for different subgroups is desirable and expected.[19]

Practice-based research program

Marking instructions
• Use a no. 2 pencil only. • Do not use ink, ballpoint, or felt tip pens. • Make solid marks that fill the response completely. • Erase cleanly any marks you wish to change. Correct: ● Incorrect: ✓ ⊗ ◒ ◔

Instructions:
This survey asks for your views about your health. The information will help your health care provider track how you feel and how well you are able to do your usual activities. Answer every question by completely filling in the correct circle. If you are unsure about how to answer a question, please give the best answer you can.

Doctor ID				
⓪	⓪	⓪	⓪	⓪
①	①	①	①	①
②	②	②	②	②
③	③	③	③	③
④	④	④	④	④
⑤	⑤	⑤	⑤	⑤
⑥	⑥	⑥	⑥	⑥
⑦	⑦	⑦	⑦	⑦
⑧	⑧	⑧	⑧	⑧
⑨	⑨	⑨	⑨	⑨

Patient ID								
⓪	⓪	⓪	⓪	⓪	⓪	⓪	⓪	⓪
①	①	①	①	①	①	①	①	①
②	②	②	②	②	②	②	②	②
③	③	③	③	③	③	③	③	③
④	④	④	④	④	④	④	④	④
⑤	⑤	⑤	⑤	⑤	⑤	⑤	⑤	⑤
⑥	⑥	⑥	⑥	⑥	⑥	⑥	⑥	⑥
⑦	⑦	⑦	⑦	⑦	⑦	⑦	⑦	⑦
⑧	⑧	⑧	⑧	⑧	⑧	⑧	⑧	⑧
⑨	⑨	⑨	⑨	⑨	⑨	⑨	⑨	⑨

Today's date					
Mo.		Day		Year	
⓪	⓪	⓪	⓪	⓪	⓪
①	①	①	①	①	①
	②	②	②	②	②
	③	③	③	③	③
	④		④	④	④
	⑤		⑤	⑤	⑤
	⑥		⑥	⑥	⑥
	⑦		⑦	⑦	⑦
	⑧		⑧	⑧	⑧
	⑨		⑨	⑨	⑨

1. **In general**, how would you describe your health? (Fill in only **one** circle)
   ① Excellent ② Very good ③ Good ④ Fair ⑤ Poor

2. **Compared with 1 year ago**, how would you rate your health in general now? (Fill in only **one** circle)
   ① Much better now than 1 year ago ② Somewhat better now than 1 year ago
   ③ About the same ④ Somewhat worse now than 1 year ago
   ⑤ Much worse now than 1 year ago

The following items are about activities you might do during a typical day. Does your health now limit you in these activities? If so, how much?
(Fill in **one** circle on **each** line)

	Yes, limited a lot	Yes, limited a little	No, not limited at all
3. **Vigorous activities** such as running, lifting heavy objects, and participating in strenuous sports	①	②	③
4. **Moderate activities** such as moving a table, pushing a vacuum cleaner, bowling, or playing golf	①	②	③
5. Lifting or carrying groceries	①	②	③
6. Climbing **several** flights of stairs	①	②	③
7. Climbing **one** flight of stairs	①	②	③
8. Bending, kneeling, or stooping	①	②	③
9. Walking **more than a mile**	①	②	③
10. Walking **several blocks**	①	②	③
11. Walking **one block**	①	②	③
12. Bathing or dressing yourself	①	②	③

During the **past 4 weeks**, have you had any of the following problems with your work or other regular daily activities **as a result of your physical health**? (Fill in only **one** circle on **each line**)

13. Shortened the **amount of time** you spent on work or other activities	① Yes	② No
14. **Accomplished less** than you would like	① Yes	② No
15. Limited in the **kind of** work or other activities	① Yes	② No
16. Had **difficulty** performing the work or other activities (for example, it took extra effort)	① Yes	② No

PLEASE DO NOT WRITE IN THIS AREA

SERIAL #

Figure 6-4 The SF-36 health survey (RAND-36 version 1.0). (From RAND Health Sciences Program: *RAND 36-Item Health Survey 1.0*, 1992, RAND.)

During the **past 4 weeks**, have you had any of the following problems with your work or other regular daily activities **as a result of any emotional problems** (such as feeling depressed or anxious)?

(Fill in only **one circle** on **each line**)

17. Shortened the **amount of time** you spent on work or other activities	① Yes	② No
18. **Accomplished less** than you would like	① Yes	② No
19. Did not do work or other activities as **carefully** as usual	① Yes	② No

20. During the past 4 weeks, to what extent has your physical health or emotional problems interfered with your normal social activities with family, friends, neighbors, or groups?
    (Fill in only **one circle**)
    ① Not at all   ② Slightly   ③ Moderately   ④ Quite a bit   ⑤ Extremely

21. How much **bodily pain** have you had during the past 4 weeks?
    (Fill in only **one circle**)
    ① None   ② Very mild   ③ Mild   ④ Moderate   ⑤ Severe   ⑥ Very severe

22. During the past 4 weeks, how much did **pain** interfere with your normal work (including work outside the home and housework)?
    (Fill in only **one circle**)
    ① Not at all   ② A little bit   ③ Moderately   ④ Quite a bit   ⑤ Extremely

These questions are about how you feel and how things have been with you during the **past 4 weeks**. For each question, please give the one answer that comes closest to the way you have been feeling. How much of the time during the **past 4 weeks**....

(Fill in **one circle** on **each line**)	All of the time	Most of the time	A good bit of the time	Some of the time	A little of the time	None of the time
23. Did you feel full of pep?	①	②	③	④	⑤	⑥
24. Have you been a very nervous person?	①	②	③	④	⑤	⑥
25. Have you felt so down in the dumps that nothing could cheer you up?	①	②	③	④	⑤	⑥
26. Have you felt calm and peaceful?	①	②	③	④	⑤	⑥
27. Did you have a lot of energy?	①	②	③	④	⑤	⑥
28. Have you felt downhearted and blue?	①	②	③	④	⑤	⑥
29. Did you feel worn out?	①	②	③	④	⑤	⑥
30. Have you been a happy person?	①	②	③	④	⑤	⑥
31. Did you feel tired?	①	②	③	④	⑤	⑥

32. During the **past 4 weeks**, how much of the time has your **physical health** or **emotional problems** interfered with your social activities such as visiting with friends, relatives, etc.?
    (Fill in only **one circle**)
    ① All of the time
    ② Most of the time
    ③ Some of the time
    ④ A little of the time
    ⑤ None of the time

How true or false is each of the following statements for you?
(Fill in **one circle** on **each line**)

	Definitely true	Mostly true	Don't know	Mostly false	Definitely false
33. I seem to get sick a little easier than other people	①	②	③	④	⑤
34. I am as healthy as anybody I know	①	②	③	④	⑤
35. I expect my health to get worse	①	②	③	④	⑤
36. My health is excellent	①	②	③	④	⑤

Figure 6-4, Cont'd For legend see opposite page.

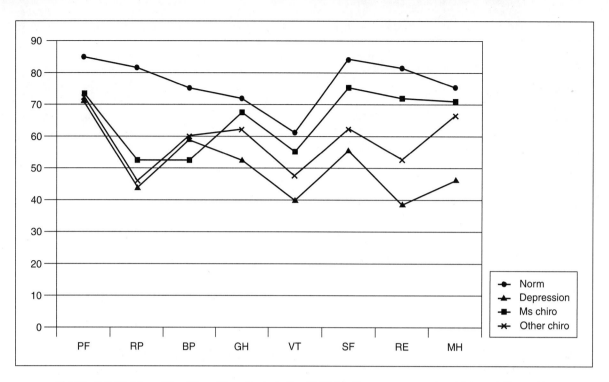

Figure 6-5 SF-36 profiles. (From Ware JE et al: *The SF-36 health survey: manual and interpretation guide,* Boston, 1993, The Health Institute. Hawk CK, Morter MT Jr: The use of measures of general health status in chiropractic patients: a pilot study, *Palmer J Res* 2(2):39-45, 1995.)

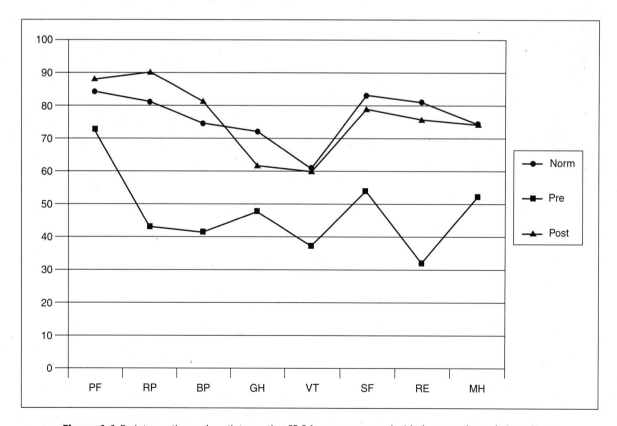

Figure 6-6 Preintervention and postintervention SF-36 scores compared with the normal population. (From Hawk C, Long C, Azad A: Chiropractic care for women with chronic pelvic pain: a prospective single-group intervention study, *J Manipulative Physiol Ther* 20:73-79, 1997.)

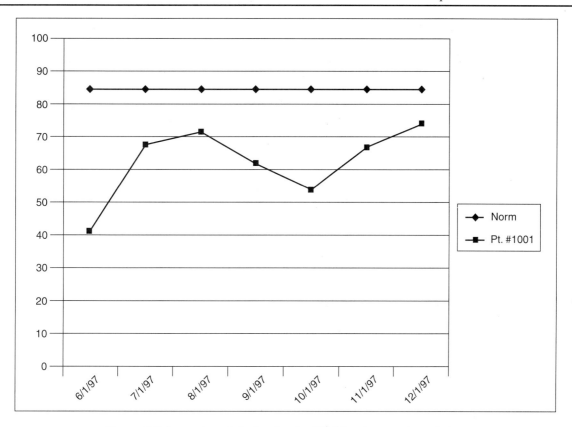

Figure 6-7 Comparison of single subscale of SF-36 to the normal population.

Other Instruments

Numerous patient-based instruments are available, but because of the amount of time required to complete, score, and interpret them, most clinicians prefer to use the minimum number of questionnaires required to measure the characteristic(s) of interest. Use of nonspecific and quality-of-life measures such as those described earlier in detail should be combined with use of a condition-specific measure to maximize information available for outcomes assessment.

More instruments are available for musculoskeletal conditions than for nonmusculoskeletal ones, probably because musculoskeletal conditions are difficult to characterize through physiologic measures and they cause considerable impairment in quality of life and activities of daily living. Although many patient-based instruments exist for assessing various conditions, very few are used widely, thoroughly tested for reliability, validity, and clinical responsiveness, or feasible for most clinicians to use, in terms of training re-

quired for interpretation and time needed for administration. Of those instruments available, the aspect of clinical responsiveness is rarely assessed.

Because the purpose of this chapter is to assist clinicians in monitoring patient outcomes, only selected instruments demonstrated to be sensitive to clinical change in a specific nonmusculoskeletal condition and likely to have wide application in chiropractic practice are mentioned. The first instrument is the Beck Depression Inventory, a brief instrument for assessing presence and degree of clinical depression (patients with chronic pelvic pain were shown to have a statistically significant decrease in their depression score after 6 weeks of chiropractic care).[30,43,44] The other instrument is the headache disability inventory, which is useful for tension and migraine headaches and reflects clinical changes to a greater degree than a VAS for pain for patients with migraine headaches.[45]

In addition, Table 6-4 provides an overview of a number of other condition-specific instruments, with citations for where they can be obtained.

Table 6-4 *Condition-Specific Instruments**

Condition	Instrument	Citation
Arthritis	Arthritis impact measurement scales 2 (AIMS2)	AIMS2 User's Guide: Boston University Arthritis Center, *Arthritis Rheum* 23:146, 1980; 25:1048, 1982; 35:1, 1992.
Angina	Seattle angina questionnaire	Medical Outcomes Trust, 20 Park Plaza, Suite 1014, Boston, MA, 02116; telephone: 617-426-4046
	Angina form 9.1†	Pryor DB et al: Determination of prognosis in patients with ischemic heart disease, *J Am Coll Cardiol* 14:1016-1025, 1989.
Asthma	Adult asthma quality of life questionnaire Pediatric quality of life questionnaire	Medical Outcomes Trust, 20 Park Plaza, Suite 1014, Boston, MA, 02116; telephone: 617-426-4046
Autonomic nervous system	Autonomic nervous system response inventory (ANSRI)	Waters WF et al: The autonomic nervous system response inventory (ANSRI): prediction of psychophysiological response, *J Psychosom Res* 33(3):347, 1989.
Cataract	Cataract form 1.1†	Steinberg EP et al: Variations in cataract management: patient and economic outcomes, *Health Serv Res* 25(5):727-731, 1990.
COPD	COPD form 15.1†	Robert A. Bethel, MD
Chronic sinusitis	Chronic sinusitis form 12.1†	Sanford R. Hoffman, MD
Depression	Beck depression inventory	Beck AT et al: An inventory for measuring depression, *Arch Gen Psychiatry* 4:561, 1961.
	Zung depression index	Zung WWK: A self-rating depression scale, *Arch Gen Psychiatry* 12:63, 1965.
Diabetes	Diabetes form 2.1†	Kravitz R et al: Differences in the mix of patients among medical specialties and systems of care, *JAMA* 267:1617, 1992.
Headache	Headache disability inventory	Jacobsen G et al: The Henry Ford Hospital headache disability inventory (HDI), *Neurology* 44:837, 1994.
	The headache scale	Hunter M: The headache scale: a new approach to the assessment of headache pain based on pain descriptions, *Pain* 16:361, 1983.
HIV	MOS-HIV health survey	Medical Outcomes Trust, 20 Park Plaza, Suite 1014, Boston, MA, 02116; telephone: 617-426-4046
Hypertension	Hypertension/lipid form 5.1†	John M. Flack, MD, MPH, Richard H. Grimm, Jr, MD, PhD, Duke University

Table 6-4   *Condition-Specific Instruments*—cont'd*

Condition	Instrument	Citation
Prostatism	Prostatism form 4.1†	Fowler FJ et al: Symptom status and quality of life following prostatectomy, *JAMA* 259:3018-3022, 1988
Sleep	Pittsburgh sleep quality index	Buysse DJ et al: The Pittsburgh sleep quality index: a new instrument for psychiatric practice and research, *Psychiatr Res* 28:193, 1989.
	Sleep diary for chronic pain patients	Haythornthwaite JA et al: Development of a sleep diary for chronic pain patients, *J Pain Symptom Manage* 6(2):65, 1991.
Stress	Daily stress inventory	Brantley PJ et al: A daily stress inventory: development, reliability, and validity, *J Behav Med* 10(1):61, 1987.
Vertigo	Dizziness handicap inventory	Jacobson GP et al: The development of the dizziness handicap inventory, *Arch Otolaryngol Head Neck Surg* 116:424, 1990.

* Information compiled by Charles Woodfield, DC, RPh.
† Available from the Health Outcomes Institute, 2001 Killebrew Drive, Suite 122, Bloomington, MN, 55425.

As patient-based outcomes assessment continues to be an important part of evidence-based care, more instruments will be evaluated for their reliability, validity, and sensitivity to clinical change. Using the principles of appropriate instrument selection, administration, and interpretation provided in this chapter will help chiropractic clinicians make valuable contributions to this movement by employing such instruments where available, developing new ones where they are not available, and reporting their results to the scientific community.

STUDY GUIDE

1. Describe a patient-based approach.
2. Name three reasons patient-based measures are an important part of evidence-based practice.
3. What appropriate procedures must be followed in a patient-based study to maintain objectivity and minimize bias?
4. Name three basic rules for applying a pencil-and-paper instrument in a single patient study.
5. What is the SF-36 health survey?
6. What is the most important distinction to make when selecting an instrument to determine pain?
7. Is disability a subjective phenomenon?
8. Describe the Visual Analog Scale (VAS).
9. What is the Pain Disability Index? When would this instrument best be used?
10. What is the Global Well-Being Scale and what is its best use?
11. Which of the above is appropriate for use with children?
12. Which pencil-and-paper instrument would be most appropriate to use to assess the presence and degree of clinical depression?
13. Name a useful tool for evaluating patients with a complaint of headache.
14. What does the dizzyness handicap inventory assess? How?

REFERENCES

1. Mootz RD, Phillips RB: Chiropractic belief systems. In Cherkin D, editor: *Chiropractic in the United States: training, practice and research,* St Louis, Mosby (in press).
2. Kelner M, Hall O, Coulter I: *Chiropractors: do they help?* Toronto, 1980, Fitzhenry and Whiteside.
3. Street RL, Gold WR, McDowell T: Using health status surveys in medical consultations, *Med Care* 32(7):732, 1994.
4. Goertz CMH: Measuring functional health status in the chiropractic office using self-report questionnaires, *Top Clin Chiro* 1(1):51, 1994.
5. Thier SO: Forces motivating the use of health status assessment measures in clinical settings and related clinical research, *Med Care* 30(suppl):15, 1992.
6. Deyo RD, Patrick DL: Barriers to the use of health status measures in clinical investigation, patient care, and policy research, *Med Care* 27(suppl):S254, 1989.
7. Parkerson GR, Broadhead WE, Tse CKJ: Quality of life and functional health of primary care patients, *J Clin Epidemiol* 45(11):1303, 1992.
8. Jenkinson C, Coulter A, Wright L: Short form 36(SF36) health survey questionnaire: normative data for adults of working age, *Br Med J* 306:1437, 1993.
9. Keating JC: The placebo issue and clinical research, *J Manipulative Physiol Ther* 10(6):329, 1987.
10. Nyiendo J et al: *Health status as an outcome measure for low back pain patients,* 1992, Arlington, Va, Proceedings International Conference on Spinal Manipulation.
11. Greenland S et al: Controlled clinical trials of manipulation: a review and a proposal, *J Occup Med* 22(10):670, 1980.
12. Fletcher A et al: Quality of life measures in health care, II: design, analysis, and interpretation, *British Med J* 305:1145, 1992.
13. Tait RC, Chibnall JT, Krause S: The pain disability index: psychometric properties, *Pain* 40:171, 1990.
14. Foundation for Chiropractic Education and Research, *Spinal Manipulation,* 9(1) 1993.
15. Deyo RA, Diehl P, Patrick DL: Reproducibility and responsiveness of health status measures, *Control Clin Trials* 12:142S, 1991.
16. Vernon H, Mior S: The neck disability index: a study of reliability and validity, *J Manipulative Physiol Ther* 14:1409, 1991.
17. Hawk C et al: A study of the reliability, validity, and responsiveness of a self-administered instrument to measure global well-being, *Palmer J Res* 2(1):15, 1995.
18. Shekelle PG et al: A brief introduction to the critical reading of the clinical literature, *Spine* 19(185):2928S, 1994.
19. Ware JE et al: *The SF-36 health survey: manual and interpretation guide,* Boston, Mass, 1993, The Health Institute.
20. Hawk C, Long CR, Boulanger K: Development of a practice-based research program, *J Manipulative Physiol Ther* 21(3):149, 1998.
21. Hoiriis KT, Owens EF, Pfleger B: Changes in general health status during upper cervical chiropractic care: a practice-based research project, *Chiro Res J* 4(1):18, 1997.
22. McDowell I, Newell C: *Measuring health: a guide to rating scales and questionnaires,* New York, 1987, Oxford University Press.
23. Maxwell C: Sensitivity and accuracy of the visual analogue scale: A psycho-physical classroom experiment, *Br J Clin Pharmacol* 6:15, 1978.
24. Wewers ME, Lowe NK: A critical review of visual analogue scales in the measurement of clinical phenomena, *Res Nurs Health* 13:227, 1990.
25. Mantha S et al: A proposal to use confidence intervals for visual analog scale data for pain measurement to determine clinical significance, *Anesth Analg* 77:1041, 1993.
26. Scott J, Huskisson EC: Graphic representation of pain, *Pain* 2:175, 1976.
27. Clarke PRF, Spear FG: Reliability and sensitivity in the self-assessment of well being, *Bull Br Psych Soc* 17:55, 1964.
28. Miller MD, Ferris DG: Measurement of subjective phenomena in primary care research: the visual analogue scale, *Fam Pract Res J* 13(1):15, 1993.
29. Triano JJ et al: A comparison of outcome measures for use with back pain patients: results of a feasibility study, *J Manipulative Physiol Ther* 16:67, 1993.
30. Hawk C, Long C, Azad A: Chiropractic care for women with chronic pelvic pain: a prospective single-group intervention study, *J Manipulative Physiol Ther* 20:73, 1997.
31. Lipscomb B, Ling FW: Chronic pelvic pain, *Med Clin North Am* 79:1411, 1995.
32. Chibnall JT, Tait RC: The pain disability index: factor structure and normative data, *Arch Phys Med Rehabil* 75:1082, 1994.
33. Pollard CA: Preliminary validity study of pain disability index, *Precept Mot Skills* 59:974, 1984.
34. Tait RC et al: The pain disability index: psychometric and validity data, *Arch Phys Med Rehabil* 68:438, 1987.
35. Gronblad M et al: Relationship of the pain disability index (PDI) and the oswestry disability questionnaire (ODQ) with three dynamic physical tests in a group of patients with chronic low-back and leg pain, *Clin J Pain* 10:197, 1994.
36. Tait RC, Pollard CA, Margolis RB et al: The pain disability index: psychometric and validity data, *Arch Phys Med Rehabil* 68:438, 1987.
37. Gronblad M et al: Intercorrelation and test-retest reliability of the pain disability index (PDI) and the oswestry disability questionnaire (ODQ) and their correlation with pain intensity in low back pain patients, *Clin J Pain* 9:189, 1993.
38. Jerome A, Gross RT: Pain disability index: construct and discriminant validity, *Arch Phys Med Rehabil* 72:920, 1991.
39. Ware JE, Sherbourne CD: The MOS 36-item short-form health survey (SF-36), I: conceptual framework and item selection, *Med Care* 30(6):473, 1992.
40. World Health Organization: Constitution of the world health organization, *Basic documents,* Geneva, Switzerland, 1948, WHO.

41. Hawk CK, Morter MT Jr: The use of measures of general health status in chiropractic patients: a pilot study, *Palmer J Res* 2(2):39, 1995.
42. RAND Health Sciences Program: *RAND 36-Item Health Survey 1.0,* San Diego, 1992, RAND.
43. Beck AT, Steer RA, Garbin MG: Psychometric properties of the Beck depression inventory: twenty-five years of evaluation, *Clin Psychol Rev* 8:77, 1988.
44. Beck AT et al: An inventory for measuring depression, *Arch Gen Psychiatry* 4:53, 1961.
45. Jacobsen GP et al: Headache disability inventory (HDI): short-term test-retest reliability and spouse perceptions, *Headache* 35:534, 1995.

CHAPTER 7

Instrumentation and Imaging

Christopher Kent, DC, FCCI

Objective assessment of the somatic and visceral components associated with vertebral subluxation may be accomplished by employing appropriate instrumentation. Imaging procedures may be useful in the evaluation of spinal biomechanics and pathology, and the information obtained from imaging studies may assist the chiropractor in determining if a relationship exists between spinal abnormalities and visceral dysfunction in a given patient.

I have classified instrumentation according to whether it is used predominantly to evaluate somatic function or autonomic activity that may be associated with visceral abnormalities, which is sometimes an arbitrary distinction.

Somatic Assessment: Electromyography

Electromyography (EMG) is the technique of recording electric potentials associated with muscular activity. Needle electrodes may be inserted in the muscle being monitored, or surface electrodes may be placed on the skin overlying the muscles being studied. Both techniques have been used for the examination of paraspinal and peripheral muscle function. However, surface EMG (SEMG) and needle EMG are not interchangeable procedures.[1-4]

Although needle techniques are more popular in medical practice than surface electrode techniques, the literature indicates that surface techniques demonstrate superior reliability.[5-12] In addition to being more reliable, the noninvasive nature of the test makes it more appropriate for the evaluation of abnormal paraspinal muscle activity associated with vertebral subluxation.

Several models and definitions have been proposed for vertebral subluxation. These models have been reviewed elsewhere.[13] A recent definition was adopted by the Association of Chiropractic Colleges (ACC), which states[14]:

> A subluxation is a complex of functional and/or structural and/or pathological articular changes that compromise neural integrity and may influence organ system function and general health.

As Lantz[15] noted, "Common to all concepts of subluxation are some form of kinesiologic dysfunction and some form of neurologic involvement."

Paraspinal muscle dysfunction is generally accepted as a clinical manifestation of vertebral subluxation.[16,17] Traditional chiropractic analysis includes examination of the paraspinal tissues for taut and tender muscle fibres. D.D. Palmer[18] expressed the relationship between tone and the dynamics of health and disease as follows:

> Life is an expression of tone. Tone is the normal degree of nerve tension. Tone is expressed in function by normal elasticity, strength, and excitability . . . the cause of disease is any variation in tone.

Surface EMG provides objective, quantitative data concerning the changes in paraspinal muscle function that accompany vertebral subluxation. Specific clinical applications require an understanding of muscle physiology.

Muscle fibres may be functionally classified as fast-twitch and slow-twitch fibres. The fast-twitch fibres control phasic or fast ballistic movements. Slow-twitch fibres are responsible for maintaining tonic postural support.[19] Assessment of postural tone is useful in determining how efficiently the body is using available resources. Efficient use of energy is termed *ergotropic function.*

Appreciation of the specific features of paraspinal muscles is necessary to the understanding of somatovisceral relationships. The erector spinae muscles present some unique histologic and physiologic characteristics. One unusual characteristic is that the slow-twitch (Type I) fibres are larger in cross-section than the fast-twitch (Type II) fibres. The large fibres may be recruited at lower forces than the smaller fibres, which is an unusual recruitment pattern. Furthermore, the erector spinae muscles are composed of separately innervated, independently contracting discrete muscle fasicles. The erector spinae muscles rarely shorten beyond their length in the upright standing position. These factors must be considered when assessing SEMG patterns in the erector spinae.[20]

The role of articular mechanoreceptors in producing afferent input to the CNS and resulting reflex muscle activity has been investigated. In the context of SEMG assessment of paraspinal muscle function, articular mechanoreceptors and muscle spindles are believed to be activated during chiropractic adjustment or manipulation.[21,22] The resulting increase in mechanoreceptor activity is thought to result in reflex inhibition of spastic muscles in the affected area. This increased sensory input is also believed to result in reduced transmission of nociceptive signals, resulting is decreased pain perception.

In the context of viscerosomatic reflexes, Cole[23] stated the following:

> When the somatovisceral reflex is overactive, stimulation from any source may result in facilitation (activation) of spinal cord segments, and this is associated with an alteration of the functional capacity of the paravertebral muscles. The vasomotor reactions thus generated cannot fail to affect visceral function through relative hypoxia and the general effects of inadequate blood supply. It has been established that the effects of overactive reflexes are transmitted to structures (and functions) that are reflexly associated with the spinal segments exhibiting abnormal activity. Moreover, there is evidence that when motor reflex thresholds are chronically reduced, at least some of the preganglionic sympathetic neurons of the same spinal cord segments are maintained in a continued state of facilitation, so that reflex activity can result from a rela-

tively light stimulus. Then as the cycle of abnormal activity continues, the segmentally related structures in turn set up a chronic bombardment of impulses that maintain the spinal cord in a hyperirritable state.

Another somatic manifestation of vertebral subluxation that presents abnormal SEMG activity is dysponesis. *Dysponesis* refers to a reversible physiopathologic state consisting of errors in energy expenditure that are capable of producing functional disorders. Dysponesis consists mainly of covert errors in action potential output from the motor and premotor areas of the cortex and the consequences of that output. These neurophysiologic reactions may result from responses to environmental events, bodily sensations, and emotions. Whatmore and Kohi[24] asserted that dysponesis results in an interference with nervous system function, including emotional reactivity and the regulation of various organs in the body.

These authors reported that dysponesis can distort perception of environmental events and disturb autonomic function. Specific clinical syndromes associated with dysponesis may likely include anxiety, digestive system and circulatory system disturbances, impotence and frigidity, headache, backache, insomnia, fatigue, depression, and skin disorders.[24]

Clinical evaluation of dysponesis involves determining the resultant aberrant muscle activity. This is done using SEMG. In chiropractic practice, dysponesis may be associated with vertebral subluxation. SEMG techniques, therefore, are used to assess muscular responses to chiropractic adjustments (Figure 7-1).

Paraspinal EMG Scanning Technique

Protocols and normative data for paraspinal EMG scanning have been published.[25,26] Handheld electrodes are applied to the skin of the patient overlying the spine at 15 paired sites. EMG signals are measured in microvolts (10^{-6} V). A computer analyses these signals and compares them with a normative database. In the interpretation of SEMG scans, the following two factors are considered:

1. Amplitude. This refers to the signal level in microvolts. The higher the signal level, the greater the paraspinal muscle activity. By comparing these readings with a normative

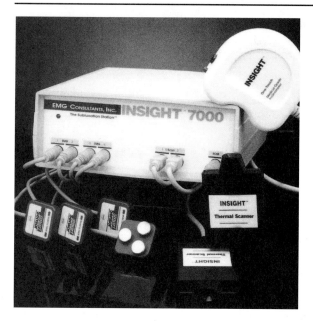

Figure 7-1 The Insight Subluxation Station uses surface electromyography, infrared skin temperature assessment, and inclinometry to assess somatovisceral relationships associated with vertebral subluxation. (Courtesy EMG Consultants, Inc, Maywood, NJ.)

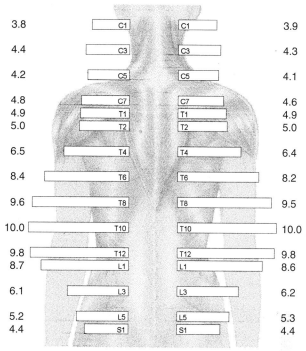

Figure 7-2 Graphic representation of normative data for paraspinal surface EMG potentials at a 25-500 Hz bandpass.

database, elevated or decreased signals can be identified.

2. Symmetry. This refers to a comparison of the left-right amplitudes at each spinal level (Table 7-1 and Figure 7-2).

Paraspinal EMG scans, taken in unison with other examination findings, may be helpful in determining the following:

1. Asymmetric contraction
2. Areas of muscle splinting
3. Severity of the condition
4. Aberrant recruitment patterns
5. Dysponesis
6. Responses to dysafferentation
7. Response to chiropractic adjustment

Construct Validity

In the absence of a universal high principle for assessment of the muscular dysfunction associated with the vertebral subluxation, the clinical efficiency of a procedure may be evaluated by determining the ability of the test to perform up to the standards predicted by a theoretic model or construct.[28] In the case of SEMG, the assumption is made that significant changes in SEMG activity will occur following chiropractic adjustment and that significant changes will not be observed with repeated assessments of controls.

Shambaugh[29] conducted a controlled study where surface electrodes were used to record paraspinal EMG activity prechiropractic and postchiropractic adjustment. Shambaugh concluded, "Results of this study show that significant changes in muscle electrical activity occur as a consequence of adjusting." In the osteopathic literature, Ellestad and others[30] conducted a controlled study that discovered that paraspinal EMG activity decreased in patients following osteopathic manipulation. Such changes were not observed in controls in either study. Therefore these studies support the construct validity of paraspinal SEMG as an outcome assessment for chiropractic adjustment.

Dynamic SEMG

Affixed surface electrodes may be employed for real-time assessment of paraspinal muscle activity throughout ranges of motion. Protocols for the

Table 7-1   *Descriptive Statistics for Paraspinal Surface Electromyography Microvolt Potentials Collected at 25-500 Hz**

	Left				Right			
	Med.	Min.	Max.	Mean (S.D.)	Med.	Min.	Max.	Mean (S.D.)
Segment								
C1	3.25	1.90	8.20	3.80 ± 1.60	3.35	1.30	10.40	3.90 ± 1.80
C3	4.10	1.30	11.40	4.40 ± 1.80	3.90	1.40	8.90	4.30 ± 1.70
C5	3.70	1.50	9.80	4.20 ± 1.80	3.80	1.60	11.30	4.10 ± 1.80
C7	4.40	1.90	10.30	4.80 ± 1.90	4.25	1.50	12.00	4.60 ± 2.00
T1	4.10	2.10	16.60	4.90 ± 2.70	4.30	1.80	16.70	4.90 ± 2.60
T2	4.30	1.60	18.80	5.00 ± 2.80	4.30	1.50	15.20	5.00 ± 2.90
T4	5.65	2.00	17.20	6.50 ± 3.00	5.80	1.80	18.50	6.40 ± 3.20
T6	7.75	2.20	21.20	8.40 ± 3.50	7.55	1.60	22.40	8.20 ± 3.50
T8	9.00	2.20	25.70	9.60 ± 6.10	8.75	1.50	27.30	9.50 ± 4.50
T10	9.25	3.20	22.80	10.00 ± 4.20	9.00	2.60	23.70	10.00 ± 4.30
T12	8.65	2.00	23.30	9.80 ± 4.50	9.60	1.50	20.20	9.80 ± 4.40
L1	8.20	2.00	26.40	8.70 ± 4.10	8.40	1.70	21.60	8.60 ± 4.00
L3	5.65	2.00	14.80	6.10 ± 3.10	5.35	1.80	16.30	6.20 ± 3.40
L5	4.75	1.50	16.30	5.20 ± 3.20	4.25	1.70	17.00	5.30 ± 3.50
S1	3.50	1.20	14.00	4.40 ± 2.70	3.55	1.20	12.80	4.40 ± 2.80

Used with permission. The data is expressed as the median, minimum, and maximum values collected and the mean ± standard deviation for each segment.
*The data collected is derived from 80 subjects. Copyright, 1996, EMG Consultants, Inc.

dynamic assessment of paraspinal muscle activity in chiropractic practice have been described.[31] A two or four channel computerized EMG scanner is used in conjunction with pregelled disposable, self-adhesive electrodes. The skin of the patient is prepared with an alcohol wipe and dried. Active electrodes are placed at similar points on each side of the paravertebral skin. Upper and lower active electrodes are employed. A ground reference electrode is placed between the active electrodes. The patient is instructed to execute the specific motion being examined, while an acquisition of EMG signal is obtained. The relative levels of EMG activity are then plotted on an amplitude and time X-Y graph. A baseline graph is recorded with the patient in the neutral position.

Paraspinal EMG scanning is a reliable tool for the quantitative assessment of paraspinal muscle activity. Altered paraspinal muscle activity is a generally accepted manifestation of vertebral subluxation. Paraspinal EMG scanning may be effectively used for objective assessment of the somatic component of somatovisceral reflexes.

Autonomic Assessments

Skin Temperature Analysis

Alterations in temperature have been associated with abnormalities in the human body since the time of Hippocrates. Hippocrates wrote, "Should one part of the body be hotter or colder than the rest, then disease is present in that part."[32]

In 1924, B.J. Palmer introduced the chiropractic profession to an instrument invented by Dossa Evins, called the *Neurocalometer*. This instrument measured paraspinal skin temperature differentials associated with vertebral subluxations.[33,34] Vlasuk[35] observed that the chiropractic profession was the first to publish information relating paraspinal temperature differentials to health and disease. The neurocalometer was followed by more sophisticated temperature sensing instruments, including computer-based infrared scanners and thermographic imaging systems.

Since the 1970s, thermography has been used as an adjunct to the assessment of a variety of visceral disorders, including stomach diseases,[36] cholecystitis[37] and other gallbladder diseases,[38] kidney disease,[39] peptic ulcer,[40] liver disease,[41] pancreatic disease,[42] coronary artery disease,[43] and viscerogenic pain.[44] Although promising, these applications have not been incorporated in general clinical practice in the United States.

Basic Principles Alterations in skin temperature patterns are associated with aberrations in the function of the autonomic nervous system, which controls the organs, glands, and blood vessels.[45] It is responsible for relating the internal environment of the patient to the dynamics of the outside world. One important function of the autonomic nervous system is temperature regulation. When the outside environment is cool, the body will attempt to conserve heat, resulting in constriction of the arterioles in the skin. When the outside environment is warm and the body seeks to eliminate heat, vasodilation of the arterioles in the skin will result. In a healthy patient, skin temperature patterns will be constantly changing but symmetric because a healthy body is constantly adapting to the environment.

Vertebral subluxations result in thermal asymmetries and/or fixed patterns. The levels of thermal asymmetry are not necessarily the levels of subluxation and may change with time.[46,47] The value of skin temperature instrumentation is in determining the overall degree of autonomic abnormality and the response of the patient to the adjustment.

Two mechanisms have been proposed that relate to altered skin temperatures: the segmental and the nonsegmental.

The Segmental Model According to the segmental model, sensory irritation by the recurrent meningeal nerve may result in a sympathetic response of vasoconstriction. This will produce thermal asymmetry in the thermatome affected. A thermatome is similar to a dermatome but refers to a region of temperature change rather than sensation.[48] When this mechanism is operative, the level of the thermal asymmetry is often the same as the level of subluxation or is close to it. Some clinicians report that chronic subluxations or prolonged organic disease may be associated with segmental responses. When a handheld thermocouple type instrument is used, a break or sharp deflection of the meter needle may be observed.[49] Segmental facilitation of the lateral horn cells of the spinal cord may produce similar changes.[50]

The Nonsegmental Model Sensory innervation of the intervertebral discs and facet joints is not only segmental but also is nonsegmental through the paravertebral sympathetic trunk.[51,52] Therefore a subluxation at any level of the spine may produce thermal changes throughout the entire spine. Depending on the degree of chronicity, these changes may be fluctuating or fixed into a pattern.

Clinical Analysis Two factors are considered in the analysis of thermal differentials: symmetry and pattern.[53] Symmetry refers to the difference in temperature between the left side and the right side at similar points along the spine. Specific temperatures vary greatly from person to person. Actual temperatures also vary in the same person from moment to moment. However, the differences in temperature from side to side are maintained within strict limits in healthy persons. Uematsu and others[45] determined normative values based on 90 asymptomatic normal individuals and proposed the following:

> These values can be used as a standard in assessment of sympathetic nerve function, and the degree of asymmetry is a quantifiable indicator of dysfunction. . . . Deviations from the normal values will allow suspicion of neurological pathology to be quantitated and therefore can improve assessment and lead to proper clinical management.

Patterns B.J. Palmer developed and used a system of skin temperature analysis called the *pattern system*.[54] Miller[55] described the basic premise of pattern analysis as follows:

> Persons free of neurological interference tend to display skin temperature readings which continually change, but when the vertebral subluxation and interference to normal neurological function appear on the scene, these changing differentials become static. They no longer display normal adaptability, and at this time the patient is said to be 'in pattern.'

Stewart and others[56] have developed algorithms that permit computer-aided pattern analysis of skin temperature differentials. Comparisons between graphs are made to determine the degree of similarity.

Instrumentation

Dual Probe Instruments Dual probe instruments are used to measure differences in temperature between like points on each side of the spine. The first chiropractic instruments employed thermocouples as the temperature sensing elements. The neurocalometer (NCM) comprises two sets of thermocouples and a sensitive galvanometer. By placing the thermocouples in probes that straddle the spine, imbalances in skin temperature at like points may be detected. Following the development of the neurocalometer, the capability of recording these temperature differences on a strip chart was added. The instrument with the strip chart recorder was termed the *neurocalograph.* Similar instruments are available today. Dual probe instruments are also available that employ thermisters and infrared radiation detectors. Such instruments may interface with computers for display and mathematical analysis.[57]

Single Probe Instruments Single probe instruments may be used to collect temperature readings of equal paraspinal points or to evaluate differences in temperature along different spinal levels.[58] A different rationale is applied to interpreting the findings of single probe instruments such as the dermathermograph (DTG). Cold readings, indicating vasoconstriction, are considered clinically significant. However, as in the pattern system, the areas of vasoconstriction do not necessarily indicate the level of subluxation. Korr[50] developed the concept of segmental facilitation, where excess sympathetic stimulation may cause vasoconstriction of the arterioles in the skin. Stillwagon[7] noted that after a sensory neuron synapses with the sympathetic nervous system, preganglionic sympathetic fibers can ascend or descend several levels before producing a vasomotor response. Vasoconstriction may also occur as a result of sympathetic responses to recurrent meningeal nerve irritation.

Acute subluxations may produce the opposite response, or *vasodilation.* The mechanisms involved may include neuroactive substances such as histamine and prostaglandins and antidromic stimulation of dorsal roots resulting in the release of substance P, causing vasodilation.[34]

Thermography Thermography is the technique of producing an image that displays temperature variations as differing colors or shades of gray. Three main types of thermographic systems are currently available.[57, 58]

Liquid Crystal Thermography Liquid crystal thermography employs flexible plastic sheets containing liquid crystals. Liquid crystals are cholesterol esters whose optical properties change with temperature. Different temperatures are seen as different colors. In practice, the flexible plastic sheet is mounted in an assembly that is held on the body part being examined. The image may be recorded on photographic film.

Low Resolution Electronic Thermography Low resolution electronic thermography uses a multichannel thermal sensing instrument called the *Visi-Therm.* The instrument consists of a handheld wand containing an array of infrared sensors. The sensor array is passed over the patient, and a computer produces a color image of the thermal emissions from the body part being examined. Temperature measurements and comparative graphs may also be produced.[59]

Electronic Telethermography Electronic telethermography involves a camera containing infrared sensors and a scanning apparatus. The camera is aimed at the body part being examined. The output of the camera is processed by a computer, and a color or black-and-white image is displayed on a video monitor. Temperature differences are represented by different colors or shades of gray.[58]

Reliability and Validity Because vasomotor activity should be a dynamic process, levels of asymmetry will change from session to session unless a chronic subluxation is present. Even though the levels change, a patient with acute or subacute subluxation will usually have approximately the same number of levels out of range, although the levels may change. Temperature patterns on a patient change from moment to moment unless chronic subluxation is present. This may incorrectly lead the examiner to believe that the instrument or procedure is not reproducible.

Plaugher and others[60] studied the interexaminer and intraexaminer reliability of a thermocouple-type skin temperature differential instrument. Nineteen pain-free female college students were examined. Concordance was evaluated using the Kappa statistic. The Kappa statistic is used to express the reliability of nominative data, for example, presence or absence of an abnormality. The higher the Kappa, the greater the agreement.

In the Plaugher study, all Kappas were statistically significant. Mild-to-moderate reliability was reported in the C2-T2 area, and substantial agreement was found in the T4-T8 region. Fair-to-excellent agreement was found between examiners.

Uematsu and others[45] addressed the clinical utility of skin temperature analysis as follows: "While the absolute values may vary with time . . . the delta Ts (temperature differences) obtained from anatomically matched homologous regions are extremely stable and reproducible." In a technical report describing computerized paraspinal skin temperature scanning, Schram and others[61] concluded that the system provides an effective and reliable means for monitoring temperature changes that may occur following chiropractic spinal adjustments.

Diakow and others[62] examined 10 subjects to determine if a relationship existed between thermographic findings and clinical indicators of spinal dysfunction, including fixation, tenderness, and skin rolling. The authors concluded that convincing evidence exists that thermography could provide objective evidence of spinal segmental dysfunction.

Brand and Gizoni[63] gathered thermographic data from 18 patients before and after chiropractic adjustment. Significant changes were observed following the adjustment.

Clinical Observations Although large controlled studies of skin temperature changes resulting from chiropractic care are lacking, the procedure is based on a sound physiologic rationale. Furthermore, acceptable reliability has been shown for various methods of skin temperature assessment.

The following clinical observations have emerged from users of paraspinal skin temperature analysis and may serve as the seed concepts for more formalized research:

1. In normal (unsubluxated) patients, thermal patterns will be constantly changing and will exhibit acceptable symmetry.
2. In acute and subacute subluxations, some levels will be out of range but the pattern will vary.
3. In chronic subluxations, the pattern will be fixed and levels out of range will be present.
4. Levels of asymmetry often do not relate to the level of primary subluxation.
5. Chronic organ dysfunction (visceroautonomic) may result in a focal segmental asymmetry (Figure 7-3).

Galvanic Skin Resistance

In addition to techniques of skin temperature measurement, sweat gland activity is another indicator of sympathetic function. Sympathetic stimulation causes increased sweat gland activity, which results in less resistance to the flow of an electric current. Therefore sweat gland activity may be assessed by passing a small electric current through the skin to measure resistance. Terms used to describe this procedure include *ESR (electric skin resistance), GSR (galvanic skin response),* and *electrodermatography.* Korr, Thomas, and Wright[64] summarized the physiologic rationale for evaluating patterns of electrical skin resistance in patients:

1. ESR is related to the activity of the sweat glands.
2. Interruption or retardation of the flow of impulses over sympathetic pathways to an area causes a marked elevation of resistance in that area.
3. Stimulation of sympathetic pathways either locally or systemically lowers the resistance.

Korr and Goldstein[65] observed that segmental differences in sweat gland activity are related to segments with reduced motor reflex thresholds. Areas of reduced skin resistance were often hyperesthetic. They concluded that in segments with chronically reduced motor reflex thresholds, at least some of the preganglionic sympathetic neurons of the same segment are also maintained in a state of facilitation (lowered thresholds).

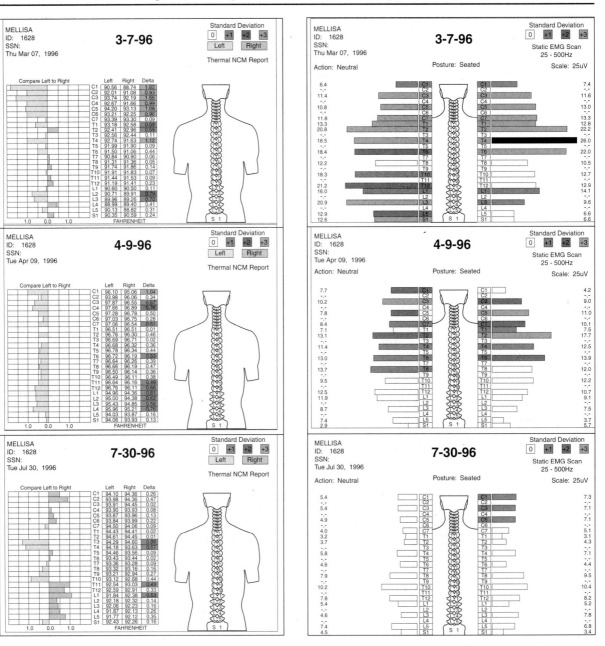

Figure 7-3 Case presentation showing changes in somatic and autonomic activity in a 6-year-old girl whose chief complaint is asthma. **A,** Infrared thermal scans. The autonomic nervous system regulates the organs and glands of the body. A person may have disturbances in the autonomic nervous system and experience no pain. By measuring skin temperature, we can monitor autonomic function. See how the chiropractic patient's skin temperature balance improved as she continued with chiropractic care. She was taking daily medication and had many hospital visits because of asthma. After 8 weeks of chiropractic care, she was finished with all medication and for the first time in her young life, she felt what it was like to be healthy. The number of shaded squares below the column titled, "Delta," reveals the number of levels of abnormality. The improvement in the scans measure the positive changes in her nervous system with chiropractic care. **B,** Surface EMG scans. When muscles contract, they emit an electric signal. The more they contract, the higher the signal. Surface EMG measures that signal. Muscle control is regulated by the motor nervous system. Through time with chiropractic care, the patient's surface EMG scans improved as did her health. Notice how the signals are progressively lower with better balance and symmetry. By monitoring the nervous system, we can better understand how a patient is responding to chiropractic care. (Courtesy Drs. Stuart and Theresa Warner.)

The results of investigations employing skin resistance methods to evaluate manifestations of visceral disease or segmental dysfunction have yielded equivocal results. This may be partly because of variations in technique and interpretation.

Korr[66] reported the results of a preliminary investigation to determine if paraspinal skin resistance patterns were related to visceral disease. Two classes of patients were evaluated. One group of patients had a history of myocardial infarction and demonstrated low resistance areas over two or more of the upper four thoracic vertebrae. In one patient, such areas were observed 3 weeks before coronary occlusion. The second group of patients had duodenal cap ulcers. These individuals had low resistance areas at the T5-T8 areas.

In a later work, Korr[67] stated that after examining hundreds of patients, the following occurred:

Each had a rather characteristic pattern that remained fairly constant; the size of the areas might vary but the segmental distributions retained the individual's characteristic pattern. We could identify the subject from his ESR—electrical skin resistance chart—almost as readily as one can from fingerprints . . . Repeatedly it has been demonstrated that the distribution of low skin resistance—that is, areas of sympathetic nerve activity—correspond quite well to the actual nerve distribution of the lesioned segment in the spine.

These conclusions are refuted by other investigators using skin resistance measurements. Bauch and Hartig[68] concluded that the electrodermatogram was unreliable as an independent or differential diagnostic method. They reasoned that because of nervous system overlap, segmental localization was imprecise and therefore not organ-specific. The authors noted that the asymmetry of the conductivity between the two sides of the body was a phenomenon that could not be explained.

Plaugher and others[69] investigated the interexaminer reliability of a galvanic skin resistance device for the detection of low resistance areas along the spinal column in relatively asymptomatic subjects. Only modest levels of concordance were found. The authors suggest that the unevenness of data generated in certain spinal regions necessitates further investigation before reaching conclusions about the usefulness of this instrument in a clinical setting.

A possible explanation for these conclusions is offered by Korr[67] in the following:

You must not look for perfect correspondence between skin resistance and the distribution of the pathologic disturbance, because an area of skin which is segmentally related to a particular muscle does not necessarily overlap that muscle. With the latissimus dorsi, for example, the myofascial disturbance might be over the hip but the reflex manifestations would be in much higher dermatomes because this muscle has its innervation from the cervical part of the spinal cord.

Ellestad and others[30] reported statistically significant changes in paraspinal skin resistance in patients with back pain who received osteopathic manipulative treatment (OMT). Specifically, skin resistance decreased following OMT. The authors suggested that this may be because of a greater degree of relaxation. It was also reported that SEMG activity decreased following OMT.

In addition to assessing segmental autonomic function, skin resistance measurements may be used as indicators of general autonomic activity. Such measurements are often taken at the fingertips. This procedure is frequently used in biofeedback training to teach relaxation techniques.

A small study by Giesen, Center, and Leach[69a] used electrodermal measurements to assess autonomic nervous system activity in hyperactive children receiving chiropractic care. Behavioral assessments were also used to evaluate outcomes. The authors concluded that chiropractic care has the potential to become an important intervention for children with hyperactivity. Because of equivocal findings and a scarcity of published research in the chiropractic literature, the acceptance of skin resistance instrumentation in general clinical practice has been limited. Additional research to explore its potential value in assessing autonomic dysfunction associated with vertebral subluxation should be encouraged.

Other Instrumentation

Heart Rate Variability Variability in heart rate reflects the vagal and sympathetic function of the autonomic nervous system and has been used as a monitoring tool in clinical conditions characterized by altered autonomic nervous system function.[70] Spectral analysis of beat-to-beat variability is a simple, noninvasive technique to evaluate autonomic dysfunction.[71]

Heart rate variability analysis has been used to assess diabetic neuropathy and to predict the risk of arrythmic events following myocardial infarction.[72] The technique has also been used to investigate autonomic changes associated with neurotoxicity,[73] physical exercise,[74] anorexia nervosa,[75] brain infarction,[76] angina,[77] and panic disorder.[78]

Normative data on heart rate variability have been collected.[79-81] This technology appears promising for assessing overall fitness. Gallagher and others[82] compared age matched groups with different lifestyles. These were smokers, sedentary persons, and aerobically fit individuals. They found that smoking and a sedentary lifestyle reduced vagal tone, whereas enhanced aerobic fitness increased vagal tone. Dixon and others[83] reported that endurance training modifies heart rate control through neurocardiac mechanisms.

In occupational health, the effects of various stresses of the work environment of heart patients and asymptomatic workers may be evaluated using heart rate variability analysis.[84]

The role of heart rate variability assessment in chiropractic patients with confirmed or suspected somatovisceral disorders has yet to be defined.

EEG and Brain Mapping B.J. Palmer was the first chiropractor to evaluate the relationship between brain waves, peripheral nerve function, and vertebral subluxation. These investigations, which began in the 1930s, employed an instrument developed at the Palmer School of Chiropractic called the *electroencephaloneuromentimpograph.*[57]

Electroencephalographic changes have been reported following chiropractic adjustments.[85] Chiropractic adjustments may alter cerebral blood flow.[86-88] The reputed effects of chiropractic care on brain function have been reported. Walton[89] observed increased IQ, improved behavior, better grades, and enhanced athletic ability in learning impaired children following chiropractic care. Thomas and Wood[90] described the abrupt improvement in mental and motor deficits in a 14-year-old girl following upper cervical chiropractic care. Because certain EEG characteristics have been related to intelligence and neural efficiency,[91-93] EEG procedures may be useful in

demonstrating the effects of chiropractic adjustments on brain function (Figure 7-4).

Imaging Procedures

Radiography B.J. Palmer closely followed the progress of the fledgling science of diagnostic imaging, which began with the discovery of x-rays by Roentgen in 1895. In 1910, the Palmer School of Chiropractic purchased a Scheidel-Western x-ray machine.[94] B.J. Palmer's original goals were to "verify or deny palpation findings and to verify or deny proof of the existence of vertebral subluxations."[95] He later discovered that x-rays could also provide information concerning developmental variants and spinal pathologies that could affect the chiropractic care of an individual (Figure 7-5).

Relation of Spinal Abnormalities to Visceral Disease
Somatovisceral relationships have been described in the medical literature of the early twentieth century and related to minor curvatures affecting specific levels of the spine. Winsor[96] examined 50 cadavers with disease in 139 organs, and found "curve of the vertebrae" belonging to the same sympathetic segments as the diseased organs 128 times. In 10 organs, an adjacent segment was involved.

Similar findings were reported in living patients by Ussher,[97] who suggested that the spinal abnor-

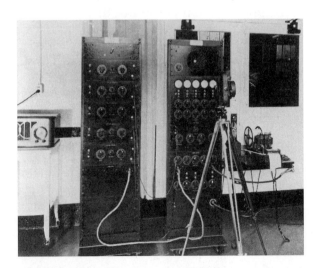

Figure 7-4 The electroencephaloneuromentimpograph used in the B.J. Palmer Chiropractic Clinic. (Courtesy Palmer College of Chiropractic Archives.)

mality could be the cause of the attendant visceral disorder. Radiography could be used to assess alterations in spinal curves and malpositioning of a vertebra, and Ussher urged "a careful neurological examination assisted by roentgenograms of the spine" when needed for differential diagnosis.

Several authors have reported a relationship between spinal osteophytes and visceral disease. Bruckman[98] discussed the relationship between cervical spondylosis and coronary infarction. Snyder, Chance, and Clarey[99] reported the presence of exostoses of the seventh or eighth thoracic vertebrae in 90% of postmortem examination in patients with gallbladder disease. These findings were confirmed by Burchett,[100] who examined 61 hospital patients radiographically. Segmental vertebral lipping between the seventh and tenth thoracic segments was found in 88% of patients with gallbladder disease. In patients with stomach disease, Burchett also noted the presence of spinal osteophytes at T9-T11 in 82% of patients and at T5-T7 in 45% of patients. 64% of patients with pancreatic disease demonstrated osteophytes, mostly at T8-T10. 31% of patients with duodenal disease had osteophytes at T9-L2.

Giles[101] examined the lumbosacral spines of three elderly cadavers to determine the anatomic relationships between osteophytes and autonomic nerves and ganglia. Giles concluded that motion segment osteophytosis may affect viscera through the autonomic nervous system.

Although the relationship of spinal abnormalities to visceral disorders is not clear, correlation of radiographic, instrumentation, and clinical findings may enable the chiropractor to better define this relationship in a given patient.

Computed Tomography Computed tomography, also referred to as *CT* or *CAT scanning,* is an imaging technique that produces axial (cross-sectional) images of body structures using x-radiation. Computer techniques may be used to produce images in other planes. The procedure was developed in Great Britain by Godfrey Hounsfield in 1972.[102] In most CT scanners, a moving x-ray tube produces a fan-shaped beam of radiation. Sensitive electronic detectors record the amount of radiation passing through the body part under examination. The information from the detector array is processed by a computer. An image is displayed on a cathode ray tube, which may be recorded on photographic film.[103]

CT may be used to image somatic and visceral structures, particularly when respiratory, cardiac, and arterial motion makes short scanning times necessary. Unfortunately, the potential of CT in the assessment of viscerosomatic relations has not yet been established.

Magnetic Resonance Imaging (MRI) Magnetic resonance imaging (MRI) provides high resolution images of the body without exposure to ionizing radiation. In chiropractic practice, MR imaging may be useful in the detection and evaluation of vertebral subluxations, disc lesions, neoplasms, and brain, cord, and nerve lesions.[104] Applications for visceral imaging are limited because of artifact associated with respiratory motion, cardiac action, and arterial pulsation.

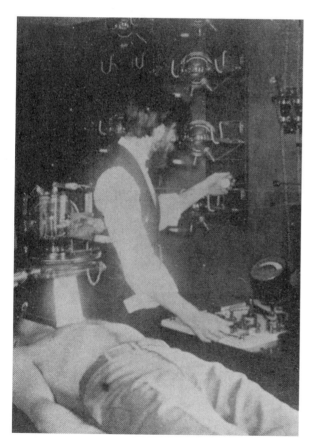

Figure 7-5 B.J. Palmer with an early x-ray machine. (Courtesy Palmer College of Chiropractic Archives.)

Pick[116] used MRI to demonstrate changes in the size and shape of the ventricles of the brain following manipulation of the cranium (Figure 7-6).

Functional Magnetic Resonance Imaging (fMRI)
Unlike conventional MRI, which discloses only anatomy and pathology, functional magnetic resonance imaging (fMRI) is a noninvasive neuroimaging technique that demonstrates alterations in brain physiology. When nerve cells are activated, increase in oxygen consumption occurs. Therefore by observing changes in the magnetic

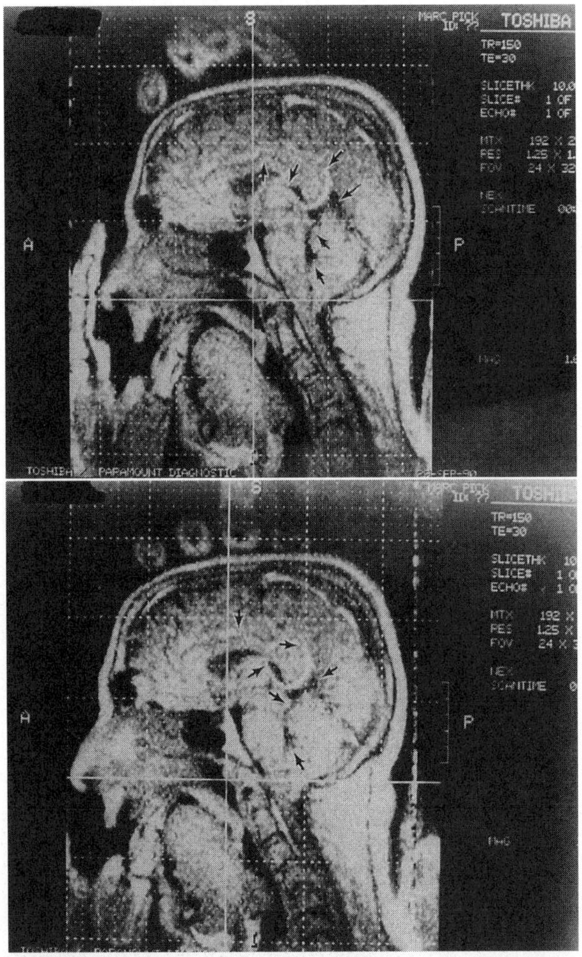

Figure 7-6 Midsagittal MRI performed at magnification 1.60; the *arrows* depict areas of investigational focus. **A,** First MRI scan performed with the investigator's contacts positioned but without the application of cranial manipulative force. **B,** Second MRI scan performed during the investigator's application of firm manipulative pressure toward the opposing contact point. (From Pick MG: Cranial Manipulation, *JMPT* 17:3, 1994.)

properties of hemoglobin, alterations in brain activity may be visualized.

The technique relies on the relationship between neuronal synaptic activity, energy metabolism, and blood circulation. During neuronal stimulation, a subtle change in signal intensity is attributed to a local change in blood oxygenation and blood flow. Changes in the oxygenation state of hemoglobin are induced by task activation. In response to activation, the MRI signal intensity increases as a result of an increase in blood flow and oxygen.[104]

Brain activation patterns have been recorded using visual, sensorimotor, and auditory stimuli, and superior cognitive processes.[105-109]

Gorman[110-111] has described alterations in visual function that resolved following manipulation and hypothesized that the favorable clinical responses were because of increased blood flow to the retina and brain. Furthermore, chiropractic care has been associated with favorable changes in children with learning disorders and attention deficit-hyperactivity disorder.[69a, 112-115]

Terrett[117] has suggested that the favorable clinical results following manipulation of the cervical spine may be because of resolution of ischemic penumbra. This is a condition in which cerebral blood flow is inadequate to maintain normal function but is not diminished at the stage where cell death occurs. The affected areas of the brain are said to be in a state of *hibernation*. Terrett conjectured that restoration of normal cerebral blood flow will result in restoration of normal function in the hibernating cells.

Functional MRI may be a useful technology for studying the effects of chiropractic adjustment on brain function (Figure 7-7).[118]

Summary

Some instruments such as surface EMG and skin temperature measurement devices are practical for use in clinical practice. These instruments provide objective, quantifiable information concerning the somatic and autonomic manifestations of vertebral subluxation.

For various reasons, other instruments discussed are not in widespread clinical use within the chiropractic profession. Galvanic skin resistance techniques have produced equivocal find-

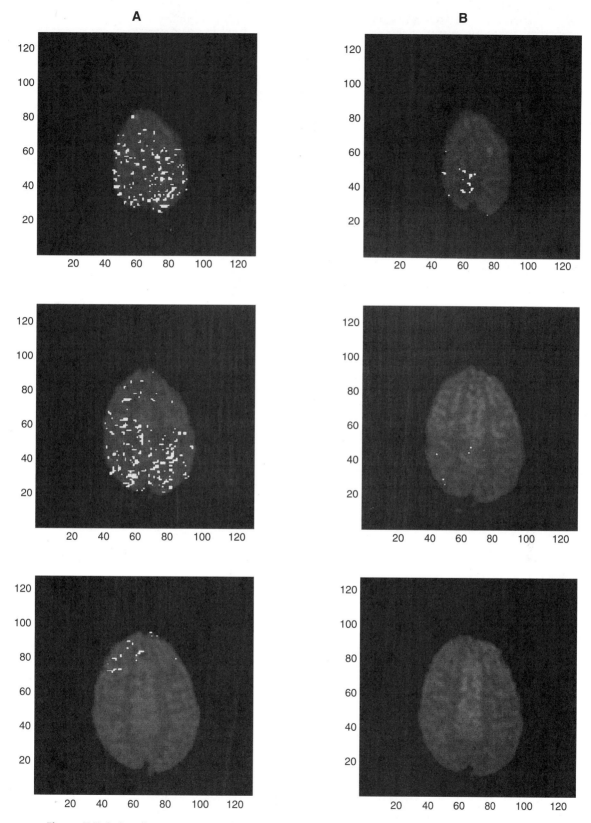

Figure 7-7 A, Preadjustment. **B,** Postadjustment. Because ankle tension is used as a clinical indicator for vertebral subluxation, the task of voluntary unilateral ankle motion was selected for preadjustment and postadjustment functional MRI evaluation. Preadjustment, generalized areas of activation *(white regions)* are seen in the upper and lower slices. After chiropractic adjustment, the regions of signal alteration are much smaller and appear to be unilateral. Chiropractic adjustments may lead to improved neural efficiency, evidenced by fewer and more specific foci of activation.

ings. Heart rate variability is acknowledged as a valid assessment of vagal-sympathetic tone but has not been widely accepted by the chiropractic profession. The high cost, complexity, and limited availability of functional MRI limits it to the research laboratory.

Many chiropractors employ spinal radiography and other imaging procedures in clinical practice. These doctors are urged to review these films in a different way. In addition to biomechanical findings, spinal pathology, and developmental varia-

tion, the possibility that spinal abnormalities may be associated with visceral disease should be considered.

Comparing the results of instrumentation and imaging examinations with clinical findings enables the chiropractor to assess somatovisceral relationships more effectively. Instrumentation may also be used to evaluate the progress of these individuals throughout a course of chiropractic care.

STUDY GUIDE

1. What does electromyography measure?
2. Name four of the findings that may be available to the clinician through the use of SEMG.
3. What is a dynamic SEMG?
4. Name two instruments used for the detection of surface temperature changes in a chiropractic clinical setting. Why would their findings be important?
5. Describe what is meant by being in pattern.
6. What does a cold reading by a single probe instrument indicate? Will it show you where the subluxation is?
7. What is the Kappa statistic?
8. What is heart rate variability and what does it indicate?
9. Can EEG readings be changed by a chiropractic adjustment? How?
10. What was the electroencephaloneuromentimpograph and how was it used? To what cur-

rently available technology is it most closely related in purpose?
11. In what year did Roentgen discover x-rays? When was the Palmer School's first x-ray unit installed?
12. Why would a chiropractor x-ray a patient and when?
13. What relationship might spinal osteophytes have to visceral disease in a patient? Does their location on the vertebra matter?
14. Name a major positive aspect of using MRI. Is it more useful for hard or soft tissue? What does functional MRI show us? Why would that be useful?
15. Describe a situation in which imaging performed in your office might be showing you a probable visceral problem at the dis-ease and the disease level in a patient.

REFERENCES

1. Brown WF: *The physiological and technical basis of electromyography,* Stoneham, Mass, 1984, Butterworth publishers.
2. Desmedt J, editor: *New developments in electromyography and clinical neurophysiology,* New York, 1973, S Karger.
3. Kimura J: *Electrodiagnosis in diseases of nerve and muscle,* Philadelphia, 1985, FA Davis.
4. Basmajian JV: *Muscles alive,* Baltimore, 1979, Williams & Wilkins.
5. Haas M, Panzer DM: Palpatory diagnosis of subluxation. In Gatterman M, editor: *Foundations of chiropractic subluxation,* St Louis, 1995, Mosby.
6. Spector B: Surface electromyography as a model for the development of standardized procedures and reliability testing, *JMPT* 2(4):214, 1979.
7. Komi P, Buskirk E: Reproducibility of electromyographic measurements with inserted wire electrodes and surface electrodes, *Electromyogr* 10:357, 1970.
8. Giroux B, Lamontagne M: Comparisons between surface electrodes and intramuscular wire electrodes in isometric and dynamic conditions, *Electromyogr Clin Neurophysiol* 30:397, 1990.
9. Andersson G, Jonsson B, Ortengren R: Myoelectric activity in individual lumbar erector spinae muscles in

sitting. A study with surface and wire electrodes, *Scand J Rehabil Med* 3(suppl):91, 1974.

10. Thompson J, Erickson R, Offord K: EMG muscle scanning: stability of hand-held electrodes, *Biofeedback Self-Regul* 14(1):55, 1989.

11. Cram JR, Lloyd J, Cahn TS: The reliability of EMG muscle scanning, *Int J Psychosom* 41:41, 1994.

12. Lofland KR et al: Assessment of lumbar EMG during static and dynamic activity in pain-free normals: implications for muscle scanning protocols, *Biofeedback Self-Regul* 20(1):3, 1995.

13. Kent C: Models of vertebral subluxation: a review, *J Vertebr Sublux Res* 1(1):11, 1996.

14. Association of Chiropractic Colleges: Position paper #1, July, 1996.

15. Lantz CA: The subluxation complex. In Gatterman MI, editor: *Foundations of chiropractic subluxation*, St Louis, 1995, Mosby.

16. Janse J, Houser RH, Wells BF: *Chiropractic principles and technic*, Chicago, 1947, National College of Chiropractic (reprinted 1978).

17. Schafer RC: *Basic chiropractic procedural manual*, Arlington, Va, 1984, American Chiropractic Association.

18. Palmer D: *The chiropractor's adjustor*, Portland, 1910, Portland Publishing House.

19. Cram J: EMG muscle scanning and diagnostic manual for surface recordings. In Cram J, editor: *Clinical EMG for surface recordings*, vol 2, Nevada City, Calif, 1990, Clinical Resources.

20. Dolan P, Mannion AF, Adams MA: Fatigue of the erector spinae muscles. A quantitative assessment using frequency banding of the surface electromyography signal, *Spine* 20(2):149, 1995.

21. Gillette RG: A speculative argument for the coactivation of diverse somatic receptor populations by forceful chiropractic adjustments, *Man Med* 3:1, 1987.

22. Zusman M: Spinal manipulative therapy: review of some proposed mechanisms, and a new hypothesis, *Aust J Physiother* 32:89, 1986.

23. Cole WB: The body economy. In Hoag JM, Cole WV, Bradford SG, editors: *Osteopathic medicine*, New York, 1969, McGraw-Hill.

24. Whatmore GB, Kohi DR: Dysponesis: a neurophysiologic factor in functional disorders, *Behav Sci* 13(2):102, 1968.

25. Kent C, Gentempo P: Protocols and normative data for paraspinal EMG scanning in chiropractic practice, *J Chiropr Res Clin Investig* 6(3):64, 1990.

26. Kent C, Gentempo P: Normative data for paraspinal surface electromyographic scanning using a 25-500 Hz bandpass, *J Vertebr Sublux Res* 1(1):43, 1996.

27. Kent C: Surface electromyography in the assessment of changes in paraspinal muscle activity associated with vertebral subluxation: a review, *J Vertebr Sublux Res* 1(3):15, 1997.

28. Patrick DL, Deyo RA: Generic and disease-specific measures in assessing health status and quality of life, *Med Care* 27(3 suppl):S217, 1989.

29. Shambaugh P: Changes in electrical activity in muscles resulting from chiropractic adjustment: a pilot study, *JMPT* 10(6):300, 1987.

30. Ellestad S et al: Electromyographic and skin resistance responses to osteopathic manipulative treatment for low-back pain, *JAOA* 88(8):991, 1988.

31. Kent C, Gentempo P: Dynamic paraspinal surface EMG: a chiropractic protocol, *J Chiropr Res* 2(4):40, 1993.

32. Adams F, translator: *The genuine works of hippocrates*, Baltimore, 1939, Williams & Wilkins.

33. Palmer BJ: *Precise posture constant spinograph comparative graphs*, Davenport, Iowa, 1938, Palmer School of Chiropractic.

34. Kyneur JS, Bolton SP: Chiropractic instrumentation—an update for the 90s, *Chiropr J Aust* 21(3):82, 1991.

35. Vlasuk SL: Chiropractic and thermography: a historic perspective, *ACA J Chiro* 26(11):42, 1989.

36. Rozanov AE, Sukhanova VF: Diagnostic value of thermography in stomach diseases, *Vestn Khir* 122(4):11, 1979.

37. Giorgadze KL et al: The radiodiagnosis of acute and chronic cholecystitis, *Vrach Delo* (11):22, 1989.

38. Herskowitz L, Tilley J: Thermographic patterns in patients with gallbladder disease, *JAOA* 75(4):428, 1975.

39. Mazo EB, Abu-Talib Zaretskii VV, Chemisova GG: Thermography in the diagnosis of kidney neoplasms, *Urol Nefrol (Mosk)* (6):15, 1982.

40. Chuzhina ES, Svetlichnyi VL: Liquid-crystal thermography in the diagnosis of peptic ulcer, *Lik Sprava* (2):81, 1992.

41. Bhatia M et al: Abdominal thermography in infantile and childhood liver disease, *South Med J* 69(8):1045, 1976.

42. Miroshnikov MM et al: Use of the thermovision method study of diseases of the pancreas, liver, and biliary tract, *Vestn Khir* 112(4):15, 1974.

43. Ben Eliyahau D, Lawson W: Noninvasive detection of coronary artery disease by infra-red thermography, *J Manipulative Physiol Ther* 17(4):272, 1994.

44. Kobrossi T, Steiman I: Thermographic investigation of viscerogenic pain: a case report, *J Can Chiro Assoc* 34(3):125, 1990.

45. Uematsu S et al: Quantification of thermal asymmetry, part 1: normal values and reproducibility, *J Neurosurg* 69:552, 1988.

46. Duff SA: *Chiropractic clinical research: interpretation of spinal bilateral temperature differentials*, San Francisco, 1976, Paragon.

47. Sherman L: *Neurocalometer, neurocalograph, neurotempometer*, Davenport, Iowa, 1966, Research as applied to eight BJ Palmer Chiropractic Clinic cases. Palmer School of Chiropractic.

48. Leach RA: *The chiropractic theories*, Baltimore, 1994, Williams & Wilkins.

49. Herbst RW: *Gonstead chiropractic science and healing art*, Mt Horeb, Wis, 1968, Sci-Chi Publications.

50. Korr IM: Clinical significance of the facilitated state, *JAOA* 54:277, 1955.

51. Nakamura S et al: Origin of nerves supplying the posterolateral portion of lumbar intervertebral discs in rats, *Spine* 21(8):917, 1996.

52. Suseki K et al: Innervation of the lumbar facet joints. Origins and functions, *Spine* 22(5):477, 1997.

53. Wallace H, Wallace J, Resh R: Advances in paraspinal thermographic analysis, *Chiro Res J* 2(3):39, 1993.

54. Palmer BJ: *Chiropractic clinical controlled research,* Davenport, Iowa, 1951, Palmer School of Chiropractic.

55. Miller JL: Skin temperature differential analysis, *Int Rev Chiro (Science)* 1(1):41, 1964.

56. Stewart MS, Riffle DW, Boone WR: Computer-aided pattern analysis of temperature differentials, *J Manipulative Physiol Ther* 12(5):345, 1989.

57. Kent C, Gentempo P: Instrumentation and imaging in chiropractic: a centennial retrospective, *Today's Chiro* 24(1):32, 1995.

58. Kent C, Daniels J: Chiropractic thermography: a preliminary report, *Int Rev Chiro* 27(7):4, 1974.

59. Stillwagon G, Stillwagon K: Early observations of the Visi-Therm, *Today's Chiro* 14(6):38, 1985.

60. Plaugher G et al: The inter- and intraexaminer reliability of a paraspinal skin temperature differential instrument, *J Manipulative Physiol Ther* 14(6):361, 1991.

61. Schram SB, Hosek RS, Owens ES: Computerized paraspinal skin surface temperature: a technical report, *J Manipulative Physiol Ther* 5(3):117, 1982.

62. Diakow PRP et al: Correlation of thermography with spinal dysfunction: preliminary results, *J Can Chiro Assoc* 32(2):77, 1988.

63. Brand NE, Gizoni CM: Moire contourography and infrared thermography: changes resulting from chiropractic adjustments, *J Manipulative Physiol Ther* 5(3):113, 1982.

64. Korr IM, Thomas PE, Wright HM: Patterns of electrical skin resistance in man, *J Neural Trans* 17:77, 1958.

65. Korr IM, Goldstein MJ: Dermatomal autonomic activity in relation to segmental motor reflex threshold, *Fed Proceed* 7:67, 1948 (abstract).

66. Korr IM: Skin resistance patterns associated with visceral disease, *Fed Proceed* 8:87, 1949.

67. Korr IM: *The segmental nervous system as a mediator and organizer of disease processes,* The Physiologic Basis of Osteopathic Medicine. The Postgraduate Institute of Osteopathic Medicine and Surgery, 73:1970.

68. Bauch K, Hartig W: Electrodermatographic examination of segmental sweat secretion in the diagnosis and differential diagnosis of internal diseases, *Acta Neurovegetativa* 30:536, 1973.

69. Plaugher G et al: The interexaminer reliability of a galvanic skin response instrument, *J Manipulative Physiol Ther* 16(7):453, 1993.

69a. Giesen J, Center D, Leach R: An evaluation of chiropractic manipulation as a treatment of hyperactivity in children, *J Manipulative Physiol Ther* 12:353, 1989.

70. van Ravenswaaij-Arts CM et al: Heart rate variability, *Ann Intern Med* 118(6):436, 1993.

71. DeDenedittis G et al: Autonomic changes during hypnosis: a heart rate variability power spectrum analysis as a marker of sympatho-vagal balance, *Int J Clin Exp Hypn* 42(2):140, 1994.

72. Kautzner J, Camm AJ: Clinical relevance of heart rate variability, *Clin Cardiol* 20(2):162, 1997.

73. Murata K, Landrigan PJ, Araki S: Effects of age, gender, heart rate, tobacco and alcohol ingestion on R-R interval variability in human ECG, *J Auton Nerv Syst* 37:199, 1992.

74. Nakamura Y, Yamamoto Y, Muraoka I: Autonomic control of heart rate during physical exercise and fractal dimension of heart rate variability, *J Appl Physiol* 74(2):875, 1993.

75. Petretta M et al: Heart rate variability as a measure of autonomic nervous system function in anorexia nervosa, *Clin Cardiol* 20(3):219, 1997.

76. Korpelaineu JT et al: Abnormal heart rate variability as a manifestation of autonomic dysfunction in hemispheric brain infarction, *Stroke* 27(11):2059, 1996.

77. Kamalesh M et al: Reproducibility of time and frequency domain analysis of heart rate variability in patients with chronic stable angina, *Pacing Clin Electrophysiol* 18(11):1991, 1995.

78. Yeragani VK et al: Decreased heart rate variability in panic disorder patients: a study of power-spectral analysis of heart rate, *Psychiatry Res* 46(1):89, 1993.

79. O'Brien IA, O'Hare P, Corrall RJ: Heart rate variability in healthy subjects: effect of age and the derivation of normal ranges for tests of autonomic function, *Br Heart J* 55(4):348, 1986.

80. Toyry J et al: Day-to-day variability of cardiac autonomic regulation parameters in normal subjects, *Clin Physiol* 15(1):39, 1995.

81. Sato N et al: Power spectral analysis of heart rate variability in healthy young women during the normal menstrual cycle, *Psychosom Med* 57(4):331, 1995.

82. Gallagher D, Terenzi T, de Meersman R: Heart rate variability in smokers, sedentary, and aerobically fit individuals, *Clin Auton Res* 2(6):383, 1992.

83. Dixon EM et al: Neural regulation of heart rate variability in endurance athletes and sedentary controls, *Cardiovasc Res* 26(7):713, 1992.

84. Kristal-Boneh E et al: Heart rate variability in health and disease, *Scand J Work Environ Health* 21(2):85, 1995.

85. Hospers L: *EEG and CEEG studies before and after upper cervical or SOT Category II adjustment in children after head trauma, in epilepsy, and in "hyperactivity,"* Arlington, Va, 84: 1992 Proceedings of the National Conference on Chiropractic & Pediatrics.

86. Risley W: Impaired arterial blood flow to the brain as a result of a cervical subluxation: a clinical report, *J Am Chiro Assoc* 32(6):61, 1995.

87. Haldeman S: The influence of the autonomic nervous system on cerebral blood flow, *J Can Chiro Assn* 18(2):6, 1974.

88. Terrett AGJ: The cerebral dysfunction theory. In Gatterman MI, editor: *Foundations of chiropractic subluxation,* St Louis, 1995, Mosby.

89. Walton EV: The effects of chiropractic treatment on students with learning and behavioral impairments due to neurological dysfunction, *Int Rev Chiro* 29 (4-5):24, 1975.

90. Thomas M, Wood J: Upper cervical adjustments may improve mental function, *Man Med* 6(6):215, 1992.

91. Ertl J: *The Louisiana study of learning potential by brain wave analysis,* Shreveport, La, 1976, Neural Evaluation.

92. Ertl J: *Neural efficiency and human intelligence,* final report, Proj No 9-0105, 1969, US Office of Education.

93. Ertl J: Fourier analysis of evoked potentials and human intelligence, *Nature* 230(5295):525, 1971.

94. Canterbury R, Krakos G: Thirteen years after Roentgen: the origins of chiropractic radiology, *Chiro Hist* 6:25, 1986.

95. Palmer BJ: *The bigness of the fellow within,* Davenport, Iowa, 1949, Palmer School of Chiropractic.

96. Winsor H: Sympathetic segmental disturbances, II, *The Medical Times* 49:267, 1921.

97. Ussher NT: Spinal curvatures—visceral disturbances in relation thereto, *Calif West Med* 38:423, 1933.

98. Bruckman W: Spondylotic change of the cervical spine and coronary infarction, *Deutsche Medizinische Wochenschrift* 44:1740, 1956.

99. Snyder GE, Chance JA, Clarey JK: Postmortem studies of viscerosomatic relationships, *JAOA* 65(5):995, 1966.

100. Burchett GD: Segmental spinal osteophytosis in visceral disease, *JAOA* 67(6):675, 1968.

101. Giles L: Paraspinal autonomic ganglion distortion due to vertebral body osteophytosis: a cause of vertebrogenic autonomic syndromes? *J Manipulative Physiol Ther* 15(9):551, 1992.

102. Eisenberg RL: *Radiology: an illustrated history,* St Louis, 1992, Mosby.

103. Kricun R, Kricum ME: Computed tomography. In Kricun ME, editor: *Imaging modalities in spinal disorders,* Philadelphia, 1988, WB Saunders.

104. LeBihan D et al: Functional magnetic resonance imaging of the brain, *Ann Intern Med* 122:296, 1995.

105. LeBihan D et al: Activation of human primary visual cortex during visual recall: a magnetic resonance imaging study, *Proc Natl Acad Sci USA* 90:11802, 1993.

106. Hinke RM et al: Functional magnetic resonance imaging of Broca's area during internal speech, *Neuroreport* 4:675, 1993.

107. Rueckert L et al: Magnetic resonance imaging functional activation of left frontal cortex during covert word production, *J Neuroimaging* 4:67, 1994.

108. Rao SM et al: Functional magnetic resonance imaging of complex human movements, *Neurology* 43:2311, 1993.

109. Belliveau JW et al: Functional mapping of the human visual cortex by magnetic resonance imaging, *Science* 254:716, 1991.

110. Gorman RF: The treatment of presumptive optic nerve ischemia by manipulation, *J Manipulative Physiol Ther* 18:172, 1995.

111. Gorman RF: Monocular vision loss after closed head trauma: immediate resolution associated with spinal manipulation, *J Manipulative Physiol Ther* 16:138, 1993.

112. Phillips C: *Case study: the effect of using spinal manipulation and craniosacral therapy as the treatment approach for attention deficit-hyperactivity disorder,* 57, 1991 Proceedings of the National Conference on Chiropractic and Pediatrics.

113. Anderson C, Partridge J: Seizures plus attention deficit hyperactivity disorder, *Intern Rev Chiropr* 49:35, 1993.

114. Barnes T: A multi-faceted approach to attention deficit hyperactivity disorder: a case report, *Intern Rev Chiropr* 51:41, 1995.

115. Barnes T: Attention deficit hyperactivity disorder and the triad of health, *J Clin Chiropr Ped* 1(2):59, 1996.

116. Pick MG: A preliminary single case magnetic resonance imaging investigation into maxillary frontal-parietal manipulation and its short-term effect upon the intracranial structures of an adult human brain, *J Manipulative Physiol Ther* 17:168, 1994.

117. Terrett AGJ: The cerebral dysfunction theory. In Gatterman MI, editor: *Foundations of chiropractic subluxation,* St Louis, 1995, Mosby.

118. Kent C, Vernon LF: *Case studies in chiropractic MRI,* Arlington, Va, 1998, International Chiropractors Association.

CHAPTER 8

Pelvic Pain and Pelvic Organic Dysfunction

James E. Browning, DC

Mechanically Induced Pelvic Pain and Organic Dysfunction

Anecdotal reports of chiropractic treatment being successfully used in the management of disorders of pelvic organic function date back to the early years of the profession.[1,2] Of all the organic disorders that have been reported to benefit from chiropractic intervention, pelvic pain and various disturbances of bladder, bowel, gynecologic, and sexual function are among the most frequently described.[2] Although isolated symptoms of pelvic pain and various disturbances of pelvic organ function have been identified as clinical entities responding to chiropractic treatment, these same disorders have also been found to exist as components of a recently described disorder known as the mechanically induced *pelvic pain and organic dysfunction (PPOD) syndrome.*[3] Most reports describing the resolution of single-symptom pelvic organic dysfunction occurring in response to chiropractic intervention have detailed the presence of multiregion spinal articular dysfunction as a possible etiology of the patient's complaints. These findings had prompted a therapeutic approach that had been directed at multiple regions of the spine. By contrast, the mechanically induced PPOD syndrome is characterized by clinical features that implicate impairment of lower sacral nerve root function occurring as a result of a mechanical lesion of the lumbar spine. Accordingly, the therapeutic emphasis of this disorder is largely confined to correcting a localized disorder thought to be the etiologic agent of a neurogenically induced pelvic organic dysfunctional state.

This chapter will highlight recent reports describing the effects of chiropractic intervention on single symptom/disorder pelvic organic dysfunc-

tion and present the diagnostic and therapeutic protocols this office has successfully used for identifying and managing the variant forms of the mechanically induced PPOD syndrome.

Single Symptom/Disorder Pelvic Organic Dysfunction

Urologic Dysfunction

Enuresis is defined as the involuntary discharge of urine. Although urinary loss can occur at any age, the term enuresis is generally used to reference urinary loss occurring in a child 5 years of age or older, and urinary incontinence refers to the loss of normal urinary control in an adult. Clinically, enuresis can be classified as primary or secondary. Primary enuresis represents urinary loss in a child who has not yet developed normal urinary control. These individuals have never been consistently dry for more than 1 to 2 weeks. Secondary enuresis occurs in a child who, after having initially developed normal urinary control, reverts to a state of uncontrolled urinary discharge. Although accounts of the successful treatment of nocturnal enuresis by spinal manipulation abound,[4,5] little evidence in the indexed literature exists in support of this claim.[6-9] Of the evidence available, two case reports and a controlled clinical trial suggest a positive therapeutic response to spinal manipulation, and one prospective study failed to find any significant improvement in enuretic children treated by spinal manipulation.

Blomerth[4] described the resolution of primary nocturnal enuresis in an 8-year-old boy by manipulation of the lumbar spine. Enuresis had been occurring an average of 6 nights per week despite the fact that the boy had already been receiving chiropractic care and undergoing spinal manipulation to the cervical and thoracic spines for the treatment of asthma. Interestingly, manipulation of the lumbar spine had to be performed before a change in his enuretic state occurred. After a single manipulation to the lower lumbar spine, the boy's mother reported a complete cessation of his nocturnal urinary loss. During the next 3½ years, however, enuresis recurred on three separate occasions. All three episodes were associated with minor sports injuries and were accompanied by relatively mild low back pain. Subsequent to each recurrence, however, further manipulation to the lower lumbar spine quickly restored normal urologic function.

A single subject, time-series design involving a 14-yr-old boy undergoing spinal manipulation for the treatment of primary nocturnal enuresis was described by Gemmell and Jacobson.[6] The patient had suffered continuous bed-wetting, never experiencing a dry night. Earlier treatment included the use of an alarm system in an attempt to condition the patient to awake before wetting the bed. However, this procedure proved to be of little help. Clinical examination, with the exception of local tenderness over the L5 spinous process and articular dysfunction detected at the L5-S1 motion unit, was completely within normal limits. A 2-week pretreatment baseline phase, during which placebo adjustment consisting of gentle massage to the low back, was followed by 4 weeks of toggle recoil manipulation to the L5-S1 articulation at a frequency of 1 to 2 times per week. After the initial 4 weeks of care, two additional treatments were then given 1 week apart. After the first treatment, the patient reported the onset of nocturnal urinary control. Normal urologic function continued throughout the initial 4-week treatment phase. However, when the treatment frequency was reduced to one time per week, urologic function gradually declined. Unfortunately, the patient was not available for follow-up, and no further information could be obtained.

Leboeuf and others[7] described a prospective outcome study in which 171 enuretic children were treated with spinal manipulation during parental monitoring of the number of enuretic nights. All patients underwent a pretreatment baseline period of 2 weeks before the onset of treatment. Treatment included specific chiropractic adjustments to the areas of aberrant spinal movement as detected at each visit through observation and palpation by fifth-year chiropractic students and was administered until the child's parent recorded fewer than 2 wet nights over 2 weeks while the child was on unrestricted fluid intake. Success of treatment was defined as a reduction of 50% or more in the number of wet nights per week between the initiation of treatment and the final follow-up. A reduction of less than 50% in the number of wet nights per week was considered failure. The median number of wet nights per week at the onset of the study was 7.0. After the 2-week pretreatment baseline, before the initiation of treatment, the number of wet nights had spontaneously decreased to 5.6. By the end of treatment, the number of wet nights per week had dropped to 4.0. Overall, only 15.5% of subjects were found to have met the criteria for success.

More recently, Reed and others[10] demonstrated the effectiveness of chiropractic treatment in managing primary nocturnal enuresis under controlled conditions in a group of 46 5- to 13-year old children. After recording a 2-week pretreatment baseline, 31 subjects were placed in the treatment group, and 15 subjects served as controls. Fifth-year chiropractic students assessed all patients for the presence of spinal segmental dysfunction at a minimum of every 10 days. Patients in the treatment group underwent short-lever, high-velocity manipulation of the Palmer Package adjusting technique, and those subjects serving as controls received a sham adjustment with the use of a nontensioned Activator. Treatment was delivered over a 10-week period, while data was collected for an additional 2 weeks. Similar to the Leboeuf and others[7] study, success was defined as a reduction of 50% or more in the frequency of bed-wetting nights in comparing the pretreatment and posttreatment periods. The pretreatment mean wet-night frequency of 9.1 nights per 2 weeks for the treatment group dropped to 7.6 nights for 2 weeks at the conclusion of the study, and the pretreatment mean wet-night frequency of 12.1 for the control group increased to 12.2. Overall, 25% of the treated subjects experienced a 50% or greater reduction of wet nights, and none of the control subjects experienced such a reduction. Although the results of this study did not reach statistic significance, they do suggest a trend toward the effectiveness of chiropractic treatment for primary nocturnal enuresis.

Enuresis associated with spinal bifida occulta has also been reported to respond to chiropractic intervention.[11] Borregard described a case in which a 13-year-old boy with spina bifida occulta sought treatment for complaints of bilateral knee pain and had a history of recurring urinary tract infections accompanied by frequent bouts of diurnal and nocturnal enuresis. Enuresis was precipitated by a strong urge to void that would initiate uncontrollable detrusor contraction. His urologic dysfunction was associated with impaired sensory perception of vesical filling so that he was unaware of bladder distention and as a result could not voluntarily initiate micturition more than once a day. Earlier cystoscopic evaluation had confirmed the presence of an atonic bladder. Treatment consisting of pelvic blocking procedures and respiratory assist manipulation resulted in a gradual return of normal sensory perception of vesical filling so that he regained the ability to initiate the micturition reflex and prevent uncontrolled urinary loss.

Several patients with enuresis and urinary incontinence who had component symptoms of the mechanically induced PPOD syndrome have also been shown to resolve under chiropractic care.[12-16] In these cases, urinary loss was one of many accompanying symptoms of bladder, bowel, gynecologic, and sexual dysfunction that had responded to distractive decompressive manipulation of the lumbar spine.

Enterologic Dysfunction

Falk[17] described a case of constipation accompanied by a loss of the normal urge to defecate that had its onset in conjunction with an episode of low back pain. The patient had no prior history of low back pain or bowel dysfunction. Clinical examination revealed significant lumbar paravertebral muscular spasm and tenderness at the lumbosacral junction. Side posture manipulation delivered to the lower lumbar spine elicited initial improvement in bowel function after 3 days. Treatment was continued for 6 weeks, during which time progressive improvement occurred in his low back pain and bowel dysfunction. After 6

weeks of care, mild low back pain persisted; however, constipation had completely resolved. Subsequent to this episode, the patient experienced several exacerbations of his low back condition. Occurring with each exacerbation was a simultaneous return of constipation, which as before resolved following side posture manipulation of the lumbar spine.

Irritable bowel syndrome (IBS) has also been reported to respond to spinal manipulation. Wagner and others[18] described a case in which a 25-year-old woman visited the doctor with a 5-year history of abdominal pain, cramping, and diarrhea. Clinical examination revealed multiple levels of articular fixation affecting the cervical, thoracic, and lumbar spines, and thoracolumbar scoliosis. Spinal manipulation of the affected articulations was followed by a resolution of symptoms after a single treatment.

As is the case with symptoms of urologic dysfunction, disturbances of enterologic dysfunction in the mechanically induced PPOD patient have also shown resolution by distractive decompressive manipulation of the lumbar spine.[13-16]

Gynecologic and Sexual Dysfunction

Chronic pelvic pain and dyspareunia have been shown to respond to chiropractic intervention by several case reports[12,13,15,16,19] and two small-scale prospective studies.[14,20]

Browning[14] demonstrated improvement in chronic pelvic pain and dyspareunia in six women meeting predetermined criteria indicating the presence of the mechanically induced PPOD syndrome. All women reported experiencing chronic pelvic pain at multiple sites and had numerous additional symptoms of bladder, bowel, gynecologic, and sexual dysfunction that were also assessed and monitored during the course of the study. Patients were treated with distractive decompressive manipulation of the lumbar spine following a predetermined protocol in which the patients received daily treatment. Treatment frequency was diminished according to the patient's response and was terminated when clinical assessment failed to detect continued improvement in the patient's condition over a 2-week period. After the termination of treatment, the patient's response was determined by a self-assessment questionnaire. All six patients reported experiencing improvement in all areas of pelvic pain. Five of the six patients reported that all areas of pelvic pain had either greatly improved or completely resolved; only one patient reported slight improvement in her pelvic pain.

Hawk and others[20] have also demonstrated a reduction in chronic pelvic pain as a result of distractive decompressive manipulation of the lumbar spine in 18 women who met predetermined criteria. They underwent flexion distraction decompressive manipulation of the lumbar spine for a 6-week period. Treatment was administered at an initial frequency of 3 times per week during the first 2 weeks, then twice a week for the duration of the 6-week intervention period. Patients completed outcome measures at baseline before the initiation of treatment and at 6 weeks after the administration of all scheduled treatment. Outcome measures used included the Pain Disability Index (primary outcome measure), visual analog scale for pain, RAND-36 health survey, and Beck Depression Inventory. The mean improvement in the Pain Disability Index was 13 and 4 cm in the visual analog scale. Mean improvement in the Beck depression inventory was 6.1 points, and all 8 subscales of the RAND-36 health survey increased in value. These results demonstrated a positive response to distractive decompressive manipulation of the lumbar spine in women with chronic pelvic pain.

Stude[21] detailed the resolution of dysfunctional uterine bleeding in a 40-year-old woman seeking treatment for 3 months of low back and bilateral lower extremity pain and bleeding abnormalities. Treatment consisting of spinal manipulation and distractive decompressive manipulation was applied to the thoracolumbar and lower lumbar spinal regions. Within 1 day of the first treatment, uterine bleeding had diminished to mild vaginal spotting and low back and lower extremity pain had been significantly reduced. After her second treatment, all symptoms completely resolved. Approximately 1 year later, uterine bleeding returned. However, with this occurrence no accompanying symptoms of low back or lower extremity pain occurred. Treatment administered in a similar fashion resolved her complaints in 2 weeks.

Symptoms associated with premenstrual tension syndrome have also shown improvement under chiropractic care.[22] A 35-year-old woman with a history of chronic premenstrual distress sought chiropractic evaluation. Her reported symptoms of crying spells, headache, forgetfulness, dizziness, abdominal cramping, heart-pounding, low back pain, breast tenderness, and abdominal bloating were assessed before and after a trial of spinal manipulation. After 12 weeks of spinal manipulation therapy administered to the patient's regions of intersegmental hypomobility, all symptoms, with the exception of backache and dizziness, were reported to have improved or resolved.

Although not extensively studied, the potential benefits of chiropractic care in the treatment of dysmenorrhea have been suggested by several case reports[23,24,25,26] and two small controlled studies[27,28] that used questionnaires to document the relief of menstruation-related symptoms. In one case report, a 25-year-old woman with a long history of dysmenorrhea underwent spinal manipulation administered to areas of articular fixation that had been identified in the sacrum, ilia, and lower lumbar spine.[24] Combined with the application of soft-tissue therapy, this treatment had the effect of decreasing the frequency and intensity of abdominal and back pain associated with menstruation. In another case, a retrospective review of the treatment of a 28-year-old woman revealed a significant reduction in low back pain and premenstrual symptoms after 2 months of care.[29]

In a prospective controlled clinical trial, 14 women meeting inclusion criteria including a history of primary dysmenorrhea for at least 1 year, menstrual pain beginning the day before or just after the onset of menstruation, pain rated as moderate or severe, and a regular menstrual cycle were treated using the Toftness system of chiropractic. All patients were treated during menstruation over a 3-month period. In contrast to 12 women undergoing sham intervention that consisted of identically applied treatment but administered to a diagnostically inert region, the treated women demonstrated significant improvement in several outcome measures determined by a Menstrual Distress Questionnaire.[27] Symptoms demonstrating the greatest improvement tended to be of a more physical nature. Included in this category were pain intensity, headaches or dizziness, activity limitation, etc. Those symptoms showing no significant improvement tended to be more of an emotional or psychologic nature, including depression, mood swings, and crying spells.

Kokjohn and others[30] may have identified a possible mechanism behind the reduction of back and/or abdominal pain and menstrual distress in women with dysmenorrhea undergoing spinal manipulation. By measuring the circulating plasma levels of the prostaglandin metabolite 15-keto-13, 14-dihydroprostaglandin before and after the administration of spinal manipulation and correlating these findings with perceived abdominal and back pain measured by a visual analog scale and Menstrual Distress Questionnaire, the authors found a significant and immediate reduction in perceived pain and plasma levels of KDPGF2a. Although these findings suggest a possible mechanism by which spinal manipulation may be effective in relieving the pain and distress associated with primary dysmenorrhea, a similar reduction in plasma KDPGF2a in the sham treated group indicated the need to resolve the question of a placebo effect.

Similar to most symptoms of bladder and bowel dysfunction associated with the mechanically induced PPOD syndrome, chronic pelvic pain, dysfunctional uterine bleeding, and dysmenorrhea have also shown resolution with distractive decompressive manipulation of the lumbar spine.[12-16]

The Mechanically Induced Pelvic Pain and Organic Dysfunction Syndrome

Characterization of the PPOD Syndrome

Of the handful reports that have detailed the effects of chiropractic intervention on disturbances of pelvic organ function, most have described a therapeutic approach designed to normalize articular dysfunction that had been found at multiple regions of the spine. In these cases, full spine manipulative intervention had been used in the treatment of individuals with a narrow range of symptoms reflecting various states of pelvic organic dysfunction. By contrast, the mechanically induced PPOD syndrome is characterized by a wide range of symptoms of pelvic organic dysfunction thought to be caused by an exclusively isolated region of articular dysfunction of the

lumbar spine.[31] Although the etiology of this disorder is thought to be a mechanical lesion of the lumbar spine with secondary impairment of lower sacral nerve root function, its clinical presentation is emphasized by various combinations of symptoms of pelvic pain and disturbances of bladder, bowel, gynecologic, and sexual function.[32] Although this disorder has been found to occur in both sexes, women appear to be much more frequently affected than men.[13,33] Although no specific data exists on the incidence or ratio of gender of PPOD patients presenting to the chiropractor, the author's experience in a general private practice setting is that the ratio of female to male involvement is on the order of 9:1.

Historic Features of the PPOD Patient

When eliciting the history of the mechanically induced PPOD patient, careful chronologic review directed at profiling the evolution of symptom development and progression usually reveals a temporal relationship between the onset or worsening of individual PPOD symptoms and some mechanical stress to the patient's low back. Not in frequently, the onset of individual PPOD symptoms can be clearly traced to a mechanical insult to the patient's lumbar spine. In some cases, however, preexisting PPOD symptoms (relative to the onset of the episode of low back pain and seemingly bearing no obvious relationship to the patient's lumbar spine) may have become more severe in response to a mechanical stress to the lumbar spine, whether distinct back pain had been an accompanying symptom of the PPOD-provoking event. When viewed over time, the history of these patients may reveal a pattern of symptom progression demonstrating individual PPOD symptoms becoming progressively more numerous and severe.[32]

Severely involved long-standing PPOD patients typically reveal a long history of recurrent low back pain that may have completely resolved during the interval stages. Although the back pain component of their overall disorder may not have been of a sufficient degree to prompt previous evaluation or treatment, often times these individuals' associated pelvic organic dysfunction had progressed to a point at which they had undergone various (sometimes numerous) diagnostic and surgical procedures in an attempt to resolve these complaints. Frequently, however, these procedures in an attempt have provided little short-term or no real improvement in the condition for which they had been performed.[13,34] Commonly encountered examples of failed symptomatic surgical treatment include a hysterectomy, hernioplasty, or laparoscopy for the complaints of pelvic pain, a suprapubic urethrovesical suspension for urinary incontinence, and a coccygectomy for coccygeal or paraanal pain.[3]

Although the clinical presentation of the mechanically induced PPOD patient is highlighted by various disturbances of bladder, bowel, gynecologic, and sexual function that at times may be quite severe, most PPOD patients seek chiropractic care as a result of complaints related to a mechanical disorder of the low back.[3] As a result, the presence and extent of PPOD involvement is often identified incidentally by the probing inquisition of an astute diagnostician. Without a thorough appreciation of the clinical features and variant signs of the mechanically induced PPOD syndrome, the unsuspecting clinician is likely to overlook even the most pronounced symptoms of pelvic pain and pelvic organic dysfunction as they relate to a mechanical disorder of the lumbar spine.[3]

Lower Sacral Neurology

The lower sacral nerve roots (primarily S2, S3, and S4) give rise to several individual nerves that, along with their respective branches, provide extensive neurologic connections to structures located throughout the pelvis.[35] These nerves are extremely important in maintaining normal pelvic organ function. For example, muscular branches derived from the level of S4 are distributed to the levator ani, coccygeus, and external anal sphincter. These structures provide the vast majority of the support to the pelvic floor and as such, are intimately involved in maintaining normal urinary and anorectal continence. In addition however, the lower sacral nerve roots also serves as the origin of the pudendal and pelvic splanchnic nerves.

In its course, the pudendal nerve gives off a branch called the *inferior rectal nerve* that supplies a muscular branch to the external anal sphincter and distributing sensory fibers to the lower portion of the rectum, the skin surrounding the anus, and the distal third of the vagina. The pu-

dendal nerve then divides into the dorsal nerve of the penis (or clitoris) and a larger branch called the *perineal nerve*. From its point of origin in the pelvic floor, the dorsal nerve runs anteriorly to supply sensory fibers to the distal half of the penile shaft and the clitoris. The perineal nerve then divides into the posterior scrotal or labial nerve, which distributes sensory fibers to the posterior two thirds of the scrotum or labia majora and a muscular branch that innervates the muscles in the anterior half of the pelvic floor that include the bulbospongiosus, ischiocavernosus, transverse perinei profundus, transverse perinei superficialis, urethral sphincter, and portions of the external anal sphincter and levator ani. In addition, the muscular branch to the bulbospongiosus gives off a twig, called the *nerve to the urethral bulb*, which supplies the corpus spongiosum and then extends to terminate in the mucous membrane of the urethra.[35]

The pelvic splanchnic nerves mediate parasympathetic control over the various pelvic organic structures by visceromotor fibers to the distal third of the colon, rectum, wall of the urinary bladder, ureters, renal pelvis, lower portion of the uterus, upper region of the cervix, and vagina. Inhibitory fibers supply the vesicle sphincter. Vasodilator fibers supply the testes, prostate, seminal vesicles, vas deferens, uterus, ovaries, fallopian tubes, greater vestibular glands, and erectile tissue of the penis and clitoris. Secretomotor fibers supply the seminal vesicles, vas deferens and ejaculatory ducts.[36,37] In addition, the pelvic splanchnic nerves also mediate a visceral afferent supply through fibers that have their origin in the muscular wall of the structure that they innervate. These nerves represent the afferent limb of the pelvic parasympathetic reflex arc and as such are extremely important in regulating normal pelvic organ function.[36] It is by the connections made through the pudendal, pelvic splanchnic, and unnamed nerves supplying the pelvic floor supportive musculature that mechanical insult to the lower sacral nerve roots can result in the wide range of disturbances of pelvic organ function commonly found in the mechanically induced PPOD syndrome.

Clinical Features of the PPOD Patient

Disturbances that have been attributed to mechanically induced impairment of lower sacral nerve root function include pelvic pain (inguinal, suprapubic, paraanal, coccygeal, rectal), urinary frequency, urgency, dribbling, incontinence, difficulty, sluggishness, retention, nocturia, enuresis, dysuria, infection, loss of ability to perceive vesicle filling, constipation, diarrhea, excessive flatus, painful anal sphincter spasm, encopresis (fecal incontinence), mucorrhea, uncontrollable spontaneous bowel discharge, loss of ability to perceive rectal filling, spontaneous miscarriage, painful and irregular menstruation, vaginal spotting (atrophic vaginitis), persistent vaginal discharge, menstrual migraine, genital pain and/or paresthesias (vulvodynia), decreased genital sensitivity, anorgasmy, dyspareunia, deficient precoital and coital lubrication, pelvic pain during orgasm (anorgasmalgia), loss of libido, and impotence.*

Although these patients typically revealed any number and combination of accompanying PPOD symptoms, certain disorders tended to be more frequently encountered. For example, within the pain syndrome category, the symptoms of inguinal, coccygeal, or rectal pain were most common. Urological impairment included the disorders of urinary frequency, urgency, dribbling or incontinence, sluggishness, retention, and impairment of ability to perceive vesicle filling as the most frequently experienced complaints. Enterologic dysfunction is most often reflected by symptoms of constipation, diarrhea, excessive flatus, and impairment of ability to perceive rectal filling. Gynecologic and sexual dysfunction usually manifested as symptoms of dyspareunia (superficial or deep), decreased genital sensitivity or anorgasmy, genital pain and/or paresthesias, loss of libido, painful and irregular menstruation, and vaginal discharge.[32]

Frequently, the patient's pain symptoms are of a bilateral nature, although not necessarily symmetrically bilateral. For example, in the absence of obvious bilateral lower extremity radicular pain or paresthesias, the PPOD patient may visit the chiropractor with low back and unilateral lower extremity pain and/or paresthesias. However, on detailed evaluation, the presence of contralateral inguinal pain or gluteal pain or paresthesias is revealed. One of the more consistent features regarding inguinal pain, as typically found in the mechanically

induced PPOD patient, is whether inguinal pain (either unilateral or bilateral) will have superior intensity on the side of the patient's dominant lower extremity pain and/or paresthesias.[32] Most PPOD patients revealed a clear correlation between the overall extent and severity of their presenting PPOD complaints and the degree of impairment of lower sacral neurologic function as detected on clinical examination.

The Clinical Diagnosis of the Mechanically Induced Pelvic Pain and Organic Dysfunction Syndrome

Establishing a diagnosis of mechanically induced PPOD is a three-step procedure for chiropractors. The first step is identifying the presence of symptoms that are characteristic or representative of mechanically induced impairment of lower sacral nerve root function. Although superficially this may appear to be a rather straightforward exercise, accomplishing it may not be that easy.[3] Because most PPOD patients consult with the chiropractor because of a low back and/or leg pain syndrome, their primary interest is in resolving issues relating to their complaints. As a result, many of these individuals tend to avert questioning into what they perceive as an unrelated intrusion into the areas of urologic, enterologic, gynecologic, and sexual function.[3,16] Furthermore, the all too common routine of casually assessing these patients for changes in pelvic organic function by inquiring if they have noted any changes in bladder or bowel function, does little more than reinforce the thoughts that no likely relationship exists between the origin of their current complaints and any accompanying disturbances of pelvic organic function.[3,32] This is especially true of patients whose presenting symptoms include long-standing PPOD involvement. These patients, having been told that their disturbances result from some local organic disorder despite being recalcitrant to all prior local therapeutic attempts, commonly believe that their ongoing difficulties represent a permanent condition caused by an internal disorder bearing no relationship to their current spinal complaints.[32] As a result, their denial of the presence of any change in bladder or bowel function in response to a nonchalant assessment of pelvic organ activity by the doctor, typically reflects a perception that no relative change in bladder, bowel, gynecologic, or

---

*3,12-16,33,34,38-46

sexual function has occurred. Accordingly, the only effective means of adequately assessing these patients for the presence of any of the over 36 individual symptoms characteristic of the mechanically induced PPOD syndrome is by questioning them for the presence of each symptom individually (Table 8-1).

After having profiled the symptomatic presentation of the suspected mechanically induced PPOD patient, the clinician then attempts to establish the presence of a lower sacral radiculopathy. As is the case in diagnosing a radiculopathy involving any other nerve root, the detection of sensory, motor, or reflex changes consistent with that of the nerve root in question is of primary importance. In terms of assessing lower sacral nerve root function, this includes the identification of sensory impairment within the boundaries of the lower sacral nerve root dermatomes, either anteriorly over the external genitalia or posteriorly over the gluteal musculature, establishing the presence of muscular paresis of the anal sphincter, and detecting abnormalities of anal reflex function.

However, because obvious impairment of lower sacral neurologic function, as revealed by standard neurologic assessment, is generally equivocal in all but the more severely involved PPOD patients, clinicians must give greater consideration to the less conventional but more frequently encountered and clinically reliable characteristics of lower sacral nerve root impairment.[32] In this regard, the recognition of myotomic or dermatomic pain patterns consistent with a lower sacral radiculalgia, establishment of the presence of palpatory hyper-

pathia over specific somatic regions corresponding to the S2 and S3 nerve roots, confirmation of nerve root involvement by pain provocation procedures, and induction of pelvic pain on straight leg raise become invaluable diagnostic signs.[3,32] Somatosensory evoked potential (SSEP) testing of the pudendal nerve has also been found to be helpful in identifying the presence of lower sacral nerve root impairment.[47] Frequently, mechanically induced PPOD patients demonstrating a normal clinical neurologic examination will reveal abnormalities on pudendal nerve SSEP testing.

Lower Sacral Radicular Pain

The pain associated with a lower sacral radicalgia is most often myotomic and usually described as aching pain in the muscles, sometimes with a sharp, cramping, or burning quality. When present, lower sacral dermatomic pain is usually described as a painful hypersensitivity involving the genital region, making touch or any type of contact exquisitely painful. In women, this pain often involves the labia, either unilaterally or bilaterally and may frequently extend to the clitoris or radiate intravaginally. In men, lower sacral dermatomic pain is usually found to involve the distal half of the penile shaft or glans. More frequently, however, men will complain of orchialgia described not in dermatomic terms but in myotomic terms as an intense aching, as if the testicle were under pressure from being squeezed.

The myotomic and dermatomic pain distribution associated with an S2 and S3 radiculalgia has

Table 8-1   *Symptoms of Mechanically Induced Pelvic Organic Dysfunction*

Bladder Dysfunction	Bowel Dysfunction	Gynecologic and Sexual Dysfunction
Frequency	Constipation	Miscarriage
Urgency	Diarrhea	Vaginal discharge
Dribbling	Excessive flatus	Vaginal spotting
Incontinence	Anal sphincter spasm	Painful and irregular menstruation
Difficulty	Encopresis	Menstrual migraine
Sluggishness	Mucorrhea	Decreased genital sensitivity
Retention	Loss of rectal sensory	Decrease or loss of orgasm
Nocturia	perception	Dyspareunia
Dysuria	Spontaneous bowel discharge	Genital pain and paresthesias
Infection		Pelvic pain on orgasm
Enuresis		Deficient precoital and coital lubrication
Loss of vesical sensory		Depressed libido
perception		Impotence

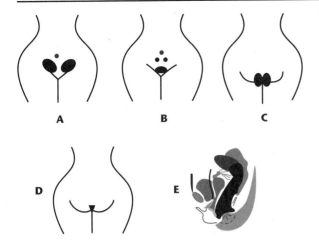

Figure 8-1 Mechanically induced pelvic pain. **A.** Inguinal. **B,** Suprapubic, **C,** Paraanal. **D,** Coccygeal. **E,** Rectal.

an anterior and posterior component. An S2 radiculalgia has the distinct ability of producing pain in the pelvis and leg. The anterior distribution of S2 myotomic pain includes the ipsilateral inguinal region, which in women is commonly perceived as involving the area of the ovary. In men, inguinal pain may be perceived as resulting from a developing inguinal hernia. The posterior distribution of S2 myotomic pain includes the inferior gluteal region, posteromedial thigh, medial popliteal fossa, and postermedial leg. The anterior distribution of S2 dermatomic pain includes the ipsilateral labia or scrotum, and the posterior distribution extends from the posteromedial gluteal region into the posteromedial thigh and postermedial leg. Pain associated with an S3 radiculalgia is entirely in the intrapelvic region. The anterior distribution of S3 myotomic pain includes the ipsilateral suprapubic region, and the posterior distribution includes the paraanal area. The anterior distribution of S3 dermatomic pain includes the most medial genital region, and the posterior distribution is felt superficially over the gluteal musculature within the boundaries of the S3 dermatome. Figure 8-1 demonstrates areas of pelvic pain commonly found in the mechanically induced PPOD patient.

Lower Sacral Palpatory Hyperpathia

The procedure of identifying the presence of palpatory hyperpathia over somatic regions corresponding to specific spinal nerve roots shares

some similarities with the nerve tracing techniques commonly employed as a diagnostic aid during the early years of the chiropractic profession.[1] Hyperpathia is a painful or exaggerated response to a stimulus. Palpatory hyperpathia is a painful response to palpation over somatic regions corresponding to a specific nerve root. In a patient who visits the doctor with a severely acute or chronically irritated lumbosacral radiculopathy, this effect is readily demonstrated as the presence of exquisite pain on mild palpation within the myotomic distribution of the affected nerve root. This same phenomenon also occurs, however, within the myotomic distribution of an S2 or S3 radiculopathy. Although these areas of somatic hyperpathia are fairly specific for individual nerve root syndromes, the presence of palpatory hyperpathia over regions corresponding to the S2 and/or S3 nerve roots is extremely helpful in establishing the presence of a lower sacral radiculopathy.

The assessment of somatic areas for the presence of palpatory hyperpathia is most accurate when done with the patient standing erect because loading the lumbar spine seems to enhance the presence of somatic hyperpathia associated with mild nerve root syndromes. Most PPOD patients do not reveal the presence of palpatory hyperpathia over all somatic regions corresponding to a specific nerve root. However, most severely involved long-standing PPOD patients do tend to reveal involvement of most, if not all, of the regions of palpatory hyperpathia corresponding to a specific nerve root. Although areas of somatic hyperpathia have not been mapped for all of the individual nerve root syndromes, they have been mapped for the lumbosacral nerve roots. Figure 8-2 shows the distribution of areas of somatic hyperpathia of the L4 through S3 nerve roots.[34]

Pain Provocation Examination

The pain provocation examination is a procedure used to help confirm and distinguish the presence of a neurogenically mediated somatic hyperpathia of spinal origin from that of a local disorder such as myalgia or tendonitis. With the patient standing erect with knees straight and feet spaced at shoulder width, the areas of somatic hyperpathia are reassessed using moderate sustained digital pressure or thrust palpation during alternating

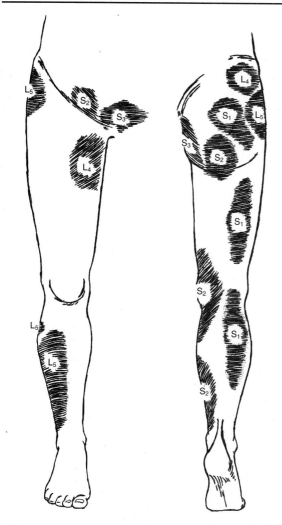

Figure 8-2 Areas of sciatic nerve root somatic hyperpathia after herlin.

right and left lateral bending movements of the lumbar spine. During this procedure, the patient is asked to report whether the pain provoked with palpation is increasing, decreasing, or remaining constant in its intensity. A positive response to the pain provocation examination occurs when the pain provoked with palpation is obviously altered in its intensity (either increasing or decreasing) during left and/or right lateral bending of the lumbar spine. This indicates a spinal origin of the corresponding somatic hyperpathia. A negative response to the pain provocation examination occurs when no apparent change occurs in the intensity of provoked pain during left or right lateral bending of the lumbar spine.

Induced Pelvic Pain on Straight Leg Raise

Induced pelvic pain on straight leg raise is probably the single most important and clinically reliable sign of lower sacral nerve root impairment of spinal origin. It manifests itself in two forms, a primary form (Browning's sign) and an enhanced form.[3] In its primary form, pelvic pain is induced during the performance of the standard straight leg raise. As lower extremity radicular pain may overshadow any accompanying pelvic pain during the performance of the straight leg raise, the patient is asked specifically to concentrate on identifying pain that develops anywhere within the anterior or posterior regions of the pelvis. The induction of pain usually occurs at a high angle of elevation, generally between 70 and 100 degrees. In severe cases, however, it can occur as low as between 15 and 30 degrees of elevation. Induced pelvic pain is usually described as being sharp, burning, or cramping in nature but at times may be expressed as an intense ache. The pattern of induced pelvic pain on straight leg raise is variable. Typically, however, any combination of inguinal, suprapubic, paraanal, coccygeal, rectal, or genital pain or paresthesias may occur. In its enhanced form, inguinal or suprapubic palpatory hyperpathia is obviously altered in its intensity during the performance of the straight leg raise. Most often, pelvic pain induced on straight leg raise (in either form) will be distinctly intensified. On occasion, however, it will be diminished.

The final consideration in diagnosing the presence of mechanically induced pelvic pain and organic dysfunction involves excluding the possibility of an intraabdominal cause of the patient's complaints. Although many internal disorders can result in the production of abdominal and/or pelvic pain and/or various disturbances of pelvic organic function, certain features and clinical findings can help differentiate mechanically induced from intraabdominal PPOD in most patients. (Table 8-2 contrasts the features of mechanically induced and intraabdominal PPOD.)

PPOD Patient Typing

Once the diagnosis of mechanically induced pelvic pain and organic dysfunction has been established, the patient is typed according to the ex-

Table 8-2 *Differential Diagnosis of Mechanically Induced Versus Intraabdominal PPOD*

	MIPPOD	IAPPOD
Onset or aggravation of PPOD associated with mechanical stress to lumbar spine	Often	Infrequent
PPOD associated with low back and/or leg pain and/or paresthesias	Usually	Occasionally
PPOD symptoms	Usually of wide variety and often involve multiple pelvic organs	Less numerous and more specific to organic pathology
Pelvic pain aggravated by stress provocation of the lumbar spine	Yes	No
Pelvic pain induced on straight leg raise	Yes	No
Sensory alteration in lower sacral nerve root dermatomes	Yes	No
Palpatory hyperpathia over somatic regions corresponding to the S2 and/or S3 nerve roots	Yes	Occasionally
Confirmation of nerve root involvement by pain provocation examination	Yes	No
Fever and/or abdominal rigidity and/or rebound pain	No	Maybe
Laboratory and urine findings	Negative or nonspecific	Dependent on pathology

MIPPOD = mechanically induced PPOD.
IAPPOD = intraabdominal and pelvic PPOD.

tensiveness and severity of PPOD complaints and impairment of lower sacral neurological function. In my experience, patient typing can be effectively used to determine the most appropriate treatment protocol and represents the most efficacious use of distractive decompressive manipulation in treating the mechanically induced PPOD patient.

Type I PPOD Patient Type I mechanically induced PPOD patients are those who seek care for symptoms that are predominantly representative of a pain syndrome. In most cases, these patients have low back and/or leg pain, pelvic pain, and either no changes in pelvic organic function or relatively mild disturbances of bladder, bowel, gynecologic, or sexual function. The most common accompanying disturbances of pelvic organic function include mild urinary frequency and urgency, relatively mild constipation or diarrhea, painful and/or irregular menstruation, or dyspareunia and/or anorgasmy. Other disturbances of pelvic organic function may occur but are less com-

monly encountered in the typical Type I PPOD patient.

On neurologic examination, the Type I PPOD patient usually demonstrates relatively mild and minimal impairment of lower sacral neurologic function. Clinically, these patients may reveal palpatory hyperpathia over specific somatic regions corresponding to the S2 and S3 nerve roots, usually over their anterior and more proximal distribution, a positive pain provocation examination, and pelvic pain induced with straight leg raise in either its primary or enhanced form.[3] Type I PPOD patients may also demonstrate relatively mild sensory impairment, especially to the modality of light touch, within the boundaries of the lower sacral nerve root dermatomes. These changes are most readily detected anteriorly over the ipsilateral labia or scrotum or posteriorly over the gluteal musculature.[32] Obvious impairment of lower sacral nerve root reflex or motor function is not a feature commonly found in the typical Type I PPOD patient.

Type II PPOD Patient Type II PPOD patients are those who seek clinical advice predominantly for symptoms of pelvic organic dysfunction. These patients generally complain of low back and/or leg pain and reveal more severe and widespread disturbances of pelvic pain and pelvic organic dysfunction. Although low back and/or lower extremity pain or paresthesias are usually accompanying symptoms in the mechanically induced PPOD patient, severe impairment of pelvic organic function has also been found in PPOD patients who have no history of low back pain.[15] When the clinician contrasts the symptoms of pain and pelvic organic dysfunction, the clinical profile of the Type II PPOD patient is dominated by symptoms of pelvic organic dysfunction. Clinically, Type II PPOD patients reveal greater neurologic involvement and on examination they generally demonstrate more extensive and significant impairment of lower sacral neurologic function. Typically, these patients may reveal the presence of more extensive palpatory hyperpathia, which may include the following:

- Posterior and more distal distribution of the specific somatic regions corresponding to the S2 and S3 nerve roots
- A more extensively involved and distinctly positive pain provocation examination
- The induction of pelvic pain on straight leg raise (in either form), usually occurring at multiple sites and perhaps a lower angle of elevation
- The typical Type II PPOD patient usually reveals more significant, extensive, and sometimes bilateral impairment of sensory function within the boundaries of the lower sacral nerve root dermatomes.

Although the presence of more significantly disturbed pelvic organic function represents a greater degree of neurologic impairment, mild-to-moderately involved Type II PPOD patients may not necessarily reveal obvious impairment of lower sacral reflex or motor function. This seemingly contradictory state may be explained by the presence of a lower sacral nerve root sensory deficit of a sufficient degree to impair the somatic sensory and sensory-dependent autonomic reflex activity mediated by the lower sacral nerve roots and underscores the importance of looking to the less conventional but more frequently encountered and clinically reliable signs of lower sacral nerve root involvement on clinical examination.[16] In addition to the findings outlined, severely involved, long-standing Type II PPOD patients tend to reveal obvious and sometimes severe impairment of lower sacral reflex or motor function.

The Application of Distractive Decompressive Manipulation

After having typed the PPOD patient, the appropriate treatment protocol may be determined. Technically, distractive manipulative intervention of the lumbar spine is administered in a similar manner for the Type I and Type II PPOD patient. The initial treatment frequency, however, is determined by patient typing and represents the most efficacious use of distractive decompressive manipulation in treating the mechanically induced PPOD patient.[32] Type I PPOD patients initially receive treatment at a frequency of three times per week. Type II PPOD patients, except when mechanically induced PPOD is found in the presence of an unstable spondylolisthesis or transitional vertebra, are initially treated daily. Each patient, after being placed in a prone position on the distraction table, is tested for tolerance to the procedure according to the guidelines of Cox.[48] For those patients for whom a prone position does not afford adequate curve reduction of the lumbar spine to allow for proper distraction, an abdominal roll is positioned beneath the midlumbar spine. Once the patient has demonstrated adequate tolerance to distraction during the testing procedure, distractive manipulation may begin.

From the outset of treatment, Type I PPOD patients may be treated with or without the application of the ankle cuffs. The decision of whether to use the ankle cuffs during the initial phase of treatment depends largely on the acuteness of the patient's back pain component of their overall disorder. Although Type I PPOD patients may demonstrate adequate tolerance to distraction testing (performed without the application of the angle cuffs), the initial effects of postdistractive inflammation may preclude the use of the cuffs during the initial phase of care. By contrast, ankle cuffs are never used on Type II PPOD patients during the initial phase of care. Because Type II patients by definition have more pronounced disturbances of pelvic organic function, when the clinician accurately monitors changes in pelvic organ function and therefore the patient's response, they should administer the procedure in a manner that minimizes the exacerbating effects of postdistractive inflammation.[32] Fortunately, because distractive manipulation is a low-velocity procedure, its immediate effects and the patient's tolerance to the procedure can be easily monitored during its application.

This may be accomplished by asking each patient, before distracting the lumbar spine, to report whether at any time during the application of the procedure they are experiencing increasing pain in the back, buttocks, front of the pelvis, or legs. This does not refer to the relatively mild static discomfort typically felt in these areas during distraction but rather to pain that is perceived to increase progressively in its intensity during the continued application of the procedure. If this effect is noted, distraction is terminated and any augmentive ancillary therapeutic procedures are then applied.[32]

The phenomenon of posttreatment inflammation is frequently observed in patients being treated with distractive manipulation when they appear with signs and symptoms of a typical lumbosacral radiculopathy, an initial increase in back and/or to leg pain and paresthesias that occurs after the first few treatments. This same type of response frequently occurs in the Type I and Type II PPOD patient,[32] however, in addition to experiencing an increase in the intensity of the back and/or leg pain component of the overall disorder, the Type I and Type II PPOD patient usually demonstrates an exacerbation of the initial PPOD symptoms and/or additional PPOD symptoms that are characteristic of lower sacral nerve root irritation or compression.[16] This initial posttreatment reaction in treating the Type I and Type II PPOD patient is typical, usual, and expected and does not herald the onset of an iatrogenically induced acute cauda equina syndrome but rather profiles the clinical course of an adequate or exceeding reaction, as described by Dvorak and others.[49] In most cases, however, this posttreatment reaction occurs only after the first few treatments or occasionally during the first few weeks of care.[16] Although this effect is common during the initial phase of treating the mechanically induced PPOD patient, it may also occur as a result of me-

chanically stressing the lumbar spine during initial PPOD patient examination. When the exacerbating effects of posttreatment inflammation stop, the ankle cuffs may then be used in the treatment of the Type II PPOD patient.

The technical procedure of applying distractive manipulation, although somewhat modified from the Cox protocol[48] in treating lumbar disc lesions, is the same for the Type I and Type II PPOD patient. The stabilization contact is made one to two segments above the level of the lesion to be treated. By keeping the stabilization contact further above the level of involvement, greater control exists in minimizing the degree of posttreatment inflammation. This is especially important in treating Type II PPOD patients because excessive irritation from the effects of posttreatment inflammation can result in more significant disturbances of pelvic organic function, making accurate assessment of the patient's response much more difficult. After positioning the contact hand, stabilization is achieved by applying a moderate downward and cephalad counterforce sufficient to traction the integument of the lumbar spine to the point of elastic noncompliance. While sustaining the stabilization counterforce, the flexion lock on the distraction table is released and a gradual downward distraction of the lumbar spine is produced by gently lowering the caudal segment of the instrument approximately 2 to 3 inches during an interval of 2 to 3 seconds.

During this procedure, additional counterforce is gently applied to balance the small degree of caudal migration that occurs during the act of distracting the lumbar spine. On reaching full flexion, joint decompression is maintained for 2 to 3 seconds by simultaneously sustaining caudal flexion of the lumbar spine and at the same time maintaining sufficient cephalad counterforce to anchor the spine and prevent caudal migration. The caudal segment of the instrument is then freed from flexion and allowed to return to its neutral position at the same time that the stabilization contact is released. This process is then repeated and performed for an overall approximate treatment time of 2 minutes or to the patient's tolerance as described above.

Postdistractive Procedures

After the clinician completes distraction of the lumbar spine, augmentive ancillary therapeutic procedures to assist in minimizing the effects of postdistractive inflammation and reactive muscular spasm may be used. Although a number of different therapeutic modalities may be employed, electrical muscle stimulation augmented with cryotherapy or thermotherapy applied in the following manner has been found to be effective in these cases. During the acute and subacute phases of treating a mechanically induced PPOD patient, pulsed muscle stimulation and cryotherapy are applied to the paraspinal musculature of the lumbar spine for approximately 15 to 20 minutes. Not uncommonly, however, PPOD patients reveal active trigger-point involvement in the quadratus lumborum musculature. In these patients, electrode placement is modified to include stimulation of this muscle. Stimulation intensity is decided at the point where the patient reports robust but comfortable contraction in conjunction with a rapid rate of stimulation.

At the point of care when postdistractive inflammation stops, as evidenced clinically by a lack of pain increase after treatment, the use of cryotherapy in the office after manipulation and at home by the patient is replaced with thermotherapy. In addition, the waveform on the muscle stimulator is modified to deliver a surge type of contraction. Stimulation rate is set at a moderate frequency, while the intensity is raised as high as the patient can comfortably accommodate. This modification assists in facilitating further reduction in reactive muscular spasm as well as minimizing the tendency toward spinal deconditioning precipitated by the need for strict recumbence.

After the initial application of treatment, each patient is fitted with a semirigid lumbosacral appliance of sufficient length to span the abdominal cavity from the lower costal margin to the level of the anterior superior iliac spine. Type I patients are asked to wear the support while they are awake, except while performing their exercises and during the home application of cryotherapy or thermotherapy. Type II PPOD patients are asked to initially wear their support 24 hours and follow similar exceptions regarding their exercises and applying cryotherapy or thermotherapy.

Exercise and Home Instructions

The exercises initially prescribed the mechanically induced PPOD patient are of prime importance in facilitating their response and allowing for accurate monitoring of their progress. In the current clinical environment, with its strong emphasis on early ambulation and the incorporation of muscle strengthening programs in the treatment of back pain patients, a seemingly growing trend exists toward using these guidelines in the treatment of all nonspecific back pain patients regardless of accompanying symptoms or cause. Although this routine may be of benefit in treating patients with simple mechanical back and/or leg pain, it should not be used in the early management of the mechanically induced PPOD patient. These patients typically appear with back and/or leg pain as their primary complaints, however, the overriding clinical concern depends on identifying and assessing the severity of any accompanying symptoms of pelvic organic dysfunction. Often times, after having triaged the patient's complaints, PPOD symptom management takes precedence over the initial complaints of back and leg pain. This initial exercise regime is essential and should be entirely inclusive of gentle, nonweight-bearing stretching maneuvers to avoid provoking excessive postexercise inflammation that could cause further reactive muscle spasm and aggravating existing or inducing additional PPOD complaints.

Accordingly, each patient is prescribed nonweight-bearing lumbar curve-reducing and muscle-stretching exercises, typically consisting of the knee-to-chest and pelvic-tilt maneuvers that initially are to be performed no more than three times per day. Once the patient demonstrates that these exercises can be tolerated without provoking any increase in PPOD symptoms, the exercise frequency may be increased. The emphasis of these exercises is on preventing progressive contraction of the paraspinal musculature, which if allowed to occur, may initiate trigger-point activation in the erector spinae or quadratus lumborum musculature. Weight-bearing spinal conditioning or strengthening exercises, especially those involving repetitive or sustained bending and/or twisting at the waist or vigorous nonweight-bearing conditioning exercises such as the prone hyperextension maneuvers, should not be prescribed until the patient has reached a point of PPOD stability within the parameters of restricted day-long, weight-bearing activity. Once the patient has demonstrated tolerance of extended weight-bearing activity, exclusive of prolonged sitting and repetitive or sustained bending, lifting, and twisting, spinal conditioning or strengthening exercises may then be initiated.

The transition to full weight-bearing activity and the addition of spinal stabilization exercises should be done gradually and carefully, with attention directed at assessing the patient's PPOD tolerance to increasing spinal stress. Patients who demonstrate an increase of their current PPOD symptoms should have their exercises modified or reduced in frequency and/or duration until the exacerbating effects of postexercise irritation no longer occur. Those reporting the recurrence of previously resolved PPOD symptoms or the development of newly acquired PPOD symptoms should have their spinal stabilization exercises eliminated. These individuals' exercise regimen needs to be reassessed and modified to avoid the return of any previous PPOD symptoms or the onset of additional ones. Some PPOD patients, typically the more severely involved and long-standing Type II patients or those with various congenital or acquired anomalies affecting the lumbar spine, may never reach a level of stability at which they can tolerate the inclusion of spinal stabilization exercises. These patients' exercise tolerance and requirements need to be assessed and prescribed individually, avoiding any exacerbation of PPOD-related complaints. These patients often require permanent restrictions and/or ongoing supportive treatment to sustain their improved clinical state.

The use of cryotherapy in the home care of the mechanically induced PPOD patient is for pain relief and control of posttreatment and postexercise inflammation. As is common in treating the mechanically induced PPOD patient, the initial effects of posttreatment inflammation reduce the patient's ability to tolerate weight-bearing and increase the potential for postexercise inflammation. Accordingly, to assist in minimizing these effects, patients are advised to apply cryotherapy to their low back for 20 to 30 minutes, while lying prone with a pillow positioned beneath their waist every 2 to 3 hours, and after each performance of their exercises. Furthermore, all PPOD patients are asked to remain completely nonweight-bearing until the diathesis of posttreatment inflammation has substantially diminished to a point at which their initial PPOD symptoms have significantly improved. Once this point is reached, the transition to normal weight-bearing activity is initiated by gradually ambulating individuals for short periods as they wear their lumbosacral support and avoid mechanically stressful positions and activities such as sitting, bending, lifting, and twisting. Assessment of the patient's tolerance to progressively increasing levels of restricted weight-bearing activity is accomplished by observing them for a reappearance or exacerbation of PPOD symptoms. Those patients who endure limited weight-bearing with-out provoking any increase in PPOD symptoms are gradually ambulated for longer periods and are carefully allowed to resume increasing levels of weight-bearing activity, while keeping within their tolerance level by avoiding a return or exacerbation of PPOD symptoms. In uncomplicated Type I PPOD patients, the necessity for strict recumbence usually ranges from a few days to 1 to 2 weeks and in uncomplicated Type II PPOD patients, recumbence is usually required for an average of 2 to 3 weeks.[32] Cases that are complicated by aggravating factors may require longer periods of recumbence and/or the use of formal restrictions to modify weight-bearing activity for varying periods. Table 8-3 summarizes the protocols of treating the Type I and Type II PPOD patient.

Aggravating Factors

As is the case in treating patients who suffer from typical spinal and spinal-related pain syndromes, mechanically induced PPOD patients frequently exhibit various acquired or congenital anomalies that may alter their response, thereby necessitating a modification in the standard treatment protocol. If problematic, these disorders may alter their response so that improvement may occur more slowly; the overall outcome may be less favorable; and they may suffer frequent exacerbations during the course of care and/or recurrences after maximum therapeutic benefit has been attained, necessitating ongoing supportive treatment at varying intervals to sustain their improved clinical state.[32] Table 8-4 highlights suggested treatment modifications for various anomalies that have been found to be helpful in managing the mechanically induced PPOD patient.

Assessing PPOD Patient Response

As mentioned earlier, most Type I and Type II PPOD patients undergoing distractive decompressive manipulation of the lumbar spine exhibit the

Table 8-3 *Treatment Protocols for Type I and Type II PPOD Patients*

	Type I PPOD	Type II PPOD
Initial treatment frequency	3 times a week	1 time a day with the exception of when found with unstable spondylolisthesis or transitional vertebra
Stabilization contact	1-2 segments above the level of lesion	Minimum of 1-2 segments above the level of lesion
Ankle cuffs	May be initially used	Not used until the diathesis of postdistractive inflammation has resolved
Treatment duration	2 minutes or to patients' tolerance	2 minutes or to patients' tolerance
Augmentive electrotherapy and cryotherapy	For postdistractive inflammation and reactive muscular spasm as indicated	For postdistractive inflammation and reactive muscular spasm as indicated
Lumbosacral appliance	Used during weight-bearing hours	Used 24 hours a day
Strict recumbency	Usually a few days; occasionally 1-2 weeks	Average of 2-3 weeks

Type I PPOD = Type I mechanically induced pelvic pain and organic dysfunction syndrome.
Type II PPOD = Type II mechanically induced pelvic pain and organic dysfunction syndrome.

effects of posttreatment inflammation, characterized by an increase in the severity of existing PPOD complaints and/or by the onset of additional PPOD-related symptoms. Although this posttreatment reaction during the initial phases of treatment may be considered the rule rather than the exception, cases exist in which little or no significant posttreatment effects occur. These patients are usually nonacute in their presentation and of the Type I or mild Type II variety. Their response tends to be more rapid overall and uncomplicated by any significant difficulty associated with transitioning from being recumbent to full, normal weight-bearing activity. In addition, these patients are usually able to accommodate the addition of spinal stabilization exercises without difficulty during reconditioning of their muscular system.

Typically, however, the response of a mechanically induced PPOD patient is gradual and at times may become quite erratic. In addition to experiencing the effects of posttreatment inflammation during the initial phases of care, these patients frequently report exacerbations of symptoms associated with the transition from recumbence to full weight-bearing activity. In the more

severely involved Type II PPOD patients or those with aggravating factors affecting the stability of the spine, exacerbations can be provoked by excessive weight-bearing activity in general but especially with activities involving sitting, bending, lifting, and twisting. Accordingly, ambulating the PPOD patient to full, normal weight-bearing needs to be done gradually and incrementally, allowing for complete tolerance to restricted weight-bearing activity in the absence of PPOD symptom provocation.

Potential Complications

Potential complications in managing the mechanically induced PPOD patient can be categorized into the following three areas:

1. Acute cauda equina syndrome
2. Impending acute cauda equina syndrome
3. Trapezius or posterior cervical myofascial pain syndrome

Because the mechanically induced PPOD syndrome represents varying degrees of cauda equina impairment, clinicians discriminating between cases of acute cauda equina impairment requiring

Table 8-4 *Treatment Modifications for Various Anomalies*

Anomaly	Treatment Modification
Spondylolisthesis in Type II PPOD patient	Follow Type I protocol; ankle cuffs are never used; stabilization contact is kept to a minimum of 2-3 segments above the level of lesion
Scoliosis	May require extended use of a semirigid appliance and/or ongoing restrictions
Sacral base unleveling (generally 5 mm or greater)	Requires incremental corrections at 2-3 week intervals after PPOD stability has been achieved
Degenerative disc disease	May require longer initial period of recumbency, continued use of the appliance, and ongoing restrictions
Transitional vertebra	Ankle cuffs are never used; stabilization contact is kept at a minimum of 2-3 segments above level of lesion; should follow Type I protocol

surgical referral and those that can be more effectively managed by manipulative procedures is necessary. Although cauda equina syndrome is generally defined as a combination of low back and bilateral lower extremity radicular pain, saddle anesthesia, and a motor weakness in the lower extremities that may progress to paraplegia[50-54] over a variable period, acute cauda equina syndrome is characterized by the sudden onset of severe back pain, sciatica, urinary retention (necessitating catheterization), motor weakness in the lower extremities, and saddle anesthesia or hypoesthesia.[55] Although recognized as a rare phenomenon in clinical practice,[3,55,56] the incidence of acute cauda equina ranges from 1 in 100,000 to 1 in 33,000 people of the general population,[57] to 1% to 16% of patients who undergo spinal surgery for disc herniation,[50,54,58,59] and in as many as 27% of patients with radiographically verified midline lumbar disc herniations.[60] Although both disorders represent impairment of cauda equina function, the distinguishing features of a Type II mechanically induced PPOD patient and one with an acute cauda equina syndrome depends on the degree of neurologic functional loss.

Table 8-5 contrasts the features of acute cauda equina syndrome as described by Mooney[57] with those of a Type I and Type II mechanically induced PPOD patient.[32] As shown, the features of an acute cauda equina syndrome include the rapid onset and/or progression of neurologic signs and symptoms, and a more pronounced degree of lower extremity muscular paresis, which may progress to paraplegia in the acute cauda equina syndrome patient. Although urinary retention and/or overflow incontinence and loss of rectal sphincter control indicate a more significant degree of neurologic impairment, these same features are commonly found in the severely involved, long-standing Type II PPOD patient and have demonstrated dramatic improvement under chiropractic manipulative treatment of a decompressive nature.[13-15] Although the acute cauda equina syndrome and Type II mechanically induced PPOD patient may seek chiropractic care with pronounced disturbances of pelvic organic function, the unstable nature of the patient with an acute cauda equina syndrome demands immediate surgical decompression.

Unlike the acute cauda equina syndrome, the impending acute cauda equina syndrome is commonly seen in clinical practice. Typically found in the long-standing Type II mechanically induced PPOD patient, the impending acute cauda equina syndrome is characterized by significant bladder and bowel dysfunction with a recent history of gradual but progressive functional deterioration. Although these patients generally respond well to the Type II PPOD treatment protocol, referral needs to be considered when sphincter control, if initially intact, becomes threatened.

The development of a trapezius or cervical myofascial pain syndrome represents a potential complication not because of any effect it may have on lower sacral nerve root function but rather because of the manner in which the clinician may choose to treat it. This disorder commonly occurs in patients who harbor latent trigger-points in the posterior cervical, scaleneous, or trapezius musculature. Because of the lack of

Table 8-5   *Differential Diagnosis of Acute Cauda Equina Syndrome Versus Types I and II PPOD Syndrome*

ACES	Type I PPOD	Type II PPOD
Rapid progression of neurologic signs and symptoms	Mild and minimal neurologic signs and symptoms	Gradually developing and progressing neurologic signs and symptoms over weeks, months, or years
Bilateral leg pain	May have unilateral or bilateral leg pain; occasionally has no lower extremity pain	May have unilateral or bilateral leg pain; occasionally has no lower extremity pain
Saddle anesthesia	May reveal mild and minimal unilateral lower sacral nerve root sensory impairment	More significant (and occasionally bilateral) lower sacral nerve root sensory impairment
Lower extremity muscle weakness that may progress to paraplegia	Occasional mild unilateral lower extremity paresis, usually confined to single myotome	May have mild unilateral (occasionally bilateral) lower extremity paresis, not tending to progress
Presence of genitourinary dysfunction with either retention or overflow incontinence	Either no changes in pelvic organ function or only mild disturbances of bladder and/or bowel function	More severe and widespread symptoms of pelvic organ dysfunction that may include retention or overflow incontinence in severe or long-standing cases
Loss of rectal sphincter control	No impairment of rectal or urinary sphincter function	May have loss of rectal and/or urinary sphincter function/control in severe or long-standing cases

ACES = acute cauda equina syndrome.
Type I PPOD = Type I mechanically induced pelvic pain and organic dysfunction syndrome.
Type II PPOD = Type II mechanically induced pelvic pain and organic dysfunction syndrome.

normal muscular mobility induced by the need for strict recumbence during the initial treatment of a mechanically induced PPOD patient, progressive tightening of the trapezius and cervical musculature can lead to activation of trigger-points within these muscular structures. Clinically, this is recognized by the development of pain and/or stiffness in the posterior cervical, suprascapular, or medial scapular regions that may or may not be accompanied by myogenic referred pain and/or paresthesias extending into the head or upper extremities. Although a number of procedures may be effectively used to resolve the symptoms associated with this type of disorder, the seated spray and stretch vapocoolent procedures advocated by Travell and Simons[61] should be avoided. Although these procedures may be helpful at releasing contracted muscles, thereby deactivating trigger-points in the trapezius or cervical musculature, the application of downward pressure while passively flexing the neck can easily strain the lumbar spine and aggravate PPOD symptoms. Accordingly, alternative approaches incorporating spinal manip-

ulation, ischemic compression, passive muscle stretching techniques, and various therapeutic procedures applied in a nonweight-bearing position have been found to be quite helpful in controlling this disorder.

▬▬▬▬▬CASE STUDIES▬▬▬▬▬

Although the following case reports will serve to illustrate many of the characteristic features commonly found in the mechanically induced PPOD patient, the signs and symptoms of accompanying lower lumbar and upper sacral nerve root impairment (contributing to the presence of lower extremity symptoms) have been minimized for purposes of clarity. The patient in case 6 reported no history of back pain and the case has been previously published.[15]

Case 1

A 15-year-old girl was seen for the complaint of low back pain that had its onset approximately 1 year earlier, unrelated to any specific traumatic event. Although her low back pain had not been constant, it had become more frequent and severe over the previous year. During this same period, she began to experience intermittent bilateral posterior thigh pain extending to the knees and bilateral inguinal pain. She noted that about 6 months earlier, she had the onset of persistent constipation, which fluctuated in its severity. In addition, menstruation, which had been regular since menarche at age 11, became painful and irregular. Approximately 4 months before being seen, menstruation abruptly stopped altogether. Although she had been evaluated by her family physician and a gynecologist, no abnormalities could be found. Clinical signs of lower sacral nerve root impairment on examination included pain distribution consistent with a lower sacral radiculopathy, the presence of palpatory hyperpathia over somatic regions corresponding to the S2 and S3 nerve roots, the induction of pelvic pain on straight leg raise in its primary and enhanced forms, a positive response to the pain provocation examination, sensory impairment within the boundaries of the right S2 and S3 nerve root dermatomes, detected posteriorly over the gluteal musculature, and diminished anal reflex activity. The lower extremity myotatic reflexes, muscular strength, and sphincter tone were all normal. Clinical diagnosis was a discogenic lumbar spine disorder with secondary bilateral lower sacral nerve root impairment and tertiary bilateral inguinodynia, constipation, and secondary amenorrhea. After her examination and before the initiation of treatment, she experienced the onset of urinary frequency and urgency in the absence of difficulty and pain. These symptoms were judged to be the result of postexamination inflammation further impairing lower sacral nerve root function.

Treatment after the Type I mechanically induced PPOD protocol resulted in a gradual resolution of her complaints. After the first few treatments, additional PPOD symptoms consisting of coccygeal pain, genital pain, and paresthesias began. After 1 week of treatment, bowel function improved so that evacuation was occurring once every 1 to 2 days. After 2 weeks of treatment, bowel function was approaching normal and menstruation, which was completely normal, had returned. After 4 weeks of care, all lower extremity and PPOD symptoms had resolved. Low back pain

persisted and was aggravated by weight-bearing activity in excess of about 1 hour. She experienced an exacerbation of her condition 5 weeks into treatment, because of excessive sitting while at school. Despite experiencing a return of her anterior pelvic pain and urologic disturbances, her menstruation occurred normally.

Further treatment after the Type I PPOD patient protocol gradually resolved all her complaints so that she was discharged from care fully improved 2½ months later. A follow-up communication with the patient's mother approximately 6 months later revealed that the patient continued to do well and had not experienced a return of any of her symptoms.

Case 2
A 54-year-old man was referred to the author for treatment of low back and left leg pain of many years standing. He reported that he had initially hurt his low back at age 16 while shoveling snow. Rest and activity limitation gradually resolved his complaints. While in his 30s, he reinjured his low back and experienced the onset of left hip and leg pain. Chiropractic treatment at that time was initially helpful, but gradually his symptoms became progressively worse. When medication and exercise failed to improve his condition, he was referred for neurosurgical evaluation.

After extensive diagnostic testing, a laminectomy was performed at the L3-4 level. Because this surgery failed to relieve him of his symptoms, he underwent additional testing and treatment without relief. Finally, because of a lack of response, his symptoms were judged to be functional, and he was referred to me for supportive treatment.

Careful historic evaluation, however, revealed that about 18 years earlier, during a time of increasing low back and left leg pain, he had developed sharp left inguinal pain. This pain had been diagnosed as resulting from a developing inguinal hernia, and as a result he underwent a left hernioplasty. Because this procedure had failed to relieve him of his pain, a second operation was performed, in which a supportive mesh was implanted. However, in addition to continuing left inguinal pain, he awoke from his second hernioplasty with persistent left testicular pain. This pain had been attributed to an atrophic left testicle. After further diagnostic testing and because of continued pain, the left testicle was removed. Unfortunately, despite removal of the testicle, phantom left testicular pain remained. These symptoms were judged to be due to poor prosthetic placement, and additional surgery had been planned.

During the same period, the patient recalled having experienced the onset of deep suprapubic pain that at times would be aggravated during micturition and a progressive loss of genital sensitivity and erectile strength so that he could achieve orgasm only after extended periods of coitus. In addition, when ejaculation occurred, it was accompanied by intense phantom left testicular pain. He had lost all sexual desire and noticed that bowel function had slowed to one evacuation every 3 to 4 days. Clinical signs of lower sacral nerve root impairment on examination included pain distribution consistent with that of a lower sacral radiculalgia, palpatory hyperpathia over somatic regions corresponding to the S2 and S3 nerve roots bilaterally, a positive pain provocation examination, and pelvic pain induced on straight leg raise in its primary form. No sensory, motor, or reflex alterations were associated with lower sacral nerve root impairment. Clinical diagnosis was a lumbosacral disc lesion with secondary bilateral S2 and S3 nerve root impairment and tertiary left inguinodynia, left orchialgia, depressed libido, impotence, cystalgia, and constipation.

Treatment following the Type I PPOD protocol resulted in a gradual resolution of his complaints. Frequently, during the application of distractive manipulation, the patient reported experiencing left inguinal, deep suprapubic, penile, and left phantom testicular pain. After the first few treatments, the patient noted the onset of urinary frequency, urgency, and postmicturition dribbling that persisted for approximately 1 week. After 2 weeks of treatment, he was aware of improved libido. In addition, bowel function had improved so that evacuation was occurring at least one time per day without difficulty. After 4 weeks of care, cystalgic and suprapubic pain had resolved and inguinal and phantom left testicular pain had all but disappeared, occurring only mildly and intermittently after prolonged sitting. Because this individual had been divorced and not sexually active during his treatment, he was unable to provide detailed information about sexual performance. Unfortunately, about 5 weeks into treatment, he reaggravated his low back condition causing a simultaneous return of all of his original PPOD

complaints. Because of profound frustration, the patient declined further treatment.

Case 3

A 48-year-old woman was seen for the complaints of long-standing low back and bilateral lower extremity pain. Low back pain had its onset at age 12 as a result of a fall on her buttocks while ice skating. Although low back pain diminished in intensity, it never completely resolved. Over time, bilateral inguinal, coccygeal, and rectal pain had developed. These pains would be distinctly aggravated during periods of increasing low back pain. Ever since menarche at age 12, menstruation had been painful, heavy, and irregular, ranging in duration from about 4 days to 2 weeks and occurring every 3 to 6 months. From the beginning, coitus had been painful and orgasm had never been possible. She became pregnant three times and delivered three normal children.

At age 25 because of worsening menstrual dysfunction, a right oophorectomy was performed. Despite this operation, pelvic pain and menstrual dysfunction continued. Gradually, bilateral lower extremity pain and paresthesias dominant on the left side developed. In addition, bladder dysfunction consisting of urinary frequency, urgency, sluggish micturition with difficulty emptying the bladder, and stress incontinence began. During the same period, chronic diarrhea and mucorrhea with intermittent periods of constipation had developed. She had given up many foods that she found to aggravate bowel function. As her condition worsened, she noticed a gradual loss of all sexual desire.

About 1 year before being seen by the author, she entered her climacteric. Menstruation ceased to occur and she developed persistent vaginal spotting because of what was diagnosed as atrophic vaginitis. Although she had undergone numerous previous evaluations for the various disturbances that had developed, no specific abnormalities could be identified. On examination, clinical signs of lower sacral nerve root impairment included pain distribution consistent with a lower sacral radiculalgia, which additionally could be provoked by orthopedic stress maneuvers, palpatory hyperpathia over somatic regions corresponding to the S2 and S3 nerve roots bilaterally, sensory impairment within the boundaries of the right S2 nerve root dermatome, detected over the gluteal musculature; a diminished left ankle jerk; and the induction of pelvic pain on straight leg raise in its primary form. Clinical diagnosis was a lumbosacral disc lesion with bilateral S2 and S3 nerve root impairment and tertiary PPOD as described earlier.

Treatment following the Type II PPOD protocol resulted in a progressive improvement of all her complaints. After her first treatment, low back, lower extremity, and pelvic pain were increased and bladder function worsened. In addition, after 1 week of care, vaginal discharge had developed. After 2 weeks of care, low back, lower extremity and pelvic pain had diminished and bladder and bowel function had improved. She had noted an improvement in genital sensitivity and dyspareunia had begun to diminish. Approximately 5 weeks into treatment, she experienced her first orgasm. Vaginal spotting resolved and she became aware of improved precoital and coital lubrication, the deficiency of which had not been apparent to her before. In addition, perineal muscle tone was noted by her and her husband to have increased. Around 2½ months after initiating treatment, her condition stabilized and she was discharged from active therapeutic care. Follow-up examination 2 months later revealed that all PPOD symptoms had remained resolved and vaginal discharge had disappeared.

Case 4

A 57-year-old woman was seen in response to a call for study participants to assess the effectiveness of chiropractic intervention in treating bladder, bowel, and sexual dysfunction. She presented wearing diapers for long-standing urinary and anorectal incontinence. She reported that although she was unable to recall the specific sequence of their onset, bilateral inguinal, suprapubic, coccygeal, and paraanal pain all had their onset during childhood. Although these symptoms continued to persist, she had not been evaluated for their presence at that time. She married at age 18 and during the next 4 years had become pregnant on 4 separate occasions. Each pregnancy had been accompanied by vaginal bleeding and all were terminated by a spontaneous miscarriage between the third and fifth months of gestation.

During this time, recurring, persistent bladder infections had begun to occur. At about age 23, she became pregnant for the fifth time. During

this pregnancy, vaginal bleeding recurred. Recumbence and activity limitation allowed her to carry this pregnancy to term, at which point a normal baby girl was born. Her next two pregnancies, although complicated by a breech presentation and toxemia respectively, resulted in the Caesarean delivery of baby boys. Her eighth and final pregnancy was complicated by bleeding abnormalities and ended in a spontaneous miscarriage at 3 months of gestation. Although she had been evaluated on numerous occasions during her many pregnancies, no specific cause could be identified for her recurring miscarriages.

About 1 year later, because of chronic pelvic pain and continued vaginal bleeding, a hysterectomy was performed. Although her bleeding abnormalities were resolved, pelvic pain persisted.

Approximately 11 years later, which was about 15 years before being seen by the author, she had injured her low back while working in a nursing home. Treatment consisting of ultrasound and physical therapy gradually resolved her complaints over a 6-month period. During this episode of low back pain, pelvic pain had increased in its intensity and urologic disturbances consisting of frequency, urgency, and stress incontinence began to occur. Over the next several years, low back pain had periodically recurred and gradually was accompanied by the development of bilateral lower extremity pain and paresthesias. Urinary incontinence had worsened and about 6 years before being seen by the author, a urologic consultation culminated in the performance of a bladder suspensory surgery. Rather than improving her clinical state, however, urologic dysfunction became more severe, developing into total urinary retention with secondary overflow incontinence. She was unable to voluntarily empty the bladder and could not initiate urethral contraction to prevent overflow incontinence. She stated that a loss of bladder and rectal sensory perception had occurred. She was trained in self-catheterization techniques that were performed three to four times per day for approximately 5 years. However, because of ongoing frustration and the inconvenience associated with having to continually catheterize herself and having to deal with recurring bladder infections associated with these procedures, she discontinued catheterizing herself altogether. As a result, bladder dysfunction resulted in total urinary retention and secondary overflow incontinence with continuous urinary leaking. She stated that she could not feel urine as it flowed over her perineum.

Bowel dysfunction had become more severe and resulted in ongoing anorectal incontinence, excessive flatus, sharp, severe rectal pain, and intermittent episodes of uncontrollable spontaneous bowel discharge occurring without any sensory awareness. These episodes would typically occur from two to six times per day. Because of the severe and continuous nature of her bladder and bowel dysfunction, she required ongoing use of diapers. Approximately 1 year later, vaginal spotting, associated with what had been diagnosed as atrophic vaginitis, developed. She was given intravaginal estrogen creams for treatment, however, their administration proved to be of little help. As a result, after several months of use, she discontinued the estrogen creams altogether.

At about this same time, a pelvic examination revealed the presence of a cystocele and rectocele. Although her bladder and bowel dysfunction had preceded the identification of these abnormalities, the cystocele and rectocele were judged to be the probable cause of her ongoing bladder and bowel complaints. Despite these findings, no specific treatment had been performed or recommended. On examination at this office, the clinical findings indicating the presence of lower sacral nerve root impairment included pain distribution consistent with a lower sacral radiculopathy, lower sacral radicular pain provoked by various orthopedic stress maneuvers, a positive pain provocation examination, palpatory hyperpathia over somatic regions corresponding to the S2 and S3 nerve roots, sensory impairment within the boundaries of the lower sacral nerve root dermatomes, and induced pelvic pain on straight leg raise occurring in its primary form.

Clinical diagnosis was a lumbosacral disc lesion with secondary impairment of lower sacral nerve root function and tertiary PPOD as described earlier. Treatment following the Type II PPOD protocol resulted in progressive improvement of her complaints. After 2 weeks of treatment, low back, inguinal, paraanal, coccygeal, and rectal pain were diminished and anorectal incontinence had lessened. At approximately 3 weeks of care, she began to experience a return of bladder-filling sensory perception along with the ability to voluntarily

initiate micturition. Although she could not yet completely empty her bladder, she could stop urine in midstream by contracting her urethral sphincter and pelvic floor musculature. Spontaneous bowel discharges had lessened in frequency and were accompanied by brief periods of sensory awareness of rectal urgency before their occurrence. After approximately 6 weeks of treatment, low back, lower extremity, and all areas of pelvic, coccygeal, and rectal pain had all but resolved. Bladder and rectal sensory awareness had returned to normal. She had regained the ability to voluntarily empty the bladder and normally restrain her previously uncontrollable bowel emissions. As a result, she was able to replace diaper dependency, which required changing from three to as many as six times per day, with ordinary pantyliners needing changing only twice daily. Vaginal spotting had resolved and genital and perineal sensitivity returned to normal. Although her improvement was remarkable, she does require ongoing treatment and activity limitations to sustain her improved clinical state.

Case 5

A 41-year-old woman was seen for low back and left leg pain of many years duration. She reported that her back pain had started as a child and had been accompanied by lower abdominal pain. Medical evaluation at that time attributed her low back and abdominal pain to constipation. Despite the prescription of exercises and dietary modifications, these pains persisted and would frequently be accompanied by left leg pain radiating to the foot. Menstruation, which had its onset at about age 16, had initially been pain-free. However, shortly after a period during which her low back pain increased, menstruation became painful and irregular, with the greatest intensity being in the inguinal region bilaterally.

She had been pregnant four times, and each pregnancy was accompanied by severe back pain. The first three pregnancies were uneventful, resulting in the normal deliveries of healthy children. The last pregnancy, however, resulted in the delivery by Caesarean section of a baby boy 2 months prematurely. Shortly thereafter, she experienced the onset of left leg pain. Spinal manipulation at that time resulted in a gradual resolution of her back and leg pain. Several years later, about 7 years before being seen by me, low back and left leg pain returned. As a result, she again underwent spinal manipulation. This attempt did not improve her condition. Gradually, her condition worsened. As a result, a few weeks before being seen by me, she obtained an orthopedic evaluation and was prescribed exercise for her condition. Because these measures failed to provide relief, she consulted me.

Detailed, historic review at that time revealed that about 20 years previously, during a time of increasingly painful low back pain, she experienced the onset of urologic disturbances consisting of urinary frequency, urgency, dribbling, and incontinence. Over time, urologic function continued to deteriorate, with the development of sluggish micturition that required forceful straining to initiate and maintain bladder emptying. In addition, sharp pain would frequently accompany micturition. During the same period, she also noted a change in the awareness of having to urinate, from the normal urge to void to a suprapubic fullness or pressure sensation that was accompanied by pelvic distention.

About 2 years before being seen by the author, bladder function had deteriorated so that micturition could only be initiated, maintained, and completed by self-administered deep bladder massage. During this time of progressive urologic dysfunction, gynecologic, sexual, and enterologic disorders also began. Pelvic pain had become more frequent and severe and would radiate to the inguinal regions, with its greatest intensity on the right. Additionally, sharp pain would frequently radiate to the coccyx, rectum, vagina, suprapubic, and outer genital areas, with its maximum intensity being felt in the clitoris. Intercourse had become intensely painful, with pelvic pain being consistently experienced in the right inguinal and suprapubic regions. Genital sensitivity had decreased so that orgasm occurred less frequently and was of a diminished intensity. Gradually, the ability to achieve orgasm completely disappeared and was accompanied by a total loss of sexual desire. The genital region had become exquisitely hypersensitive so that touch or contact of any kind was intensely painful. She had developed a strong aversion to any sexual advance by her husband and as a result had not engaged in coitus for many months.

Bowel function, which had been poor for many years, slowed to a single evacuation once every 4 to 5 days and would not occur without the use of a laxative or a suppository and forceful straining to achieve emptying. She had undergone several evaluations, however, on no occasion could any specific abnormality be identified. On examination, clinical signs of lower sacral nerve root impairment included pain distribution consistent with a lower sacral radiculalgia, which was distinctly aggravated by orthopedic stress provocation, palpatory hyperpathia over somatic regions corresponding to the S2 and S3 nerve roots, a positive pain provocation examination, sensory impairment within the boundaries of the lower sacral nerve root dermatomes; and induced pelvic pain on straight leg raise in its primary form.

Clinical diagnosis was a lumbosacral disc lesion with secondary impairment of lower sacral nerve root function and tertiary bladder, bowel, gynecologic, and sexual function as outlined earlier. Treatment following the Type II PPOD protocol resulted in progressive improvement of her back, leg, and PPOD complaints. After 2 weeks of care, she was aware of improved bladder and bowel function. Evacuation was occurring one to two times per day without the use of a laxative or need to strain. Urinary frequency, urgency, dribbling, incontinence, and pain had disappeared. She was initiating and maintaining micturition normally, without having to apply external pelvic compression. Bladder control improved so that coughing and sneezing did not result in incontinence. The awareness of having to urinate by suprapubic pressure and distention was replaced by the normal desire to void. Pelvic pain had progressively diminished and genital sensitivity returned to normal. Intercourse became pain-free and the ability to achieve normal orgasm returned. Menstruation, which occurred during the course of treatment, was without the sharp intense pelvic pain experienced previously.

Case 6

A 39-year-old woman was referred to the author for the chief complaint of chronic pelvic pain and dyspareunia. She explained that left inguinal pain began at about age 18, occurring shortly after a fall down a flight of stairs. A few months later, right inguinal pain commenced. As a result, she was hospitalized and an appendectomy had been performed. Tissue evaluation revealed a normal appendix, and right inguinal pain persisted. Menarche at age 15 had been pain-free, however, around the time of her appendectomy, menstruation became severely painful with pelvic pain occurring primarily in the inguinal region bilaterally and dominant on the left. In addition, chronic diarrhea began. As a consequence, she was rehospitalized for evaluation and treatment.

Her symptoms were attributed to an irritable bowel secondary to stress and she was released from the hospital with no change in her bowel dysfunction. About 2 to 3 years later, persistent vaginal discharge and recurrent bladder and vaginal infections began. Treatment for what were identified as local yeast and bladder infections provided only temporary relief. Also during this time, she began to experience genital pain radiating bilaterally into the labia and clitoris. The genital region became painfully sensitive to any touch or contact. Menstruation, which had been intensely painful, became even more so and was accompanied by irregularity and excessive bleeding. She was prescribed estrogen for regulation of her menstrual dysfunction but no significant improvement occurred.

At age 26, she married and became pregnant with her first child. Since the beginning, coitus had been painful and as a result of diminished genital sensitivity, orgasm had never been possible. During this pregnancy, she began to experience the onset of low back pain and intermittent bilateral posterior thigh pain and paresthesias. Her pregnancy ended in prolonged labor with the delivery of a normal, healthy boy. About 2 years later, she became pregnant for the second time. At about 3 months of gestation, vaginal bleeding began. At about 5½ months of gestation, this pregnancy was terminated by a spontaneous miscarriage. A few months later, she became pregnant for the third time. This pregnancy was accompanied by vaginal bleeding as before and ended 2 months prematurely with the birth of a girl. After this delivery, because of continuous pelvic pain and diarrhea, which had been present since age 18, and vaginal bleeding, which persisted following her third pregnancy, a laparotomy had been performed. This surgery, however, failed to reveal any abnormalities. As a result of continuing symp-

toms, a partial hysterectomy was performed several months later.

When she awoke from this surgery, total urinary retention accompanied by a complete loss of vesicle sensory perception had developed. Her inability to initiate micturition required training in self-catheterization techniques, which she had to perform every 3 hours to achieve bladder emptying. At about this same period, bowel dysfunction, which had been continuous since its onset, worsened and consisted of chronic diarrhea with pain, excessive flatus, bleeding, and mucous discharge. These symptoms were attributed to proctalgia fugax and rectal fissures. In addition, nocturnal encopresis also began occurring numerous times per week. Around 8 weeks later, left-sided inguinal pain increased in severity. As a result, surgery was performed and the left ovary was removed.

Histologic examination revealed the presence of numerous cysts. Inspection of the right ovary at that time showed no evidence of abnormality. After her oophorectomy, inguinal pain persisted on the left side. During the next year, right-sided inguinal pain increased in its intensity. A right oophorectomy was performed and ovarian cysts similar to those that had been identified in the left ovary were found. After removal of the right ovary, right inguinal pain continued. Despite the continuation of total urinary retention, stress urinary incontinence developed 4 years later. This was accompanied by the onset of recurrent bladder infections. As a result, an initial bladder suspensory surgery was performed. This improved her incontinence and infections for about 1 year. Approximately 1 year later, urinary incontinence and recurring bladder infections returned. A second suspensory surgery was performed that again provided relief of her incontinence and infections. These procedures, however, provided no improvement in her loss of vesicle sensory perception or urinary retentive state. Approximately 6 months later, she fell twice in the same week, and within 24 hours she experienced the return of urinary incontinence. A third suspensory surgery, with the addition of a supportive mesh, was performed. However, because she was unable to accept the implant, the mesh was removed and incontinence continued to persist. A second attempt at implanting the supportive mesh was made and

Table 8-6 *PPOD Symptoms at Presentation*

	D	I	N
Pelvic Pain			
Inguinal left/right	25	2	4
Suprapubic	25	2	4-6
Coccygeal	8	2	4-6
Rectal	22	2	4-6
Genital	8	2	4
Dyspareunia	13	4	6-8
Pelvic Organic Dysfunction			
Recurrent bladder infections	22	None	
Urinary retention	10	2	4
Vesicle sensory loss	10	1	4
Enuresis	2	2	4
Inability to contract urethral sphincter	10	2	4
Diarrhea	22	2	4
Excessive flatus	22	2-4	6-8
Decreased rectal sensory perception	22	1	4
Rectal bleeding	8	2	8-10
Rectal mucus discharge	22	2	8-10
Nocturnal encopresis	8	2	4
Decreased genital sensory perception	Always	4	8-10
Anorgasmy	13	4	30
Pain on orgasm	13	8	19
Loss of libido	10	5	8-10
Deficient precoital lubrication	10	8	12

D = duration in years.
I = initial improvement was noted in weeks.
N = normalization in weeks.

after this surgery, urinary incontinence was relieved. At no time, during the previous 10 years, since the onset of her urologic disorders, did any of her bladder surgeries provide any improvement in her absent vesicle sensory perception or inability to volitionally micturate. In addition, with the exception of during her pregnancies, she had never experienced any pain symptoms attributable to her low back.

On examination, the clinical signs indicating impairment of lower sacral nerve root function included pain distribution consistent with that of a lower sacral radiculalgia, which was distinctly provoked by orthopedic stress maneuvers, a slightly diminished right ankle jerk, sensory impairment within the boundaries of the right S2 and S3 dermatomes, detected posteriorly over the gluteal musculature, palpatory hyperpathia

over somatic regions corresponding to the left and right S2 and S3 nerve roots, a positive pain provocation examination; and the induction of pelvic pain on straight leg raise in its primary form. Clinical diagnosis was that of a well-defined asymptomatic central lumbosacral disc protrusion with secondary bilateral S2 and S3 nerve root impairment and tertiary PPOD as described earlier. Treatment following the Type II PPOD patient protocol provided progressive improvement in the patient's symptoms (Table 8-6). Interestingly, at no time during her many previous examinations and exhaustive diagnostic work-ups did any of her previous doctors relate the presence of any of her symptoms to impairment of lower sacral nerve root function or consider a mechanical disorder of the lumbar spine as a possible cause of her complaints.

STUDY GUIDE

1. What is a single-subject, time-series design?
2. What are the major differences between the studies of LeBoef and others and Reed and others?
3. Name five possible symptoms that may indicate PPOD syndrome. In this syndrome, where is the major subluxation usually found?
4. Describe Hawk's pelvic pain study.
5. Discuss the dysmenorrhea studies. How do they differ and why is this important?
6. Many patients only report pain to the DC when they may be suffering from multiple problems. How does Browning recommend clinicians elicit all pertinent information from patients when obtaining a history?
7. Name two nerves originating from the lower sacral nerve roots.
8. Where is the pain associated with an S3 radicalgia usually felt?
9. What is palpatory hyperpathia and why would it be important in a chiropractic examination?
10. What is the difference between a Type I and Type II PPOD patient? Why is this important? Discuss how clinicians should explain these types to patients to ensure they fully comprehend the situation.
11. Why is the pain provocation examination important in chiropractic analysis?
12. Discuss the difference between acute cauda equina syndrome and impending acute cauda equina syndrome. Why is differentiating between the two important? Where is the cauda equina found in terms of spinal levels?
13. Is it possible for patients to have the VSC that affects the lower sacral nerve roots and not see the doctor with low back pain? Why and how?
14. Many patients in the case studies already underwent multiple painful tests and surgeries before seeking chiropractic care. Because clinicians obtaining a thorough history is important, what possible connection did most or all of the previous doctors fail to discern? How is this possible?

REFERENCES

1. Palmer DD: *The science, art and philosophy of chiropractic,* Portland, 1910, Portland Printing House.
2. Leach RA: *The chiropractic theories: a synopsis of scientific research,* ed 2, Baltimore, 1986, Williams & Wilkins.
3. Browning JE: The recognition of mechanically induced pelvic pain and organic dysfunction in the low back pain patient, *J Manipulative Physiol Ther* 12:369-373, 1989.
4. Blomerth PR: Functional nocturnal enuresis, *J Manipulative Physiol Ther* 17:335-338, 1994.
5. Lines DH: Chiropractic in the 21st century: the past, the present and the future, *J Aust Chiro Assoc* 19:49-54, 1989.
6. Gemmell HA, Jacobson BH: Chiropractic management of enuresis. Time-series descriptive design, *J Manipulative Physiol Ther* 12:386-389, 1989.
7. Leboeuf C et al: Chiropractic care of children with nocturnal enuresis: a prospective outcome study, *J Manipulative Physiol Ther* 14:110-115, 1991.
8. Stavish GE: Nocturnal enuresis, *Dig Chiro Economics* 76-81, 1985.
9. Parra A, Bonci MA: Etiology, treatment and management of enuresis: a review, *ACA J Chiro* 25-28, 1989.
10. Reed WR et al: Chiropractic management of primary nocturnal enuresis, *J Manipulative Physiol Ther* 17:596-600, 1994.
11. Borregard PE: Neurogenic bladder and spina bifida occulta: a case report, *J Manipulative Physiol Ther* 10:122-123, 1987.
12. Browning JE: Pelvic pain and organic dysfunction in a patient with low back pain, response to distractive manipulation: a case presentation, *J Manipulative Physiol Ther* 10:116-121, 1987.
13. Browning JE: Chiropractic distractive decompression in the treatment of pelvic pain and organic dysfunction with evidence of lower sacral nerve root compression, *J Manipulative Physiol Ther* 11:426-432, 1988.
14. Browning JE: Chiropractic distractive decompression in treating pelvic pain and multiple system pelvic organic dysfunction, *J Manipulative Physiol Ther* 12:265-274, 1989.
15. Browning JE: Mechanically induced pelvic pain and organic dysfunction in a patient without low back pain, *J Manipulative Physiol Ther* 13:406-411, 1990.
16. Browning JE: Uncomplicated mechanically induced pelvic pain and organic dysfunction in low back pain patients, *J Can Chiro Assoc* 35:149-155, 1991.
17. Falk JW: Bowel and bladder dysfunction secondary to lumbar dysfunctional syndrome, *Chiro Technique* 2:45-48, 1990.
18. Wagner T et al: Irritable bowel syndrome and spinal manipulation: a case report, *Chiro Technique* 7:139-140, 1995.
19. Polk JR: A new approach to pelvic pain management, *Today's Chiro* 20:42-46, 1991.

20. Hawk C, Long C, Azad A: Chiropractic care for women with chronic pelvic pain: a prospective single group intervention study, *J Manipulative Physiol Ther* 20:73-79, 1997.

21. Stude DE: Dysfunctional uterine bleeding with concomitant low back and lower extremity pain, *J Manipulative Physiol Ther* 14:472-477, 1991.

22. Stude DE: The management of symptoms associated with premenstrual syndrome, *J Manipulative Physiol Ther* 14:209-216, 1991.

23. Arnold-Frochot S: Investigation of the effect of chiropractic adjustments on a specific gynaecological symptom: dysmenorrhea, *J Aust Chiro Assoc* 10:6-10; 14-16, 1981.

24. Liebl NA, Butler LM: A chiropractic approach to the treatment of dysmenorrhea, *J Manipulative Physiol Ther* 13:101-106, 1990.

25. Radler M: Dysemenorrhea-chiropractic application, *Am Chiro* 29-32, 1984.

26. Wiles M: Gynecology and obstetrics in chiropractic, *Gynecol Obstet* 24:163-166, 1980.

27. Snyder BJ, Sanders GE: Evaluation of the toftness system of chiropractic adjusting for subjects with chronic back pain, chronic tension headaches, or primary dysmenorrhea, *Chiro Technique* 8:3-9, 1996.

28. Thomason PR et al: Effectiveness of spinal manipulative therapy in treatment of primary dysmenorrhea: a pilot study, *J Manipulative Physiol Ther* 2:140-145, 1979.

29. Hubbs EC: Vertebral subluxation and premenstrual tension syndrome: a case study, *Res Forum* 2:100-102, 1986.

30. Kokjohn K et al: The effect of spinal manipulation on pain and prostaglandin levels in women with primary dysmenorrhea, *J Manipulative Physiol Ther* 15:279-285, 1992.

31. Browning JE: The mechanically induced pelvic pain and organic dysfunction syndrome: an often overlooked cause of bladder, bowel, gynecologic and sexual dysfunction, *J Neuromusculoskel Syst* 4:52-66, 1996.

32. Browning JE: Distractive manipulation protocols in treating the mechanically induced pelvic pain and organic dysfunction patient, *Chiro Technique* 7:1-11, 1995.

33. Herlin L: *Sciatic and pelvic pain due to lumbosacral nerve root compression,* Springfield, Ill, 1966, Charles C Thomas.

34. Emmett JL, Love JG: "Asymptomatic" protruded lumbar disc as a cause of urinary retention: preliminary report, *Mayo Clin Proc* 42:249-257, 1967.

35. Warwick R, Williams P: *Gray's anatomy,* ed 35 (Brit), Philadelphia, 1973, WB Saunders.

36. Hockman CH: *Essentials of autonomic function. The autonomic nervous systems: fundamental concepts from anatomy, physiology, pharmacology and neuroscience for students and professionals in the health sciences,* Springfield, Ill, 1987, Charles C Thomas.

37. Appenzeller O: *Clinical autonomic failure. Practical concepts,* New York, 1986, Elsevier.

38. Emmitt JL, Love JG: Vesical dysfunction caused by protruded lumbar disc, *J Urol* 105:86-91, 1971.

39. Rosomoff HL et al: Cystometry in the evaluation of nerve root compression in the lumbar spine, *Surg Gynecol Obstet* 117:263-269, 1963.

40. Amelar RD, Dubin L: Importance in the low back syndrome, *JAMA* 216:520, 1971.

41. Shafer SN, Rosenblum J: Occult lumbar disc causing impotence, *NY Sta J Med* 18:2465-2470, 1969.

42. Rosomoff HL et al: Cystometry as an adjunct in the evaluation of lumbar disc syndromes, *J Neurofurg* 1:67, 1970.

43. Mosdol C, Iverson P, Iverson-Hansen R: Bladder neuropathy in lumbar disc disease, *Acta Neurochir* 3:281-286, 1979.

44. Ross JC, Jameson RM: Vesical dysfunction due to prolapsed disc, *Br Med J* 3:752-754, 1971.

45. Malloch JD: Acute retention due to intervertebral disc prolapse, *Br J Urol* 37:578, 1965.

46. Yaxley RP: Letter to the editor, *Br J Urol* 38:324-325, 1966.

47. Tackmann W, Porst H, vanAhlen H: Bulbocavernosus reflex latencies and somatosensory evoked potentials after pudendal nerve stimulation in the diagnosis of impotence, *J Neurol* 235:219-225, 1988.

48. Cox JM: *Low back pain mechanism, diagnosis and treatment,* ed 5, Baltimore, 1990, Williams & Wilkins.

49. Haldeman S: *Principles and practice of chiropractic,* ed 2, pp 549-577, San Mateo, Calif, 1992, Appleton and Lange.

50. Aho AJ, Auranen A, Pesonen K: Analysis of cauda equina symptoms in patients with lumbar disc prolapse, *Acta Chir Scand* 135:413-420, 1969.

51. Choudhury AR, Taylor JC: Cauda equina syndrome in lumbar disc disease, *Acta Orthop Scand* 51:493-499, 1980.

52. McLaren AC, Bailey SI: Cauda equina syndrome: a complication of lumbar discectomy, *Clin Orthop* 204:143-149, 1986.

53. Mayer PJ, Jacobsen FS: Cauda equina syndrome after surgical treatment of lumbar spinal stenosis with application of free autogenous fat graft, *J Bone Joint Surg* 71A:1090-1093, 1989.

54. Shephard RH: Diagnosis and prognosis of cauda equina syndrome produced by protrusion of lumbar disk, *Br Med J* 2:1434-1439, 1959.

55. Kostuik JP et al: Cauda equina syndrome and lumbar disc herniation, *J Bone Joint Surg* 68A:386-391, 1986.

56. Finneson BE: *Low back pain,* ed 2, Philadelphia, 1980, JB Lippincott.

57. Mooney V: Differential diagnosis of low back disorders, principles of classification. In Frymore JW, editor: *The adult spine: principles and practice,* pp 1551-1567, New York, 1991, Raven Press.

58. Jennett WB: A study of 25 cases of compression of the cauda equina by prolapsed intervertebral discs, *J Neurol Neurosurg Psychiatry* 19:109-116, 1956.

59. O'Connell JEA: Protrusions of the lumbar intervertebral discs, *J Bone Joint Surg* 33B:8-30, 1951.

60. Walker JL, Schulak D, Murtagh R: Midline disk herniations of the lumbar spine, *South Med J* 86:13-17, 1993.

61. Travell J, Simons D: *Myofascial pain and dysfunction: the trigger point manual,* Baltimore, 1983, Williams & Wilkins.

CHAPTER 9

The Alimentary Canal: A Current Chiropractic Perspective

Charles S. Masarsky, DC • *Edward E. Cremata, DC*

When a subluxated patient visits a doctor of chiropractic (DC) with concomitant alimentary canal disorders, monitoring the gastrointestinal symptoms and signs can enhance the clinical assessment process. Furthermore, the more chiropractors know about the potential neurologic effect of the vertebral subluxation complex (VSC) on the alimentary canal, the better they can educate the patient about the possible role of chiropractic in assisting the body in the restoration and maintenance of health.

Ideally, the clinical encounter becomes an occasion for the doctor and patient to observe the wonders of the human body in its quest for homeostasis. The information in this chapter is presented in the hope of promoting this clinical ideal.

Basic Neurologic Considerations

The sympathetic nerve supply to the alimentary canal originates from spinal nerves T5-L2. After synapse at one of the prevertebral plexi, post-ganglionic sympathetic fibers generally course with blood vessels to their alimentary destinations. The parasympathetic innervation to the gut is primarily through the vagus nerves and spinal nerves S2-4.[1]

A third division of the autonomic nervous system (ANS) is described as a semiautonomous network that lies in the wall of the gastrointestinal tract, pancreas, and gallbladder—the enteric nervous system.[2] About 100,000,000 neurons exist in the enteric system, approximately the same number of neurons found in the entire spinal cord.

With this neural infrastructure available, not surprisingly, gastrointestinal motility and secre-

tion are largely locally controlled by the gut itself. However, alimentary function should not be assumed to be completely independent of sympathetic and parasympathetic influence. This would be similar to assuming that an ant has no need for a brain simply because the beheaded insect continues to walk. The doomed creature walks without environmental information; it cannot go faster to escape a predator, change direction in its search for food, or find its way back to the colony. In a similar fashion, the alimentary canal can continue to function without sympathetic and parasympathetic innervation but it will do so without information from the rest of the body. Sympathetic inhibition and parasympathetic acceleration of enteric tone are the means by which alimentary function is fully integrated with the needs of an organism's complete physical and emotional life.

For example, the nervous performer, athlete, speaker, or lawyer has experienced the profound effects of sympathetic stimulation to the gut. Gastritis and bowel dysfunction commonly accompany this intense sympathetic stimulation. These experiences are examples of the sympathetic alarm reaction, more intuitively known as the *fight-or-flight reaction*. To the extent that vertebral subluxation can increase general sympathetic tone, the alarm reaction may become hair-trigger, with resultant deleterious effects on alimentary function.

More measured sympathetic involvement in gastrointestinal function is seen in such responses as the enterogastric reflexes, in which signals from the small intestine and colon inhibit gastric motility and secretion, and the colonoileal reflex, in which signals from the colon inhibit emptying of ileal contents.[3] These reflexes are essential in allow-

137

ing the various portions of the intestinal tract to receive contents at a rate slow enough to process them appropriately.

Vertebral subluxation causing such localized reflex inhibition has been demonstrated in a study on conscious rabbits.[4] Using surgical implants, DeBoer and others[4] misaligned T6 for 2½ minutes. This procedure was intended to mimic a vertebral subluxation at that level. Recordings from implanted electrodes indicated a dramatic drop in the rabbits' gastric myoelectric activity during this subluxation-like event. Essentially, the subluxation mimic disengaged these rabbits' gastric tone from the requirements of digestion.

Parasympathetic involvement in gastrointestinal function is evident in such responses as accelerated secretion of saliva and gastric acid in response to food, or even the smell, sight, or thought of food. Normal defecation also relies on parasympathetic intensification of the peristaltic waves in the lower colon.[5] Subluxation-related disruption of the parasympathetic pathways would be expected to disturb these functions.

Sensory innervation to the alimentary canal follows various routes. The phrenic nerves supply some sensory branches to the upper portion of the peritoneum, the folds of peritoneum forming the falciform and coronary ligaments of the liver, and possibly the gallbladder.[6] For the alimentary canal at large, the most important sensory fibers are those that course with the sympathetic nerves, the parasympathetics (involving vagal and sacral pathways), and those nerves located entirely within the enteric system. Because the purely enteric pathways have no direct connection to the spinal nerves, vertebral subluxation would be expected to alter the alimentary sensorium primarily through the sympathetic, parasympathetic, and phrenic pathways.

Clinical Research: Historic Perspectives

Our current understanding of the interactions of spinal dysfunction and alimentary disorders owes a great debt to medical, osteopathic, and chiropractic research performed in the first half of the twentieth century. Osteopathic researchers were the most active of the three professions during this era, in experimental and clinical work. Louisa Burns and others[7] studied the effects of experimental spinal lesions on animals from 1907 to approximately 1948. Hyperemia, hyperchlorhydria,

petechial hemorrhages, and ulcers were found in the gastric mucosa of rabbits lesioned at T4-T7. Edema and congestion were noted in the tissues of the liver, pancreas, and stomach in at least one rabbit lesioned at T2; however, the researchers speculated that these changes were secondary to "weakness of the heart."[8]

Medical researcher Henry K. Winsor[9] studied correlations between spinal curvatures and internal organ pathology observed during 50 autopsies at the University of Pennsylvania in 1922. Stomach pathology was identified in 9 cadavers, liver disease was found in 13, gallbladder pathology was described in 5, and pancreatic disorders were observed in 5. In 28 of these 32 instances of alimentary pathology, curvature was noted in the T5-9 area.

Clarence Gonstead (1898-1978) recorded a number of clinical insights relevant to the alimentary tract during his long chiropractic career.[10] Gonstead found peptic ulcers and diarrhea to be most frequently related to upper cervical subluxation, and duodenal ulcers were more likely to involve T4-T10. Constipation was found to have multiple sites of frequent subluxation, including T3-5, T8-12, L1-4, and occasionally the upper cervical area.

In a review of a number of cases presented at several meetings of the Women's Osteopathic Club of Los Angeles, Bondies and Stillman[11] maintained that T4-10 and the upper cervical region were most often implicated in gastric and duodenal ulcers. These same levels were mentioned in relation to peptic ulcers by Hay.[12] Magoun[13] emphasized the importance of lesions of the jugular foramen. He maintained that such lesions could affect the vagus nerve and thereby contribute to various kinds of gastrointestinal disease. He reported that such patients often responded favorably to cranial manipulation.

A 1939 study by Downing[14] emphasized the importance of spinal lesions involving T8-10 in patients with nonsurgical gallbladder disease, although he noted that a complete structural examination should be performed, as with any patient.

Northup, in his 1941 paper on mucous colitis,[15] emphasized the importance of lesions at the thoracolumbar junction, although he believed that every segment from the midthoracics to the sacroiliacs should be examined, along with the upper cervical spine. He also advocated gentle manipulation of Chapman's neurolymphatic reflexes for the colon, at the lateral aspect of the thighs, after spinal manipulation.

Lindberg and others, in 1941,[16] demonstrated a correlation between spinal lesions from T6-L1 and colitis, based on analysis of 349 cases at Chicago Osteopathic Hospital.

Recent Research Developments

By the end of the 1950s, support for experimental and clinical research into the spinal-alimentary relationship appears to have diminished within the osteopathic community. Much of the recent research in this area is found in chiropractic publications.

Bowel Disorders

Irritable bowel syndrome (IBS) is characterized by abdominal pain and cramping, bloating, flatulence, and diarrhea and/or constipation.[17] Wagner and others[18] described the case of a 25-year-old woman who had IBS for 5 years. Her symptoms were primarily sharp abdominal pain and diarrhea, with a frequency of one to two episodes per week. These symptoms were exacerbated by periods of increased stress, a common observation among of IBS sufferers. Subluxation signs were clustered around the upper cervical and thoracolumbar regions. Two adjustments were administered in the first week of care, followed by 2 years of follow-up visits that occurred approximately once per month. The patient reported complete freedom from IBS symptoms during these 2 years of care.

Many cases of constipation have been described in the chiropractic literature. A case study of a 7-month-old with chronic constipation was reported by Hewitt.[19] According to the patient's mother, the child had suffered from constipation since birth. At the first doctor visit, the mother said her child's bowel movements occurred between once per day and once every 3 days. Hours of straining and crying preceded each bowel movement, and the consistency of the feces was described as similar to rabbit pellets. After chiropractic examination, gentle diversified adjusting was administered to the L5-S1, L4-5, T6-7, and occ-C1 motion segments and the coronal suture. Four such adjustments were performed over a period of 8 weeks. During this time, the child had one to two soft, effortless stools per day, with the exception of 1 week of diarrhea secondary to chicken pox. At the time of publication, this improvement was stable with 1 year of follow-up.

Eriksen[20] reported the case of a 5-year-old girl with a lifetime history of constipation. Despite medication, she was experiencing only one bowel movement per week. This promptly changed to four to six bowel movements per week after Grostic upper cervical adjusting.

Falk[21] reported the case of a 40-year-old man, whose main complaints were low back pain and left sciatica. Accompanying these problems, the patient reported constipation, an ailment he denied experiencing in the past. Side-posture adjustments at L5 resolved these conditions.

In addition to these presentations, bowel dysfunction was often a feature of the type of case reported when the patient exhibited signs of lower sacral nerve root irritation, a topic described extensively in Chapter 8.

Gastric and Duodenal Dysfunction

Manual medicine practitioners Pikalov and Kharin[22] presented a study of spinal manipulative therapy in the management of duodenal ulcer patients. A total of 16 adult duodenal ulcer patients received spinal manipulative therapy 3 to 14 times over a 5 to 22 day period in addition to standard medical treatment, while a control group of 40 cases received medical treatment only. The progress of both patient groups was monitored by clinical signs and weekly endoscopic examination. The most frequently manipulated motion segments were within the T9-T12 area. Recovery was substantially accelerated in the group receiving manipulation, with ulcer remission taking place an average of 10 days earlier than the group under traditional care. Although recent biomedical literature has focused on the role of infection in general and *Helicobacter pylori* in particular in the generation of gastric and duodenal ulcers, the apparent benefit of manipulative therapy in this study emphasized the importance of host immunity. Infection required not only the presence of the pathogen but also the vulnerability of the target tissue.

A survey on the prevalence of indigestion and heartburn in chiropractic practice was presented by Bryner and Staerker.[23] Responses were obtained from 1494 patients in 8 practices. Patients with thoracalgia were more likely to also report indigestion or heartburn. Among patients with a positive examination finding for thoracic anteriority, 69% reported dyspepsia. Interestingly, although 22% of the patients with indigestion received relief from this symptom, 76% of this group failed to inform their chiropractors of this favorable phenomenon.

Infantile Colic

Infantile colic is generally characterized by violent crying, with the legs drawn to the abdomen, presumably indicating abdominal pain.[24] Although abdominal distension and flatulence commonly accompany infantile colic, these may be related to aerophagia caused by the incessant crying. Despite these symptoms, the infants suffering from infantile colic generally eat well, thrive, and demonstrate no consistent objective signs. One proposed set of diagnostic criteria defines infantile colic as at least 3 hours of crying per day at a frequency of at least 3 days per week over a period of at least 3 weeks. Parental distress from this incessant crying may be a factor in child abuse.[25]

A prospective study of 316 infants suffering from infantile colic was conducted by Klougart and others[26] with the cooperation of some 38% of the active doctors of chiropractic in Denmark. Based on parent diaries, 94% of the cases resolved in 2 weeks or less (on an average of 3 visits); 23% of the cases resolved after a single adjustment. Citing previous research, the authors noted that spontaneous resolution of infantile colic generally takes 12 to 16 weeks. The upper cervical area was the most frequently adjusted.

In addition to the landmark prospective study by Klougart and others, a number of instructive case reports have been published. Pluhar and Schobert[27] presented the case of a 3-month-old girl with a history of 4 weeks of colicky crying. Medical intervention was not successful. The infant would sleep as little as 2 hours per day and would sometimes consume less than 5 oz of formula per day. After a single adjustment (C1, T7, and T9), the patient slept soundly for 8 hours, consumed 32 oz of formula, and exhibited a marked reduction in crying. The infant was reportedly doing well 6 weeks after this initial visit.

Hyman[28] reported the case of a 5-week-old boy with frequent episodes of gut-wrenching crying accompanied by arching of the back and flatulence, which had been occurring for 3 weeks. After the first adjustment (C1 and T9), the parents reported a reduction in frequency and intensity of crying episodes. The infant continued to progress over the next 3 weeks.

Fallon and Lok[29] presented a case that suggested a possible etiology for some instances of infantile colic. Their patient was a 3-week-old girl with a 2 day history of projectile vomiting, accompanied by colicky crying (up to 18 hours each day). Based on a previous medical diagnosis of pyloric stenosis, surgery had been recommended. The parents opted for a chiropractic consultation before surgery. Palpation of the right upper abdominal quadrant revealed a hard olive-shaped mass, consistent with hypertrophy of the pyloric muscles, thereby supporting the previous diagnosis of pyloric stenosis. A temperature difference of 3° F was noted at the styloid fossae, and attempts to motion palpate the upper cervical spine produced a loud wail from the infant. Light-force upper cervical adjusting was the only intervention, with the exception of a T4 adjustment during one visit. Cessation of the projectile vomiting and reduction in the screaming was noted by the mother at the fourth visit (eighth day of care); the temperature difference was reduced to 2° F. By the tenth visit, screaming had ceased. The authors suggested that undiagnosed pyloric stenosis may be the etiology of many cases of infantile colic.

The notion that much of the recent chiropractic clinical literature cited earlier related to pediatric patients resonates with a recent paper by Nyiendo and Olsen.[30] These investigators found that gastrointestinal problems were common primary complaints among pediatric patients seen at a chiropractic college teaching clinic.

Summary

The medical, osteopathic, and chiropractic literature on the relationship of alimentary disorders to somatic dysfunction is promising. Reasonably, when a patient's symptoms result from a primary somatic problem, one can expect that timely chiropractic care may spare the patient much danger and expense from iatrogenic complications of unneeded diagnostic and medical therapeutic interventions. However, no definite method exists to establish the primary nature of the somatic dysfunction in an initial clinical encounter. The relationship is generally verified post hoc; the presence of the VSC or other somatic dysfunction is established independently of the alimentary symptom, then the symptom is followed as care progresses.

A number of observations exist that can increase the clinician's index of suspician that a particular alimentary dysfunction is related to a somatic problem in general and a VSC in particular. Beal[31] suggested that tissue texture changes at the costotransverse area are more likely to represent autonomic involvement than other paravertebral changes. Such changes in the T5-T12 area could be associated with alimentary dysfunction.

The maneuver of Carnett is performed by having supine patients tighten the abdominal muscles by raising their head or ballooning and fixing the abdomen with a deep inhalation.[32] This maneuver protects the underlying visceral tissue with abdominal armoring. If tenderness to digital pressure is not substantially reduced by this maneuver, the origin of the abdominal pain is likely to be somatic.

Conversely, rebound tenderness is more likely to be present when the visceral tissues are involved. This is done by suddenly removing the examiner's hands after pressing on the abdomen, setting a pressure wave in motion through the patient's abdomen. Pain will often be referred to the involved visceral tissue.

When the results of rebound tenderness and the maneuver of Carnett suggest the probability of genuine alimentary pathology, medical comanagement is strongly indicated. This same indication exists in severe, acute abdominal pain or persistent fever. Although close medical-chiropractic coordination would be ideal in such cases, referral followed by mutual noninterference should be the minimal standard. Medical intervention for visceral pathology can and should coincide with chiropractic intervention for improved neurologic function. No rational basis exists for one type of practitioner to blindly disrupt the patient's relationship with another kind of practitioner.

In general, the widespread innervation of the alimentary canal makes dysfunction in this system a useful barometer of neurologic dysfunction, although it does not precisely direct the clinician to the involved motion segments. In clinical practice, alimentary symptoms can be followed using ordinal scales such as the visual analog scale (VAS). This pencil-and-paper instrument is described in Chapter 6.

STUDY GUIDE

1. What are the origins of the sympathetic and parasympathetic nerve supplies to the alimentary canal?
2. What is the enteric nervous system and how extensive is it?
3. Given the existence of the enteric nervous system, what purpose do sympathetic inhibition and parasympathetic acceleration serve in a living organism?
4. What is the colonoileal reflex?
5. Describe the work of DeBoer and others.
6. Name two structures of the alimentary canal that receive their sensory innervation from the phrenic nerve. What other major structure receives its primary innervation from the phrenic nerve?
7. In Louisa Burns's study on rabbits, what were four examples of dis-ease resulting from experimentally induced subluxations at T4-T7? The investigators speculated that these were secondary to weakness of what organ system?
8. Being aware of the limitations of the road map approach to chiropractic analysis, Gonstead found peptic ulcers and duodenal ulcers to be most frequently related to spinal lesions at _____ and _____.
9. Describe the work of Pikalov and Kharin in the management of patients with duodenal ulcers. Because of the recent popularity of *H. pylori* being a primary source of digestive tract ulcers, what is the function of host immunity in ulcer formation?
10. What are the symptoms of the condition called *infantile colic?* Describe Klougart's study.
11. In Hyman's case study, where were the areas of subluxation? Is this different from Pikalov's and Kharin's study?
12. Describe the pyloric stenosis study as reported by Fallon and Lok. What other pediatric problem is this hypothesized to be related to?
13. Describe the movement of Carnett and its importance to the chiropractic clinician.
14. What is rebound tenderness and how is it a helpful test?

REFERENCES

1. Camilleri M: Disturbances of gastrointestinal motility and the nervous system, p 267. In Aminoff MJ, editor: *Neurology and general medicine,* New York, 1995, Churchill Livingstone.
2. Guyton AC: *Basic neuroscience: anatomy and physiology,* p 348, Philadelphia, 1991, WB Saunders.
3. Guyton AC: *Basic neuroscience: anatomy and physiology,* p 349, Philadelphia, 1991, WB Saunders.
4. DeBoer KF, Shutz M, McKnight ME: Acute effects of spinal manipulation on gastrointestinal myoelectric activity in conscious rabbit, *Man Med* 3:85, 1988.
5. Guyton AC: *Basic neuroscience: anatomy and physiology,* p 352, Philadelphia, 1991, WB Saunders.
6. Warwick R, Williams PL: *Gray's anatomy:* Ed 35 (Brit), p 1037, Philadelphia, 1973, WB Saunders.
7. Burns L, Candler L, Rice R: *Pathogenesis of visceral diseases following vertebral lesions,* p 213, Chicago, 1948, American Osteopathic Association.
8. Burns L, Steudenberg G, Vollbrecht WJ: Family of rabbits with second thoracic and other lesions, *J Am Osteopath Assoc* 37:908, 1937.
9. Winsor HK: Sympathetic segmental disturbances, II, *Med Times* 49:267, 1922.
10. Plaugher G et al: Spinal management for the patient with a visceral concomitant, p 370. In Plaugher G, editor: *Textbook of clinical chiropractic: a specific biomechanical approach,* Baltimore, 1993, Williams & Wilkins.
11. Bondies OI, Stillman CJ: Notes on the diagnosis and treatment of ulcerative gastritis, *J Am Osteopath Assoc* 36:568, 1936.
12. Hay J: The importance of faulty structural relations in etiology and treatment of peptic ulcer, *J Am Osteopath Assoc* 39:162, 1939.
13. Magoun HI: Clinical application of the cranial concept, *J Am Osteopath Assoc* 47:413, 1948.
14. Downing WJ: Osteopathic manipulative treatment of nonsurgical gall-bladder, *J Am Osteopath Assoc* 39:104, 1939.
15. Northup TL: Manipulation in mucous colitis, *J Am Osteopath Assoc* 41:87, 1941.
16. Lindberg RF, Strachan WF, Koehnlein WO: The relation of structural disturbances to irritable colon ("colitis"), *J Am Osteopath Assoc* 41:253, 1941.
17. Schaefer RC: *Symptomatology and differential diagnosis: a conspectus of clinical semeiographies,* p 741, Arlington, Va, 1986, American Chiropractic Association.
18. Wagner T et al: Irritable bowel syndrome and spinal manipulation: a case report, *Chiro Technique* 7:139, 1995.
19. Hewitt EG: Chiropractic treatment of a 7-month-old with chronic constipation: a case report, *Chiro Technique* 5:101, 1993.
20. Eriksen K: Effects of upper cervical correction on chronic constipation, *Chiro Res J* 3:19, 1994.
21. Falk JW: Bowel and bladder dysfunction secondary to lumbar dysfunctional syndrome, *Chiro Technique* 2:45, 1990.
22. Pikalov AA, Kharin VV: Use of spinal manipulative therapy in the treatment of duodenal ulcer, *J Manipulative Physiol Ther* 17:310, 1994.
23. Bryner P, Staerker PG: Indigestion and heartburn: prevalence in persons seeking care from chiropractors, *J Manipulative Physiol Ther* 19:317, 1996.
24. Tanaka ST, Martin CJ, Thibodeau P: Clinical neurology, p 605. In Anrig CA, Plaugher G, editors: *Pediatric chiropractic,* Baltimore, 1998, Williams & Wilkins.
25. Miller AR, Barr RG: Infantile colic: is it a gut issue? *Pediatr Clin North Am* 38:1407, 1991.
26. Klougart N, Nilsson N, Jacobsen J: Infantile colic treated by chiropractors: a prospective study of 316 cases, *J Manipulative Physiol Ther* 12:281, 1989.
27. Pluhar GR, Schobert PD: Vertebral subluxation and colic: a case study, *J Chiro Res Clin Investig* 7:75, 1991.
28. Hyman CA: Chiropractic adjustments and infantile colic: a case study, p 65. In International Chiropractors Association, editor: *Proceedings of the national conference on chiropractic and pediatrics,* Arlington, Va, 1994, International Chiropractors Association.
29. Fallon JP, Lok BJ: Assessing the efficacy of chiropractic care in pediatric cases of pyloric stenosis, p 72. In International Chiropractors Association, editor: *Proceedings of the national conference on chiropractic and pediatrics,* Arlington, Va, 1994, International Chiropractors Association.
30. Nyiendo J, Olsen E: Visit characteristics of 217 children attending a chiropractic college teaching clinic, *J Manipulative Physiol Ther* 11:78, 1988.
31. Beal MC: Viscerosomatic reflexes: a review, *J Am Osteopath Assoc* 85:786, 1985.
32. Schaefer RC: *Symptomatology and differential diagnosis: a conspectus of clinical semeiographies,* p 783, Arlington, Va, 1986, American Chiropractic Association.

CHAPTER 10

Chiropractic Care and the Cardiovascular System

Charles S. Masarsky, DC • *Edward E. Cremata, DC*

Cardiovascular disease is one of the main causes of mortality and morbidity in the industrialized world. Cardiovascular health is one of the most important aspects of physical fitness. For these reasons, understanding the neurologic influence over cardiovascular tone is an important consideration for doctors of chiropractic (DC) who are interested in the role of subluxation correction in general and vertebral subluxation complex (VSC) correction in particular in the overall health and wellness of their patients.

Basic Neurologic Considerations

Neurologic Control of the Heart

The heart is the most sophisticated muscular organ in the human body. Even if all sympathetic and parasympathetic fibers were disconnected from the heart, it would maintain an automatic rhythm because of a series of specialized muscle fibers capable of self-excitation that are connected to a network of fibers modified for rapid conduction.[1] This rhythm originates with a body of specialized fibers in the right atrium, called the *sinus* or *sinoatrial* node. Impulses are conducted from the sinus node by internodal pathways to the atrioventricular node. From here, impulses are conducted to all parts of the ventricles by the left and right bundles of Purkinje fibers (Figure 10-1).

As impressive as this intrinsic neural structure may be, an isolated heart would not be able to adapt its function to the needs of the rest of the body. Communication by parasympathetic, sympathetic, and sensory pathways is essential for coordinating cardiac tone with the physiology of the whole organism.

The parasympathetic innervation to the heart comes from cardiac branches of the vagus nerves. The terminal fibers of these vagus branches are most numerous at the sinus and atrioventricular nodes.[2] Vagal stimulation slows the rhythm of the sinus node while simultaneously decreasing the excitability of the internodal pathways. The net result is a slowing of heart rate and some decrease in the power of heart muscle contraction. Very strong stimulation of the vagi can cause cardiac arrest for up to 10 seconds.[3]

Sympathetic innervation to the heart originates from the first five thoracic spinal nerves. These preganglionic fibers synapse at the superior cervical, middle cervical, and stellate ganglia, from which postganglionic fibers reach the heart.[4] The effects of sympathetic stimulation are essentially the opposite of those caused by parasympathetic stimulation. Maximal stimulation can almost triple heart rate, while doubling the power of cardiac muscle contraction.[5]

Sensory innervation to the heart concerned with pain impulses generally follows the sympathetic efferent pathways outlined earlier, although some pain fibers reach the heart directly from the upper thoracic spine. General visceral afferent (nonpain) innervation to the heart is by the vagus nerves.[6]

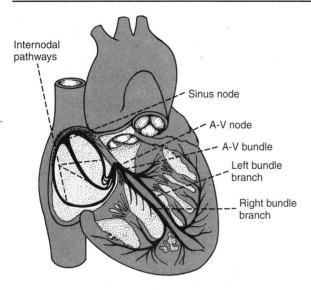

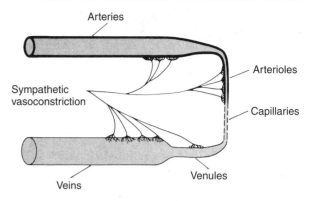

Figure 10-2 Sympathetic innervation of the systemic circulation. (From Guyton AC: *Basic neuroscience: anatomy and physiology,* p 323, Philadelphia, 1991, WB Saunders.)

Figure 10-1 The sinus node and the Purkinje system of the heart, showing also the A-V node, the atrial internodal pathways, and the ventricular bundle branches. (From Guyton AC: *Basic neuroscience: anatomy and physiology,* p 323, Philadelphia, 1991, WB Saunders.)

Neurologic Control of Vasomotor Function

Vasoconstrictor fibers are distributed from the sympathetic chain ganglia to virtually all blood vessels other than capillaries and precapillary sphincters (Figure 10-2). In the resting condition, a partial state of vasoconstrictor tone is maintained in the blood vessels throughout the body. Outside of the heart, parasympathetic efferents play little role in regulating circulation.

The major sensory innervation to the blood vessels consists of a series of stretch receptors in the walls of most of the large arteries in the neck and thorax. These stretch receptors are generally referred to as *baroreceptors* or *pressoreceptors.*

Baroreceptors are particularly abundant in the carotid bodies, located in the internal carotid arteries just above their origin from the common carotid arteries. Baroreceptor signals from the carotid bodies are conducted to the brainstem by the glossopharyngeal nerves. Baroreceptors are also quite abundant in the arch of the aorta. Signals from aortic baroreceptors are conducted to the brainstem by the vagus nerves. Normal baroreception is necessary for maintaining constant arterial pressure during postural changes; failure of

baroreception can cause postural hypotension, resulting in vertigo or syncope.

The same vagus and glossopharyngeal pathways from the aortic arch and carotid bodies also serve chemoreceptors. These receptors are sensitive to changes in oxygen, carbon dioxide, and hydrogen ion content in the blood. Although vasomotor tone is strongly influenced by these peripheral sensory inputs, central influences are also important and should not be forgotten. The initiation of exercise, cerebral ischemia, and fear will generate reflex responses in the vasomotor system.[7]

Cardiovascular Neuroanatomy and the Vertebral Subluxation Complex

Subluxation may affect the rate, rhythm, and power of heart contraction through the sympathetic efferent pathways originating from T1-T5. Cervical subluxation at any level could also affect sympathetic efferent pathways to the heart by the superior cervical, middle cervical, and stellate ganglia. These cervical ganglia being part of a continuous body, called the *paravertebral chain,* should be remembered. A subluxation does not necessarily have to be located in the cervical spine to disturb the function of these ganglia. Homewood[8] has described cases in which postpartum subluxation of the coccyx was accompanied by tachycardia. This symptom was exacerbated during bowel movements. He hypothesized that anterior subluxation of the coccyx may irritate the junction of the left and right paravertebral chain at the ganglion impar. This could create a spreading electrical disturbance up the chain, leading to disruption of cardiac rhythm by the cervical levels. This irritation would be exacerbated when a pincer effect was created by the passage of a fecal bolus anterior to the coccyx.

Afferent and parasympathetic efferent innervation to the heart could be disturbed by upper cervical subluxation, primarily because of the passage of the vagus nerve through the jugular foramen. The relationship of this foramen to upper cervical structures is discussed in Chapter 4. Upper cervical subluxation could also disturb the afferent limb of vasomotor regulation in general because the jugular foramen conducts the glossopharyngeal nerve and the vagus.

The cranial nerves exerting profound reflex influences on each other should be noted. For this reason, disturbance in cranial nerves other than the vagus and glossopharyngeal affecting cardiac function is possible. Gottesman and others[9] reported the case of a 67-year-old man with a 12-year history of trigeminal neuralgia accompanied by fainting. During admission to the hospital for one such episode, the patient suffered a cardiac arrest. After resuscitation, ECG, cardiac enzymes, and echocardiogram were all within normal limits. However, massage of the carotid sinus on the side of the trigeminal neuralgia induced a 7.5 second cardiac pause, with a sensation of faintness. The authors concluded that trigeminal nerve activity triggered cardioinhibition by some vagus or glossopharyngeal connection. Although this case is unusual, the oculocardiac reflex (bradycardia after pressure over the orbits of the eyes) is a routine demonstration of a trigeminal connection to vagus and glossopharyngeal function.[10] Because the trigeminal nerve may be vulnerable to cervical subluxation by its cervical nucleus, the trigeminal-cardiac connection offers another pathway by which the VSC may affect the heart.

The same upper cervical relationships described previously are also relevant regarding general vasomotor tone, which is influenced by baroreceptive and chemoreceptive signals carried by the vagus and trigeminal nerves. Of course, sympathetic influence over vasomotor tone can be affected by the VSC at any level through the paravertebral chain ganglia.

Blood volume, and therefore blood pressure, is sensitive to changes in the overall amount of water in the body and the osmolality of the body's fluids. The kidneys play a vital role in maintaining optimal water volume and osmolality through constant adjustments of urine output and concentration under the control of a complex network of neurohormonal feedback mechanisms.[11] When the VSC disturbs this delicate control of renal function, hypertension is one possible result.

Clinical Research: Historic Perspectives

The influence of the spinal nerves on cardiovascular function has been a chiropractic concern since the profession's earliest days. D.D. Palmer[12] described a case of "heart trouble" shortly after the Harvey Lillard case. Palmer recommended adjusting T4 for functional and organic disease of the heart and pericarditis.[13]

Henry K. Winsor,[14] a medical anatomist at the University of Pennsylvania, reported autopsy results correlating regions of spinal curvature to 20 cases of heart and pericardium pathology. Spinal curvature was found in the T1-T5 region in 18 cases, and at C7-T1 in 2 cases.

Osteopathic researcher Louisa Burns and others[15] demonstrated cardiac pathology in rabbits with experimentally induced lesions at T2. In one case, the pathology was verified by microscopic examination of the heart muscle. In a later experiment by Burns, experimental lesions at T3 were found to produce clear clinical signs of cardiac pathology in two rabbits of the same litter.[16] One of the rabbits was sacrificed and an autopsy confirmed cardiac pathology. The other rabbit underwent osteopathic manipulation to correct the T3 lesion. Clinical signs abated, and when this rabbit was later sacrificed, an autopsy revealed much less severe cardiac pathology than the rabbit with the uncorrected T3 lesion.

A later study by Burns[17] included a record of pulse tracings of the cardiac apex beat of rabbits with experimentally induced lesions of T3, T4, C1, or the occiput. Irregularities in pulse rate and intensity were found in the rabbits that were so lesioned; in some cases, these abnormalities were reversed when manipulation was performed to correct the spinal lesions. Interestingly, autopsy generally revealed notable myocardial pathology in rabbits with T3 or T4 lesions but not in rabbits with C1 or occipital lesions.

Based on years of private and academic osteopathic clinical experience, Arthur D. Becker[18] recommended close attention to lesions from T1-T6 and the upper cervical spine. He also emphasized the importance of correcting lesions of the left third, fourth and fifth ribs and soft-tissue work for the intercostal tissues at these levels. Illustrative cases included a 3-week-old infant with cyanotic spells and an 80-year-old woman with angina pectoris.

Chiropractic clinician, educator, and researcher Carl S. Cleveland, Jr.[19] published a number of pilot studies similar in some respects to the earlier osteopathic work by Burns and others. While Burns and others produced lesions in rabbits by manually administered spinal trauma, Cleveland used a surgical technique done with fluoroscopic assistance to produce measured misalignments verified by radiographs. Physiologic measures on live rabbits were correlated with postmortem findings. Heart diseases, valvular leakages, arrhythmias, and vasomotor paralysis were noted, but the exact spinal levels were apparently not reported. Cleveland did note a direct correlation between T12 subluxation and renal pathology.

Osteopathic researcher Richard Koch[20] presented a clinical series including 50 cases of organic heart disease in which the diagnosis was verified by cardiologic examination, including ECG, fluoroscopy, and chest x-ray. He also reported 100 cases of functional heart disease in which patients demonstrated clinical signs consistent with heart disease but no clear objective evidence of pathology.

In 93% of the functional group and 100% of the organic group, palpatory and roentgenographic evidence of vertebral dysfunction was noted in the T2-T6 region, with findings clustering at T4-6. In summarizing the histories of these patients, Koch found that they all experienced upper thoracic symptoms. Furthermore, the majority of these patients reported that they developed upper thoracic spine symptoms months or years before the onset of their cardiac symptoms. Koch also observed a high frequency of noncardiac conditions referable to the upper thoracic spine in these patients, including arthritis and tendonitis in the upper extremities, frozen-shoulder syndrome, and bronchial disease.

Koch also noted that general body or lower extremity exertion was less likely to precede heart attacks in these patients than upper extremity exertions (lawn-mowing, long periods of desk work or driving, ironing, carrying suitcases, etc.). Clinical improvement was noted in all cases with osteopathic manipulative therapy combined with home exercises for cervicothoracic spine flexibility. This favorable clinical response was true of patients taking heart medication and those not undergoing drug therapy.

After retrospectively reviewing 5,000 case records, Thomas Northup[21] selected those of 100 hypertensive patients who demonstrated highly favorable responses to osteopathic manipulation. Among these patients, the average reduction in pressure immediately after intervention was 33 mmHg systolic and 9 mmHg diastolic, with decreases as great as 70 mmHg systolic and 20 mmHg diastolic in a few instances.

In essential hypertension, Northup focused on spinal dysfunction at the T8-9 and upper cervical areas, along with cranial faults at the occipitomastoid junction. He found that patients with higher systolic pressure in the supine position than in the sitting position were more likely to be hypertensives complicated by nephritis; for these patients, he emphasized the importance of lower thoracic dysfunction.

Recent Research Developments

In 1975, the U.S. Department of Health, Education, and Welfare held its first interdisciplinary conference on spinal manipulation, under the auspices of the National Institutes of Neurological and Communicative Disorders and Stroke (NINCDS).[22] This conference evidenced a new level of interest in chiropractic and osteopathic research by the scientific community at large. A gradual movement towards increased funding and rigor and decreased professional isolation has characterized chiropractic, osteopathic, and manual medicine research initiatives since the NINCDS conference. For this reason, 1975 appears to be a reasonable date for the dawn of the modern research era of these fields.

Larson[23] reported palpation findings for 196 patients with diagnoses of myocardial disease in the intensive care unit (ICU) of Chicago Osteopathic Hospital. The abnormal findings clustered around T2-T5 and C2. The thoracic involvements were somewhat more frequent on the left side, with T2 involvement most commonly found with arrhythmias. When C2 involvement was found, it was almost universally on the left side.

Cox and others[24] found a significant correlation between spinal palpation findings and coronary artery disease. Musculoskeletal findings were reported for 97 patients before cardiac catheterization for angiography. In those patients with angiographically demonstrated coronary artery disease, musculoskeletal findings clustered around T4. This was especially significant when soft-tissue texture (compliance of the paravertebral and intercostal tissue at the T4 area) and range of motion (intersegmental restriction of T4 against T5 or T3) were considered. In the same year, Cox and Rogers[25] presented a study demonstrating osteophytosis of the thoracic spine in 43% of patients with coronary artery stenosis, compared with 15% in heart-healthy controls.

Myron Beal,[26] reporting on a series of approximately 100 patients with confirmed cardiovascular disease, stated that some 90% of patients had segmental dysfunction somewhere between T1 and T5 on the left side, with findings clustered at T2-T3. He also noted that the majority of such patients demonstrated left-sided dysfunction at C2. Beal maintained that hypertonicity of the deep paraspinal tissues was the most important finding and that a supine compression test was the most effective examination procedure (Figure 10-3).

An interesting biomedical observation relating *straight back syndrome (SBS)* to heart disease was investigated by Ansari.[27] SBS consists of loss of normal physiologic curvature in the upper dorsal spine, with narrowing of the anteroposterior diameter of the chest. Radiographically, SBS is determined by measuring the anteroposterior diameter of the chest by drawing a line from the anterior border of T8 to the posterior border of the sternum. This is compared with the transthoracic diameter, measured by a line connecting the inner margins of the left and right ribs at the level of the greatest width of the rib cage. The ratio of anteroposterior diameter to transthoracic diameter is expressed as a percentage. The mean of this ratio is 35% (+/− 2.3%) in patients with SBS versus 45% (+/− 3.5%) in controls. Among 55 patients with SBS, Ansari reported that 71% had valvular heart disease, with the most common form being mitral valve prolapse.

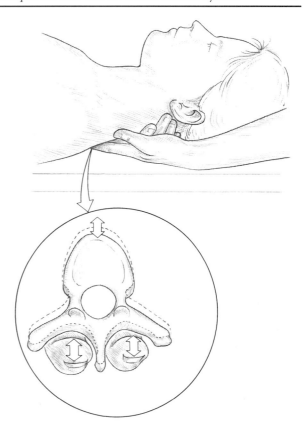

Figure 10-3 Beal's springing assessment for paraspinal facilitation rigidity associated with segmental facilitation. (From Chaitow L: *Palpation skills,* p 66, New York, 1997, Churchill Livingstone.)

Previous researchers had suggested that SBS affects the heart by mechanical pressure—a pancake or squashing effect. Ansari did not find this to be the case and instead proposed that SBS and valvular heart disease are aspects of a genetically determined fault in development.

Interestingly, SBS bears a striking similarity to the type of subluxation complex referred to in chiropractic as the *Pottenger's saucer,* or the *thoracic anteriority.*[28,29] These chiropractic sources generally define this subluxation complex as a series of extension malpositions superior to a flexion malposition. Chest pain, dyspnea, and dyspepsia are concomitant symptoms commonly reported in patients with thoracic anteriority; these same symptoms often accompany cardiac disease. This subluxation complex is commonly reported in the upper half of the thoracic spine, which has been connected with cardiovascular disorders in a number of the studies already reviewed.

Morgan and others[30] presented a study in which osteopathic mobilization techniques were compared with a sham procedure (soft-tissue massage) in treating a group of 29 hypertensive patients. Mobilization consisted of figure-8 motion of the head, with an attempt to isolate the upper cervical region, extension mobilization of T1-T5, and muscle energy technique for the mobilization of T11-L1. This study failed to demonstrate a significant decrease in systolic or diastolic blood pressure with either the mobilization or the sham procedure. If some or all of these patients had SBS, the extension mobilization used by Morgan and others may have actually exacerbated these patients.

The adrenal cortical hormone *aldosterone* is one of the components in the neurohormonal control of renal activity; it acts on the kidney to cause sodium retention. An elevated serum level of aldosterone is associated with an increased risk of hypertension. Osteopathic researcher Mannino[31] investigated the effect of Chapman's neurolymphatic reflexes on serum aldosterone levels. Chapman's reflexes are areas in the subcutaneous tissue that become tender and palpably nodular when active. Stimulation of these reflexes is thought to normalize lymphatic flow through associated organs.

Mannino selected a pair of Chapman's reflexes associated with the adrenal glands located between T11 and T12, midway between the spinous processes and tips of the transverse processes. In a group of hypertensive patients, a statistically significant drop occurred in serum aldosterone levels within 36 hours of Chapman's reflex stimulation. No significant changes in serum aldosterone levels were demonstrated in the controls. After a sham treatment, serum aldosterone levels returned to baseline in the hypertensive patients and then were reduced again with stimulation at the Chapman's reflex for the adrenals.

No significant reduction in blood pressure was noted, but the author cited previous research indicating that pharmaceutical aldosterone-blocking agents do not begin to affect blood pressure for 5 to 7 days. Mannino suggested that future studies with a longer period of follow-up may be required to determine whether a change in blood pressure eventually follows the modifications in serum aldosterone levels.

Wagnon and others[32] investigated the effect of chiropractic adjustments on serum aldosterone levels in a group of hypertensive patients. Subluxation findings clustered at the upper cervical spine, T9 and L5, were reported in a group of hypertensive patients after chiropractic analysis, including x-ray assessment, static and motion palpation, and heat-reading instrumentation. The group received Gonstead or diversified adjustments at these levels, with blood pressure and serum aldosterone measurements performed before and after the adjustment. Reduction in blood pressure was noted postadjustment for most subjects, but a return to baseline levels usually appeared within 72 hours. A statistically significant decrease in serum aldosterone levels occured postadjustment, and these levels remained substantially below baseline levels 10 days after the adjustment. Echoing Mannino, these authors suggested that long-term effects of the chiropractic adjustment on blood pressure and serum aldosterone levels could only be observed with a much longer follow-up period than the one available in their study.

Reviewing clinical literature presented over a period of 30 years by members of the International College of Applied Kinesiology, Walther[33] noted an association between disturbance of the heart meridian of acupuncture and subluxation of the T5-6 motion segment. An association has also been noted linking dysfunctions of the heart meridian and dystonia of the subscapularis muscle. This connection is interesting in view of Koch's finding that cardiac patients have a higher incidence of upper extremity problems, including frozen-shoulder syndrome.[20]

Walther[34] also cited literature by Goodheart, indicating that hypertensive patients with higher systolic blood pressure in the recumbent position than the seated position are often suffering from renal complications, implying involvement of the thoracolumbar area. This clinical finding is in agreement with the earlier publication by Northup.[21]

After an extensive literature review, Jarmel[35] concluded that increased sympathetic tone or decreased vagal tone predisposes the heart to ventricular fibrillation and sudden cardiac death. Intense vagal stimulation tends to cause vasospasm of the coronary arteries, possibly generating cardiac arrhythmias leading to sudden cardiac death. Because upper cervical subluxation can disturb vagal function and upper thoracic subluxation can disturb sympathetic innervation to the heart, Jarmel proposed that such subluxation could generate or aggravate cardiac arrhythmias that are risk factors for cardiac sudden death.

In a later study, Jarmel and others[36] demonstrated that cardiac arrhythmias in 11 asymptomatic patients noted on 24-hour Holter monitoring were improved after correction of cervical or upper thoracic subluxation. Spinal analysis largely consisted of unilateral palpatory tenderness over a spinal joint facet or the paravertebral muscles. Diversified chiropractic adjusting at a frequency of 3 visits per week for 4 weeks was the sole intervention.

Premature ventricular contractions and abnormal heart rate variability during sleep were the two arrhythmias most often noted. The authors offered the following speculation based on their findings[36]:

> Cervical or upper thoracic spinal joint dysfunction may thus act as a chronic trigger of the electrophysiologic substrate favoring the development of arrhythmias. Aggravation of cervical or upper thoracic spinal joint dysfunction may also act as an acute trigger, initiating a sequence of events resulting in sudden death.

A previous study also found electrocardiographic evidence of improvement in arrhythmia under a treatment package that included chiropractic care, dietary advice, and exercise recommendations.[37] Tachycardia and atrial flutter were among the arrhythmias found to respond to this treatment. Unfortunately, the levels of chiropractic adjustment were not noted and the dietary and exercise programs were not described.

Reviewing seminar material by chiropractic technique developer, researcher, and educator Clarence S. Gonstead from 1964-1991, Plaugher and others[38] indicated that cardiac arrhythmias were generally associated with the region T1-T4 or the upper cervicals. Gonstead also maintained that diastolic hypertension was often associated with subluxations from occiput-C5, systolic hypertension was associated with subluxations from C7-T3 and T10-L2, mixed hypertension was most often correlated with subluxations from T10-T12, and hypotension related to adrenocortical insufficiency was associated with subluxations from T8-T12.

Yates and others[39] presented a controlled clinical trial involving activator adjustments with hypertensive patients. A total of 21 hypertensive patients were randomly assigned to active treatment with adjustments in the region of T1-T5, based on Activator analysis, placebo treatment with sham adjustments with the Activator instrument set on 0 tension, and control groups with no intervention. Noting that previous studies may have been confounded by elevated initial readings because of anxiety, Yates and others used a standard psychologic questionnaire before and after the intervention. They found a statistically significant decrease in systolic and diastolic blood pressure in the active treatment group but not in the placebo-treated or control groups. Because the active and control groups did not differ in terms of anxiety reduction, this was ruled out as an explanation for the difference between groups. These findings supported the hypothesis that blood pressure reduction in hypertensives is a true physiologic effect of the chiropractic adjustment.

Plaugher and Bachman[40] published an instructive case study involving a 38-year-old man with a 14-year history of hypertension. He also reported side effects because of his two medications, including bloating sensations, depression, fatigue, and impotence. Low back pain was also reported as an incidental issue.

Examination according to Gonstead analysis protocols revealed evidence of the VSC at various levels, with signs clustering at the midcervical, upper thoracic, and middle thoracic regions. Adjustments were administered once per week. After three visits, the patient's medical doctor was able to stop one medication altogether and reduce the dosage of the other. All medication was discontinued after seven visits. After this, the frequency of visits was reduced to twice per month. Follow-up at 18 months showed that blood pressure was stabilized at normal levels without medication. Bloating, depression, fatigue, and low back pain had abated and normal sexual function had returned.

Peterson[41] reported reduction in serum cholesterol levels by more than 22% in two patients after a single chiropractic adjustment each. These adjustments were administered according to neuroemotional technique (NET) protocols, in which an attempt was made to link a patient's subluxation complex to memories of emotionally stressful events. An elevated level of serum cholesterol is associated with an increased risk of hypertension. Because spontaneous fluctuations in serum cholesterol levels average only 4.8%, Peterson maintained that spontaneous fluctuation was an unlikely explanation for these clinical results.

The results of Peterson's study are particularly interesting when considered in the light of an earlier study by Gutstein and others.[42] In this study, laboratory rats were exposed to electric stimulation of the lateral hypothalamus. Behavior during stimulation was suggestive of anxiety (hurrying and scurrying about the cage, whisker-twitching, and rapid and shallow breathing). Serum cholesterol levels increased as much as 24% during these hypothalamic stimulations. Postmortem histologic examination of the abdominal aorta and left descending coronary artery revealed pathologic changes, including plaque formation, consistent with the early stages of arteriosclerosis. Gutstein and others chose an arteriosclerosis-resistant species for this experiment, making the results all the more impressive. The authors concluded that important components of the development of arteriosclerosis were mediated through the nervous system.

Studying a group of 21 baseball players randomly assigned to either a control group or an upper cervical adjusting group, Schwartzbauer and others[43] observed changes in athletic ability and physiologic measurements. One measure of extremity microcirculation, or capillary count was made by viewing the nailbed of the right and left middle fingers through a microscope at 60× magnification. The number of capillaries visible in one microscopic field was recorded. As microcirculation to the fingers improved, more capillaries became visible. Athletes receiving upper cervical adjustments demonstrated statistically significant improvements in capillary count. The control group did not.

Connelly and Rasmussen[44] reported favorable results with three hypertensive patients, using the cranial procedures of sacro-occipital technique (SOT) developed by DeJarnette. When the patient sought treatment for hypertension, SOT protocols required special attention to the occipitomastoid suture. According to DeJarnette's writings, opening this suture was intended to decompress the jugular foramen, which therefore would reduce interference to the vagus nerve. In the osteopathic field,

Northup made the same observation regarding the occipitomastoid suture.[21]

Clinical Implications

From the perspective of chiropractic analysis, a history of cardiovascular disease does not isolate an area of subluxation with certainty. The findings recorded in the medical, osteopathic, and chiropractic literature made it clear that subluxations from the cranium to the coccyx must be considered. However, increased suspicion is certainly warranted regarding subluxation at the upper thoracic and upper cervical regions and the occipitomastoid suture. Beal's supine compression test can contribute to accurate analysis of the upper thoracic region in general,[26] and assessment of subscapularis function may be useful in monitoring the severity of the T5-T6 VSC in particular.[33]

In patients with signs consistent with renal involvement, including elevated systolic pressure in the recumbent position compared with the seated position, special attention is indicated at the thoracolumbar junction.[21] Chapman's neurolymphatic reflexes may prove a useful manual adjunct to the chiropractic adjustment in such cases.[31]

The patient with a cardiovascular history raises a number of risk-management issues for the chiropractic clinician. At a meeting of medical neurologists sponsored by the American Heart Association, Dr. William Powers of Washington University stated, "Every neurologist in this room has seen two or three people who have suffered this (cerebrovascular accident) after chiropractic manipulation."[45] This statement, quoted or paraphrased, was widely reported by the news media in the United States in February 1994. This statement is exemplary of a perennial effort by various nonchiropractic organizations to create a perception in the general public that chiropractic procedures for the cervical spine are an important risk factor for stroke.

A clear-headed review of the literature reveals that this perception is not evidence-based. Estimates of the probability of stroke after chiropractic manipulation of the cervical spine range from 1 case in 400,000 manipulations to less than 1 in 5 million manipulations.[46-51]

Terrett,[52] reviewing original sources for some

cases reported in the biomedical literature as stroke resulting from chiropractic manipulation, found that many of these cases did *not* involve a doctor of chiropractic. Terrett found that a significant number of these cases of stroke followed cervical manipulation by medical doctors, osteopaths, massage therapists, physical therapists, kung fu instructors, barbers, the patient's spouse, and even the patient.

Viewing this stunning biomedical exaggeration of danger from chiropractic cervical procedures is useful because of the established danger from certain medical procedures widely believed to be "safe." For instance, nonsteroidal antiinflammatory drugs (NSAIDs) are common first-line medical treatment for many musculoskeletal pain syndromes.[53] Yet, gastrointestinal bleeding is a widely reported complication of NSAID use, accounting for an estimated 3,200 deaths per year in the United States alone.[54] Less adverse reactions include renal dysfunction, liver damage, and central nervous system (CNS) disorders.[55,56]

Media warnings concerning the danger of chiropractic cervical manipulation appear absurd when looked at from the point of view of the published evidence. However, this should not lull the clinician into complacency. Reasonable prudence can make safe chiropractic care of the cervical spine even safer. Lauretti[57] advocated the use of nonmanipulative adjusting techniques for high-risk patients.

Manipulation generally involves a high-velocity motion of a joint past its physiologic range of motion, usually resulting in an audible cavitation noise. Many nonmanipulative techniques exist that are generally known as *nonforce adjustments.* Lauretti suggested that nonmanipulative adjusting be strongly considered when the patient has a history of dizziness, drop-attacks, diplopia, difficulties in speaking or swallowing, or ataxia. These indicators are particularly significant when provoked by cervical motion, especially rotation and extension (particularly with a latency of 15 to 30 seconds). Avoiding extremes of rotation and extension in such patients is wise, whether manipulative or nonmanipulative adjustments are used.

To the previous indicators, one might add the auscultation of bruits over the cervical or carotid arteries and a previous history of stroke and adverse reactions to cervical manipulation and current use of anticoagulant drugs.

Because the risk of stroke resulting from chiropractic care is more a phenomenon of perception than fact, the patient's perceptions should be addressed. If the patient expresses a fear of cervical manipulation, the use of a nonmanipulative adjusting technique is wise risk management.

An important aspect of patient perception was discussed by Plaugher and Bachman.[40] They noted that a patient on antihypertensive medication may experience additional lowering of blood pressure as a result of chiropractic care. Although this is beneficial in the long run, the combined effects of the drugs and the adjustments may render the patient temporarily hypotensive. A patient experiencing vertigo secondary to hypotension after a cervical adjustment may unfairly accuse the doctor of chiropractic (DC) of causing a stroke or some other form of damage. Explaining the possibility of transient hypotension to such a patient at the beginning of care can save the patient much anxiety and preserve the doctor's reputation.

As an additional risk management precaution, the DC should avoid describing a chiropractic technique as a "blood pressure control technique" or other such phrase. Describing a chiropractic technique in a way that implies cure or treatment of any disease is a slippery slope. This is especially true when the disease is a cardiovascular disorder. An offer to cure or treat disease can be seen as an implied contract that is broken when any patient fails to recover under care.

The chiropractic adjustment should never be presented as a cardiovascular treatment. What chiropractors treat, or more appropriately reduce or correct is the VSC and other subluxations, including cranial faults. These subluxations create disturbances of neurologic tone. Although subluxation and subsequent disturbed neurologic tone can provoke or aggravate a particular cardiovascular disease symptom in a particular person, it is the patient not the disease that is adjusted. The DC is justified in following blood pressure, arrhythmia, or any other cardiovascular manifestation as a general barometer of the patient's neurologic fitness but not as the actual rationale for the delivery of the adjustment.

For instance, if the T4-T5 motion segment is

found to be subluxated, it should be adjusted whether the patient's blood pressure is elevated. If the patient's blood pressure is elevated, the DC may choose to monitor it whether signs of the T4-T5 VSC exist.

Alerting patients to the potential benefit of subluxation correction for their overall health and wellness, including cardiovascular fitness, is essential. The normalization of arrhythmia in asympto-matic subjects[36] and improvement in microcirculation in healthy athletes[43] are early indicators of what future investigations may find in terms of the preventive role of the chiropractic adjustment. Hopefully, future chiropractic literature will be as rich in this arena of preventive cardiovascular health and fitness as past literature has been in the area of active cardiovascular disease.

STUDY GUIDE

1. The heart has specialized muscle fibers capable of maintaining an automatic rhythm, even in the absence of direct autonomic innervation. What are these fibers called and where are they located?
2. If the previous statement is true, why are sympathetic and parasympathetic innervation important to the heart's normal function?
3. What does vagal stimulation do to the heart? Is this sympathetic or parasympathetic?
4. Where does the major sympathetic innervation to the heart originate? Relate this to T4 syndrome.
5. Where do the preganglionic fibers of the above nerves synapse?
6. What is a baroreceptor and where would you find one?
7. Explain the baroreceptor in terms of tone. Explain this in terms of postural changes.
8. Could a postpartum coccygeal or SI subluxation generate tachycardia? How?
9. Describe the possible effects of the upper cervical VSC on the heart. How would this happen?
10. Describe the oculocardiac reflex.
11. Describe Henry Winsor's findings in relation to this chapter.
12. Describe Louisa Burns' study of genetically related rabbits with T3 subluxation. What is the importance of this study and how would you use it to educate a patient?
13. Describe Carl Cleveland Jr.'s findings regarding T12 subluxation. Why is this important in terms of patients with cardiac problems?
14. Relate Ansari's findings on SBS to the hypotheses of previous researchers.
15. Discuss Mannino's study of Chapman's reflexes on serum aldosterone levels. Which neurolymphatic reflexes did he use and at what spinal levels are they located? Why are his findings important to chiropractic?
16. Relate Walther's findings regarding the heart meridian and T5-6 subluxation to the work of Koch.
17. In Plaugher's review of Gonstead's work, what were the differences between the findings on diastolic and systolic hypertension? Although we must avoid a road map approach to subluxation and its results, what might be the significance of these findings?
18. What is the incidence of stroke following cervical manipulation as opposed to the number of deaths per year from NSAID use? Name some of the kinds of individuals who actually delivered the "chiropractic" in Terrett's study.
19. What are some indicators that could cause you to look to minimal force techniques for a patient?
20. Explain one possible effect of chiropractic adjustments on patients taking antihypertensive medication. How would you explain this to a patient?

REFERENCES

1. Guyton AC: *Basic neuroscience: anatomy and physiology,* p 323, Philadelphia, 1991, WB Saunders.
2. Warwick R, Williams PL: *Gray's anatomy,* ed 35 (Brit), p 1077, Philadelphia, 1973, WB Saunders.
3. Guyton AC: *Basic neuroscience: anatomy and physiology,* p 328, Philadelphia, 1991, WB Saunders.
4. Warwick R, Williams PL: *Gray's anatomy,* ed 35 (Brit), p 1070, Philadelphia, 1973, WB Saunders.
5. Guyton AC: *Basic neuroscience: anatomy and physiology,* p 328, Philadelphia, 1991, WB Saunders.
6. Warwick R, Williams PL: *Gray's anatomy,* ed 35 (Brit), p 1082, Philadelphia, 1973, WB Saunders.
7. Guyton AC: *Basic neuroscience: anatomy and physiology,* p 334, Philadelphia, 1991, WB Saunders.
8. Homewood AE: *The neurodynamics of the vertebral subluxation,* p 247, St. Petersburg, Fla, 1977, Valkyrie.
9. Gottesman MH et al: Cardiac arrest caused by trigeminal neuralgia, *Headache* 36:392, 1996.
10. Chusid JG: *Correlative neuroanatomy and functional neurology,* p 106, Los Altos, 1979, Lange.
11. Guyton AC: *Basic neuroscience: anatomy and physiology,* p 337, Philadelphia, 1991, WB Saunders.
12. Palmer DD: *The science art and philosophy of chiropractic,* p 18, Portland, Ore, 1910, Portland Publishing House.
13. Palmer DD: *The science art and philosophy of chiropractic,* p 951, Portland, Ore, 1910, Portland Publishing House.
14. Winsor HK: Sympathetic segmental disturbances, II, *Med Times* 49:267, 1922.
15. Burns L, Steudenberg G, Vollbrecht WJ: Family of rabbits with second thoracic and other lesions, *J Am Osteopath Assoc* 37:908, 1937.
16. Burns L: Preliminary report of cardiac changes following the correction of third thoracic lesions, *J Am Osteopath Assoc* 42:3, 1943.
17. Burns L: Tracings showing pulse changes following certain lesions, *J Am Osteopath Assoc* 44:4, 1945.
18. Becker AD: Manipulative osteopathy in cardiac therapy, *J Am Osteopath Assoc* 38:317, 1939.
19. Cleveland CS Jr: Researching the subluxation on the domestic rabbit, *Sci Rev Chiro* 1(4):5, 1965.
20. Koch RS: A somatic component in heart disease, *J Am Osteopath Assoc* 60:735, 1961.
21. Northup TL: Manipulative management of hypertension, *J Am Osteopath Assoc* 60:973, 1961.
22. Goldstein M, editor: *Monograph no. 15. The research status of spinal manipulative therapy,* Washington, DC, 1975, U.S. Department of Health, Education and Welfare.
23. Larson NJ: Summary of site and occurrence of paraspinal soft tissue changes of patients in the intensive care unit, *J Am Osteopath Assoc* 75:840, 1976.
24. Cox JM et al: Palpable musculoskeletal findings in coronary artery disease: results of a double-blind study, *J Am Osteopath Assoc* 82:832, 1983.
25. Cox JM, Rogers FJ: Incidence of osteophytic lipping of the thoracic spine in coronary artery disease—results of a pilot study, *J Am Osteopath Assoc* 82:837, 1983.
26. Beal MC: Palpatory testing for somatic dysfunction in patients with cardiovascular disease, *J Am Osteopath Assoc* 82:822, 1983.
27. Ansara A: The "straight back" syndrome: current perspective: more often associated with valvular heart disease than pseudoheart disease: a prospective clinical, electrocardiographic, roentgenographic, and echocardiographic study of 50 patients, *Clin Cardiol* 8:290, 1985.
28. Fracheboud R, Kraus S, Choiniere B: A survey of anterior thoracic adjustments, *Chiropractic* 1:89, 1988.
29. Zachman ZJ et al: Understanding the anterior thoracic adjustment: (a concept of a sectional subluxation), *Chiro Technique* 1:30, 1989.
30. Morgan JP et al: A controlled trial of spinal manipulation in the management of hypertension, *J Am Osteopath Assoc* 84:308, 1985.
31. Mannino JR: The application of neurologic reflexes to the treatment of hypertension, *J Am Osteopath Assoc* 74:25, 1975.
32. Wagnon RJ, Sandefur RM, Ratliff CR: Serum aldosterone changes after specific chiropractic manipulation, *Am J Chiropr Med* 1:66, 1988.
33. Walther DS: *Applied kinesiology—synopsis,* p 222, Pueblo, Colo, 1988, Systems DC.
34. Walther DS: *Applied kinesiology—synopsis,* p 524, Pueblo, Colo, 1988, Systems DC.
35. Jarmel ME: Possible role of spinal joint dysfunction in the genesis of sudden cardiac death, *J Manipulative Physiol Ther* 12:469, 1989.
36. Jarmel ME et al: Improvement of cardiac autonomic regulation following spinal manipulative therapy. In Cleveland C, Haldeman S, editors: *Conference proceedings of the chiropractic centennial foundation,* p 359, Davenport, Iowa, 1995, Chiropractic Centennial Foundation.
37. Lott GS et al: ECG improvements following the combination of chiropractic adjustments, diet, and exercise therapy, *J Chiro Res Clin Investig* 5:37, 1990.
38. Plaugher G et al: Spinal management for the patient with a visceral concomitant. In Plaugher G, editor: *Textbook of clinical chiropractic: a specific biomechanical approach,* p 365, Baltimore, 1993, Williams & Wilkins.
39. Yates RG et al: Effects of chiropractic treatment on blood pressure and anxiety: a randomized, controlled trial, *J Manipulative Physiol Ther* 11:484, 1988.
40. Plaugher G, Bachman TR: Chiropractic management of a hypertensive patient: a case study, *J Manipulative Physiol Ther* 16:544, 1993.
41. Peterson KB: Two cases of spinal manipulation performed while the patient contemplated an associated stress event: the effect of the manipulation/contemplation on serum cholesterol levels in hypercholesterolemic subjects, *Chiro Technique* 7:53, 1995.
42. Gutstein WH et al: Neural factors contribute to atherogenesis, *Science* 199:449, 1978.
43. Schwartzbauer J et al: Athletic performance and physiological measures in baseball players following upper cervical chiropractic care: a pilot study, *J Vertebr Sublux Res* 1(4):33, 1997.
44. Connelly DM, Rasmussen SA: The effect of cranial adjusting on hypertension: a case report, *Chiro Technique* 10:75, 1998.

45. Doctors say twist in neck can trigger a stroke: *The Washington Post,* 14 (col 1), Feb 20, 1994.

46. Jaskoviak P: Complications arising from manipulation of the cervical spine, *J Manipulative Physiol Ther* 3:213, 1980.

47. Henderson DJ, Cassidy JD: Vertebral artery syndrome, p 194. In Vernon H, editor: *Upper cervical syndrome: chiropractic diagnosis and treatment,* Baltimore, 1988, Williams & Wilkins.

48. Dvorak J, Orelli F: How dangerous is manipulation to the cervical spine? *Man Med* 2:1, 1985.

49. Patjin J: Complications in manual medicine: a review of the literature, *Man Med* 6:89, 1991.

50. Carey PF: A report on the occurrence of cerebral vascular accidents in chiropractic practice, *J Can Chiro Assoc* 37:104, 1993.

51. Klougart N, Leboef-Yde C, Rasmussen LR: Safety in chiropractic practice, part I, the occurrence of cerebrovascular accidents after manipulation to the neck in Denmark from 1978-1988, *J Manipulative Physiol Ther* 19:371, 1996.

52. Terrett AGJ: Misuse of the literature by medical authors in discussing spinal manipulative therapy injury, *J Manipulative Physiol Ther* 18:203, 1995.

53. Dillin W, Uppal GS: Analysis of medications used in the treatment of cervical disc degeneration, *Orthop Clin North Am* 23:421, 1992.

54. Fries JF: Assessing and understanding patient risk, *Scand J Rheumatol* 92:21, 1992 (suppl).

55. Carson JL, Willett LR: Toxicity of nonsteroidal anti-inflammatory drugs: an overview of the epidemiological evidence, *Drugs* 46:243, 1993 (suppl 1).

56. Saag KG, Cowdery JS: Nonsteroidal anti-inflammatory drugs: balancing benefits and risks, *Spine* 9:1530, 1994.

57. Lauretti WJ: The comparative safety of chiropractic, p 231. In Redwood D, editor: *Contemporary chiropractic,* New York, 1997, Churchill Livingstone.

CHAPTER 11

Breathing and the Vertebral Subluxation Complex

Charles S. Masarsky, DC • *Marion Todres-Masarsky, DC*

The autonomic innervation of the lungs and bronchi has much in common with the autonomic innervation of the heart, with major parasympathetic innervation from the vagus nerve and major sympathetic innervation from T1-T5.[1] However, the act of breathing is not possible with autonomic innervation alone. The somatic innervation to skeletal muscles, including the diaphragm, external intercostals, internal intercostals, sternocleidomastoids, levator scapulae, serrati, scalenes, abdominals, trapezii, latissimus dorsi, and pectoralis major and pectoralis minor, makes inspiration and expiration possible.[2,3]

In other words, breathing is a musculoskeletal act in the service of a visceral systemic requirement. More than most bodily functions, breathing straddles the somatovisceral interface. For this reason, the clinical literature linking the vertebral subluxation complex (VSC) to disturbances of breathing is important to chiropractic clinicians of all technique schools.

Chronic Obstructive Pulmonary Disease

Chronic obstructive pulmonary disease (COPD) has attracted significant attention within the chiropractic and osteopathic research communities. A paper of historic and scientific interest was presented by Miller[4] at an early interdisciplinary conference on the research status of spinal manipulative therapy, sponsored by the National Institute of Neurological and Communicative Disorders and Stroke (USA). In this study, 44 COPD patients underwent osteopathic examination. Signs of somatic dysfunction noted in this examination included asymmetry of paraspinal muscle tension, loss of intersegmental mobility, skin drag (palpatory assessment of asymmetry of local alteration in friction offered to the examiner's finger as it moves along the patient's paraspinal skin) and red reaction (visual assessment of asymmetry or unusual intensity in reactive skin hyperemia). On the basis of this evaluation, the greatest number of abnormal findings was in the T2-T5 region.

Miller's patients were randomly assigned to treatment and control groups. Both groups received standard medical interventions, including bronchodilators, postural drainage, and breathing exercises, and the treatment group also received osteopathic manipulation two times per week (the duration of care was not mentioned). Lung volumes were measured and patients filled out a questionnaire on respiratory symptoms.

The lung volume results were inconclusive; both groups improved, with no significant difference between groups. However, more patients in the treatment group reported the ability to walk greater distances, along with fewer colds, less coughing, and less dyspnea than before treatment.

A case report of a COPD patient under chiropractic care was published by Masarsky and Weber.[5] After a 2-week baseline period, diversified chiropractic adjustments were administered at various levels, usually including the upper cervical and upper thoracic regions. The frequency of visits was 3 times weekly for more than 14 months. Motorized intersegmental traction, vitamin C supplementation, cranial adjusting, and neurolymphatic reflex stimulation for the lungs and diaphragm were also included in the chiropractic regimen.

Outcome measures included lung volumes (forced vital capacity [FVC] and forced expiratory volume in 1 second [FEV-1]), a 10-point severity scale (with 1 being the mildest and 10 being the most extreme) for coughing, dyspnea and fatigue, and a daily count of laryngospasms. Up to 3 laryngospasms per week had been the norm for this patient for 17 years.

Mean scores during the last 7 months of this study were compared with the mean baseline scores. FVC increased by more than 1 L and FEV-1 increased by more than 0.3 L. Coughing intensity, dyspnea, and fatigue all decreased sharply. The patient reported no laryngospasms during the final 5 months of the study. Improved lung volumes lagged behind the subjective improvements by several months.

Asthma

A case series presented by Hviid[6] failed to gather enough data to provide calculations of statistical significance. However, the preliminary data gathered was useful. Of 17 symptomatic asthma patients, more than 75% reported subjective improvement by the eighth chiropractic visit. More than 35% were symptom-free by the eighth visit. Five of these patients demonstrated increased vital capacity.

Nilsson and Christiansen[7] published a retrospective study of 79 patients with medically diagnosed bronchial asthma. Patients who experienced significant improvement with chiropractic care tended to have less severe asthma symptoms when they sought treatment at an earlier age of onset than patients with a poor response under chiropractic care. Outcome measures included medication usage, frequency of asthma attacks, working capacity, and lung volumes.

An instructive case report involving pediatric asthma was presented by Bachman and Lantz.[8] After three Gonstead adjustments at T3, T12, and the sacrum, the 34-month-old patient experienced 8 weeks of freedom from symptoms. During the previous year, the patient had weekly asthma attacks, 20 of which were severe enough to require visits to the hospital emergency department. An exacerbation at 8 weeks followed a fall from a step ladder; this time the asthma symptoms were accompanied by nocturnal enuresis. Both sets of

symptoms resolved after three more adjustments at the same levels. After a full year of freedom from symptoms, the boy fell from a horse and experienced a return of asthma and enuresis. A single adjustment resolved this exacerbation. Bachman and Lantz reported no recurrence at 2 years of follow-up.

Three case studies involving two children and one adult with medically established diagnoses of bronchial asthma were presented by Lines.[9] All three of these cases combined chiropractic adjustments and the use of a food diary technique to identify allergens. Thoracic adjusting was used in two cases and lumbar adjusting in two cases (the techniques and analyses were not specified). At the time of the report, these patients had been free of asthma symptoms anywhere from 6 months to 2 years. Other problems including ear infections, abdominal pain, nightmares, eczema, and low back pain apparently resolved by the combination of clinical ecology and chiropractic adjustments.

Although the clinical ecology approach alone having produced these results is possible, Lines related an instance in which an asthma attack was quickly resolved after an adjustment. The author also stated that asthma patients would often self-refer for an adjustment when an attack appeared because of the immediate relief they characteristically experienced.

Peet and others[10] reported encouraging results with eight pediatric patients with medically diagnosed asthma. After 10 adjustments using chiropractic biophysics technique (CBP) protocols, this patient group demonstrated an average increase in peak flow rate of 25%. In the cases of seven of the eight children, the parents also reported a decrease in medication use.

Killinger[11] reported the case of an 18-year-old man with a 2-year history of medically diagnosed asthma. This patient's first asthma attack occurred shortly after a sports injury. At the time of the patient visit, he was experiencing daily attacks that left him exhausted. Results of medical intervention were disappointing. Palmer upper cervical (HIO) adjustments were administered 3 times over a period of 4 months; the patient was then monitored by correspondence and annual visits to the Palmer clinic over a 5 year period.

Asthma attacks dropped sharply in frequency and severity during this period. Eosinophil counts elevated at the first visit were reduced to normal levels. By the second year of the study, attacks were strictly nocturnal and relatively rare, with intervals of several months sometimes separating them. Concurrent improvement was noted in x-ray, palpation, and neurocalometer paraspinal temperature findings.

This 1995 paper was part of an effort by Killinger and others[11] to archive the huge body of clinical data collected between 1935 and 1962 at the B.J. Palmer Chiropractic Clinic. This data was once thought to have been lost or deliberately destroyed, but file cabinets containing thousands of intact patient folders from this period were recently recovered from an abandoned elevator shaft at the Palmer College campus in Davenport, Iowa. Selected cases are currently being prepared for journal publication. The asthma case previously discussed is one of the results of this effort, which uniquely combines historic and clinical research.

Nielsen and others[12] reported a randomized clinical trial of chiropractic care for adult asthma patients. Although no statistically significant differences were found between sham adjustments and actual chiropractic intervention, the sham procedure may not have been as biologically inert as these investigators had anticipated.

The sham maneuver consisted of gentle, apparently specific manual pressure, with the patient positioned on a drop table. While this light pressure was applied with one hand, the drop mechanism was simultaneously released with the other hand. Because the whole patient sample experienced improvement by the end of the study in asthma symptom severity and nonspecific bronchial hyperreactivity, or a measure of resistance to histamine-induced bronchial obstruction, the sham adjustments and the actual adjustments may have elicited healing effects.

Graham and Pistolese[13] gathered self-reported changes in impairment experienced by 81 pediatric asthma patients from a group of chiropractic practices in Michigan. The authors developed a new pencil-and-paper instrument similar in format to the Oswestry Low Back Pain Disability questionnaire, with modifications to relate the questions to breathing difficulty instead of low back pain. This new questionnaire was found to have good test-retest reliability.

Statistically significant improvements in the scores on this instrument were reported for more than 90% of these subjects 60 days after chiropractic care had commenced, compared with the prechiropractic scores. Although the lack of a gold standard pencil-and-paper instrument for asthma assessment makes assessing this new instrument's validity difficult, reduced frequency of asthma attacks and decreased perceived need for medication accompanying improvement in questionnaire scores was encouraging.

Peet[14] presented the case of an 8-year-old girl medically diagnosed with asthma 3 years before initiation of care. Interestingly, this patient exhibited no evidence of respiratory disease until she suffered a traumatic injury. This injury was severe enough to cause dislocation of the left elbow. Beclovent and Albyterol inhaler was used by this patient one to three times per day before her first visit.

Chiropractic analysis included postural assessment and x-ray examination according to chiropractic biophysics (CBP) protocols. Cervical and thoracic subluxations were identified, with the signs clustering at the upper cervical area. After eight adjustments during a period of 2½ weeks, the mother stated that the child had not used her inhaler for 2 days, her wheezing had ceased, and she could run without gasping. Postural reassessment indicated substantial improvement. Follow-up x-ray at the eleventh visit verified these improvements in subluxation signs. At the time of publication, the patient was reported to have been free of asthmatic attacks for 4 months without medication.

An important and controversial study was recently published by Balon and others[15]. After a 3-week baseline evaluation period, 91 children who had continuing symptoms of asthma despite usual medical therapy were randomly assigned to receive either actual or simulated chiropractic adjustments for 4 months. Morning peak expiratory flow was the major outcome measure. Although both groups of children exhibited improved peak flow, no significant difference existed between the groups. No significant difference between groups was noted in any of the secondary outcome measures such quality-of-life, including nighttime symptoms.

The authors offer the following possible explanations for the results of this study:

1. Patients in both groups may have responded favorably to frequent professional attention.

2. Patients in both groups may have been growing out of their symptoms at the time of the study.
3. Patients in both groups may have complied more with their medication schedules during the study than before the study.

One explanation that was not offered was that the simulated treatment was not as biologically inert as a placebo should be. Simulated treatment included several distraction and low-amplitude, low-velocity impulse maneuvers to the cervical, thoracic, and lumbopelvic areas. As in the previously cited paper by Nielsen and others,[12] Balon and others assumed that these simulated adjustments would not affect any correction of subluxation. This assumption is questionable.

Unfortunately, preintervention and postintervention palpation findings were not reported. Without this information or some other type of subluxation-based outcome measure no way of knowing whether the sham procedures inadvertently corrected subluxations exists. The development of truly inert sham procedures is a serious methodologic problem in controlled chiropractic research. Unless subluxation-based outcome measures are routinely reported in such research, the problem is unlikely to be overcome anytime soon.

An additional problem with the paper by Balon and others was recently discussed by Rosner.[16] Rosner noted that in a presentation at a convention of the American Thoracic Society 17 months before publication in the *New England Journal of Medicine,* Balon and others stated that the patients receiving real chiropractic adjustments improved in terms of nighttime symptoms to a significantly greater degree than those patients receiving the sham procedure. This finding is at variance with the data and conclusions noted in the journal paper.

Perhaps the findings presented at the American Thoracic Society were in error and were corrected before journal publication. A much more disturbing possibility is that editorial pressure was brought to bear on the authors to sanitize the paper of any findings favorable to chiropractic. Unfortunately, this discrepancy remains unexplained to date (April, 1999).

Somatic Dyspnea

Masarsky and Weber[17] reported six cases of dyspnea that resolved on correction of the VSC and related somatic dysfunctions. The term *somatic dyspnea* has been coined to refer to such clinical situations. All six patients demonstrated midthoracic fixations on motion palpation, leading the authors to suspect restriction of rib excursion and/or disturbance to the sympathetic nerve supply to the lungs and bronchi. One patient reported a clear cut association between a C2-3 correction and relief from the dyspnea she had experienced, suggesting a connection to the phrenic nerve. The most common extravertebral dysfunction associated with somatic dyspnea was at the temporomandibular joint. The nature of the association between dysfunction at this joint and somatic dyspnea is not clear.

Somatic dyspnea is a symptom, or a subjective phenomenon that is not always accompanied by measurable depression of lung volumes. However, the improved subjective ease of breathing is often rapid and dramatic. In one of the reported cases (Case #1), somatic dyspnea was recognized retrospectively. Although this patient had not mentioned difficulty in breathing during her intake history, she remarked after the adjustment, "I feel like I'm taking in more air." Follow-up examination 4 days later revealed no significant improvement in FVC or FEV-1, even though her relief from dyspnea was still marked.

This case highlights the importance of remembering that somatic dyspnea is a symptom—a subjective phenomenon. It is not always accompanied by measurable depression of lung volumes, and even rapid and dramatic relief from dyspnea does not always correlate with measurably improved ventilation. This case is also typical of many chiropractic patients in that she initiated care with a musculoskeletal pain symptom, not a respiratory one. Her dyspnea was either no longer noticed because of chronicity or was not mentioned because of its seeming irrelevance at the time of her visit to a "back doctor." The prevalence and significance of somatic dyspnea in the chiropractic patient population cannot be explored until better methods of uncovering this symptom at intake are developed; merely including the question, "Do you have difficulty in breathing?" on the case history form is apparently not adequate.

Hiccups

The bouts of uncontrollable stacatto inspiration known as *hiccups* are usually a minor annoyance. However, long-lasting bouts of sufficient severity can be debilitating and even dangerous. Homewood[18] reported that hiccup episodes can often be brought to an end by chiropractic adjustments. Subluxations are generally found in the midcervical region, presumably resulting from the motor innervation of the phrenic nerve that controls the diaphragm or in the lower thoracic area, from which the phrenic nerve receives afferent innervation.

Improved Lung Volumes in Lung-Normal Patients

A number of studies have demonstrated improved lung volumes in patients without hypoventilation after one or more chiropractic adjustments. Masarsky and Weber[19] presented a retrospective study in which FVC and FEV-1 improved in a sample of 50 chiropractic patients after one to three adjustments. The majority of these patients had no pulmonary complaints at initiation of care and demonstrated FVC and FEV-1 within normal limits at intake examination. An additional instance of spirometric improvement in a lung-normal patient appeared in a later case series published by the same authors (Case #1).[20] Diversified adjusting based on motion palpation and/or applied kinesiologic challenge was the major intervention in both of these studies.

Kessinger[21] reported FVC and FEV-1 improvement in a sample of 55 patients after they had received chiropractic care for the correction of upper cervical subluxation. These improvements were significant in the 33 patients with depressed lung volumes at their first doctor's visit and the 22 patients with initially normal lung volumes. Patients ranging from 48 to 80 years of age demonstrated a significantly greater improvement than the younger patients. These findings imply that many people, even those with normal lung volumes, are functioning well below their potential and that this suboptimal respiratory function is especially common within the middle-aged and elderly population.

The general health implications of improved pulmonary function cannot be overstated. Lung volumes have long been recognized as a biologic marker of aging. Furthermore, a recent mortality study has demonstrated that individuals with depressed FEV-1 scores are more likely to die from all causes, not just respiratory diseases, at 4 years, 15 years, and 24 years postmeasurement, when compared with those with FEV-1 scores at or above expected values.[22] This observation holds true across all adult age groups, including smokers and nonsmokers. Apparently, reduced pulmonary function is a good general indicator of a person's vulnerability to a wide variety of serious health problems. Conversely, improving pulmonary function through chiropractic care can be seen as a contribution to a person's overall vitality.

STUDY GUIDE

1. What is the major autonomic innervation to the lungs and bronchi?
2. Name six muscles that assist in respiration.
3. In Miller's study presented at the NINCDS conference, where were the greatest number of abnormal findings discovered?
4. Describe the relationship of improved lung volumes with the rate of subjective improvement in the Masarsky and Weber COPD paper.
5. Name an important finding in the Nilsson and Christiansen asthma paper.
6. Describe the changes in peak flow readings in Peet's original asthma case.
7. In the asthma case written by Killinger, describe the findings in blood work. Why is this worthy of notice to chiropractors and what would be the role of this kind of finding in future research?
8. Describe the perfect sham adjustment for use in research.
9. Describe the possible importance of trauma in relation to the histories of the subjects mentioned in the studies.
10. What is somatic dyspnea? What is the most common extravertebral finding in the Masarsky and Weber retrospective study? Hypothesize as to its significance.
11. In Kessinger's paper *Changes in pulmonary function associated with upper cervical specific chiropractic care*, which group showed the greatest improvement? Why is this significant?
12. What is an FEV-1 score? What is an FEV score?
13. How could a VSC at L5 lead to somatic dyspnea?
14. If an asthmatic patient is able to decrease use of medication after receiving chiropractic care but is unable to completely discontinue use, has chiropractic failed the patient?

REFERENCES

1. Chusid JG: *Correlative neuroanatomy and functional neurology,* p 143, Los Altos, Calif, 1979, Lange Medical Publications.
2. Guyton AC: *Textbook of medical physiology,* p 517, Philadelphia, 1976, WB Saunders.
3. Basmajian JV: *Muscles alive,* p 356, Baltimore, 1979, Williams & Wilkins.
4. Miller WD: Treatment of visceral disorders by manipulative therapy, p 295. In Goldstein M, editor: *The research status of spinal manipulative therapy,* Bethesda, 1975, National Institute of Neurological and Communicative Disorders and Stroke.
5. Masarsky CS, Weber M: Chiropractic management of chronic obstructive pulmonary disease, *J Manipulative Physiol Ther* 11:505, 1988.
6. Hviid C: A comparison of the effect of chiropractic treatment on respiratory function in patients with respiratory distress symptoms and patients without, *Bull Eur Chiropr Union* 26:17, 1978.
7. Nilsson N, Christiansen B: Prognostic factors in bronchial asthma in chiropractic practice, *Chiro J Austral* 18:85, 1988.
8. Bachman TR, Lantz CA: Management of pediatric asthma and enuresis with probable traumatic etiology, p 14. In *Proceedings of the national conference on chiropractic pediatrics,* Arlington, Va, 1991, International Chiropractors Association.
9. Lines DH: A wholistic approach to the treatment of bronchial asthma in a chiropractic practice, *Chiro J Austral* 23:4, 1993.
10. Peet JB, Marko SK, Piekarczyk W: Chiropractic response in the pediatric patient with asthma: a pilot study, *Chiro Pediatr* 1:9, 1995.
11. Killinger LZ: Chiropractic care in the treatment of asthma, *Palmer J Res* 2:74, 1995.
12. Nielsen N et al: Chronic asthma and chiropractic spinal manipulation: a randomized clinical trial, *Clin Exp Allergy* 25:80, 1995.
13. Graham RL, Pistolese RA: An impairment rating analysis of asthmatic children under chiropractic care, *J Vertebr Sublux Res* 1(4):41, 1997.
14. Peet JB: Case study: eight year old female with chronic asthma, *Chiro Pediatr* 3:9, 1997.
15. Balon J et al: A comparison of active and simulated chiropractic manipulation as adjunctive treatment for childhood asthma, *New England J Med* 339:1013, 1998.
16. Rosner AL: A walk on the wild side of allopathic medicine: going ballistic instead of holistic, *Dynamic Chiro* 17(9):10, 1999.
17. Masarsky CS, Weber M: Somatic dyspnea and the orthopedics of respiration, *Chiro Technique* 3:26, 1991.
18. Homewood AE: *The Neurodynamics of the vertebral subluxation,* p 194, St. Petersburg, Fl, 1977, Valkyrie Press.
19. Masarsky CS, Weber M: Chiropractic and lung volumes—a retrospective study, *ACA J Chiro* 20(9):65, 1986.
20. Masarsky CS, Weber M: Screening spirometry in the chiropractic examination, *ACA J Chiro* 23(2):67, 1989.
21. Kessinger R: Changes in pulmonary function associated with upper cervical specific chiropractic care, *J Vertebr Sublux Res* 1(3):43, 1997.
22. Beaty TH et al: Effects of pulmonary function on mortality, *J Chron Dis* 38:703, 1985.

CHAPTER 12

Chiropractic Aspects of Headache as a Somatovisceral Problem

Darryl D. Curl, DDS, DC

Headache

The concept of headache is as broad as the subject of pain. The student who first encounters the headache literature will immediately realize that the subject is as voluminous and interesting as it is perplexing. An extraordinary amount has been written about headaches and has interested healers, philosophers, organized religion, and the many people who suffer from headache. In the last century, at least 100,000 articles and 1500 books have been written on headache. Explanations for headache range from the divine (original sin) to the microscopic (the nitric oxide molecule).

The reader will also notice an obvious bias within the literature toward migraine. Migraine is distinctive throughout history; therefore it is easier to follow than other less glamorous varieties of headache. Although this bias cannot entirely explain the headache phenomenon, it profoundly influences our modern views regarding nearly all recurring headache.

In primitive societies, illness and pain were typically seen as punishment delivered from afar. In fact, the word *pain* comes from the Latin *poena*, meaning "penalty, fine," or "punishment." This ancient connotation, as it applies to headache, survives today in a thinly disguised and largely unmodified form. For example, the pressures and tensions of modern life are still considered routine causes of headache. In this instance, the obvious punishment is headache, which is cast on the individual externally by society's demon forces of pressure and tension.

The Scientist Versus the Clinician

When studying the history of headache, one is acutely aware of two separate, parallel trends. One represents the progression of theories, major contributors, and discoveries that gradually contribute to our accumulation of headache knowledge. Its counterpart is the practice of the average clinician. In the case of twentieth century allopathic physicians, they sought simultaneously to restore physiologic balance and eliminate bad or vitiated, consumable elements such as red wine, cheese, chocolate, preserved meats, pollution, chemical exposure, and tobacco smoke from their patients. The only troubling question for clinicians was not whether to resort to drugging, purging, surgery, hospitalization, and so on but to what degree.

The research scientist often trails established clinical practice by providing a posthoc rationale for established studies. This is particularly true of headache therapy, as science has only began a serious investigation of the mechanism of headache in the last 2 decades. Therefore not surprisingly, the contribution of science to innovative headache treatment has so far been modest. To this day, most headache treatments, including chiropractic, remain pragmatic. They are often derived from timeworn practice, such as aspirin, pain medications, and manipulation, or from common-sense methods such as in home care, massage, heat and cold compresses, improved posture, rest, and reassurance.

Early Focus on the Cervical Spine

Attempts to find answers to many of the puzzling questions about headache began to emerge in the late 1930s. Clinical and laboratory studies were initiated on a variety of fronts, many using modern concepts of experimental design. Studies examining extracranial sources of headache first emerged at this time and turned attention, albeit less focused and energetic than its pharmaceutical counterparts, to the cervical spine.

In fact, not until 1933 did researchers give serious consideration to extracranial structures as either a cause or contributor to headache. Lewis' pioneering work in this area[1] is of particular interest to upper cervical chiropractic practitioners. He stated, "The origin of headache from muscle or aponeurosis attached to the occiput can be determined by inducing such headache in the quiescent period by irritating the corresponding structures."[1]

Lewis apparently happened on a great discovery the importance of which was further strengthened approximately 30 years later. In 1996, scientists at the University of Maryland discovered a physical connection between the upper cervical muscular system and the central nervous system (CNS).[1] Their observation that the rectus capitus posterior minor (RCMP) forms a connective tissue bridge between the dorsal spinal dura at the atlantooccipital junction was observed in each of 10 specimens. They postulated that the arrangement of muscle fibers appear to function to resist infolding of the dura toward the spinal cord during head and neck extension. Any failure to do so, as conjectured, may lead to entrapment of the pain-sensitive dura, thus leading to headache. B.J. Palmer, the originator of the upper cervical technique, would have undoubtedly been heartened by these recent findings in upper cervical anatomy.[2]

Headache Theories Versus Factual Support

Incremental discoveries about the nature of headache were made during the first 30 years of the twentieth century but not until the 1980s did significant progress toward headache understanding occur. Although theories on headache proliferated, little factual data to support these theories were developing from the basic sciences or clinical studies. Often, much to the dismay of the headache sufferer, treatment proceeded with flimsy scientific rationale. In the past a woman unfortunate enough to have a persistent headache was given a hysterectomy in the hopes that her headache would cease.[3]

Difficulties with Headache Research

A time-tested rule in headache research exists, essentially stating that around 60% to 90% of headache sufferers will benefit from an experimental therapy, regardless of the type of therapy tested. Approximately 33% will benefit from placebo therapy.

Clinicians studying the effectiveness of headache therapy can be compared with scientists studying sand dunes in the midst of a windstorm. With every passing moment the subject of study (the population of headache sufferers) is shifting, taking on a new form and never holding still long enough to get a predictable picture of the problem.

The innumerable factors affecting headache such as diet, posture, daily habits, stress, over-the-counter medication, prescribed nonheadache and headache medications, and more do not exert themselves in isolation. Rather, each factor commingles; thereby the patient assumes a new form. The physiologic effects of aging continually shift headache sufferers, and the innumerable daily variables never allow them to hold still long enough for the clinician to accurately capture their specific profiles.

This problem is illustrated in the 1995 study by Boline and others.[4] Their much-publicized, randomized, uncontrolled trial compared chiropractic manipulation with amitriptyline in the treatment of tension-type headache over 6-weeks, with a follow-up at 4 weeks. The results showed that the headache outcome measures improved for both forms of intervention with no statistical significance between them. However, at the 4-week follow-up, the spinal manipulation group showed a statistically significant improvement over the group that had stopped taking the amitriptyline 4 weeks earlier. Whether chiropractic manipulation is effective in headache control is questionable.

Although the results of the study are interesting, as the authors described, they may not be because of spinal manipulation. One of the problems with this study is that headache often worsens as a result of withdrawal from amitriptyline.[5] In other words, the withdrawal of amitriptyline shifted the physiologic effects of only the group taking the drug, thereby making comparisons between the two groups problematic.

New Insight into the Headache Mechanism

Fortunately, many headaches go away without treatment. On this basis a logical nature to the timeworn traditions noted earlier exists. However, many forms of headache are progressive, with the nervous system reacting in stages as it accommodates the pain-producing mechanism to no avail.

As science has progressed in understanding the headache mechanism, clinicians are now witnessing new therapies. The pace of the new understanding has been accelerated in the last few years. Seemingly, the headache mechanism has multiple facets and cannot be explained by any singular etiology, in part because the nervous system is not a series of separate compartments each designed to handle a single problem. Headache passing through several controlling measures is now known, and at each step, it is influenced by the regulatory posture set by the CNS and the musculoskeletal system (Figure 12-1). For some patients these systems also apparently change slowly in terms of headache control.

Earliest Chiropractic Contribution to the Headache Literature

Chiropractic researchers have also studied headache. In fact, the earliest chiropractor to study headache was the founder of chiropractic, D.D. Palmer. He rationalized that disease (for example, headache) resulted from restrictions or perversions of nerve force and the cause was the vertebral subluxation. Headache's removal by the adjustment allowed the nerve force to return to equilibrium, hence the return to health, or in this case relief from headache. In May 1906, Palmer apparently impressed the physicians attending a medical society meeting with his headache cure. He wrote the following*: Dr. Martin said that he had a headache. I offered to cure it by one touch.

---

*From *Nat Chiropr J*, 1936.

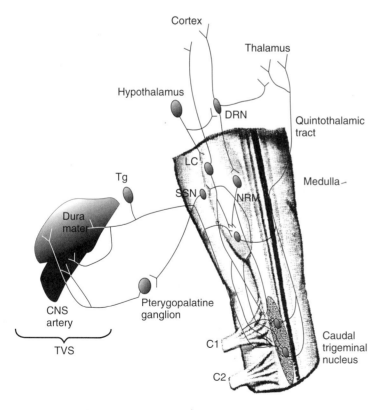

Figure 12-1 The neural elements required to maintain homeostasis in a headache-free state. The peripheral input from the trigeminovascular system that appears in the dura mater and blood vessels passes through the ophthalmic division of the trigeminal nerve and has its cell body in the trigeminal ganglion. The second-order neurons lie in the most caudal area of the trigeminal nucleus caudalis and in the dorsal horn of the upper cervical spinal cord at the C1 and C2 levels. Before the peripheral input begins its ascent to the higher CNS centers, it receives modulating stimuli from the locus ceruleus *(LC)*. These cells project via the quintothalamic tract, which decussates, before synapsing on third-order neurons in the thalamus. At this level the input is modulated by the dorsal raphe nucleus *(DRN)* and the periaqueductal gray (not shown), which in turn are modulated by the hypothalamus. Note that noxious stimuli, for example from chronic entrapment of the dura at the occiput-C1 junction, may overload the modulating mechanism. This disrupts the homeostasis and may cause the patient to have headaches. *SSN*, Superior salvatory nucleus; *TG*, trigeminal ganglion; *NRM*, nucleus raphe magnus; *TVS*, trigeminovascular system.

He accepted. I seated him in front of the audience. He showed his surprise and admitted his headache was gone. Several questions were asked for me to answer.

Chiropractic Overcomes Hindrances to Headache Research

For several decades the chiropractic profession struggled with professional development and against its allopathic counterpart, the American Medical Association (AMA), which tried to abolish chiropractic. Fortunately, chiropractic prevailed and the last time a chiropractor was jailed for defending the right to practice chiropractic in the United States was in 1974.

Merely 4 years later, the profession published its first scientific journal, *Journal of Manipulative and Physiological Therapeutics*. Within a few years, the profession created a community of academics, researchers, and scientific thinkers who began a campaign of scientific investigation into the workings and benefits of chiropractic.

Using Chiropractic Adjustment to Control Headache

The laying on of hands is unquestionably the oldest, most universally used, and probably the most appreciated means of relieving pain and suffering. Touching, massaging, and manipulating areas that are painful, tense, or tight occurs in every society. This form of care reaches its highest form in the chiropractic adjustment.

The primary impetus for the recognition of adjustive therapy is the change by chiropractic practitioners from emphasis in territorial protection and dogmatic theoretical beliefs to scientific investigation. The publication of clinical trials, scientific conferences, and experimental research papers in chiropractic have occurred more in the past decade than in the previous 90 years. However, the reason the adjustment causes the relief of headache is not clear. The type of headache and patient most likely to respond to the adjustment have yet to be defined. These questions are currently under scientific investigation and debate.

The best chiropractic studies presented in this chapter illustrate the fact that headache research is exceedingly difficult. In fact, conclusive studies on almost every aspect of headache have eluded researchers for many centuries. Not surprisingly, modern chiropractic research in this field is still in its early stages of development.

Helped by the growth of organizations, journals, and chiropractors with a particular interest in the topic, headache research has evolved into a series of categories useful for clinical evaluation of various headaches. Clinical research in headache is as important as laboratory advances; the more carefully and concisely the various types of headache are described and identified, the more likely the chiropractor is to provide accurate clinical assessment and appropriate intervention.

The chiropractic clinician is urged to be patient as progress in headache research is being made. With time, effort, and plenty of research funds, chiropractic will eventually provide clinicians with evidenced-based studies that explain the reasons their patients' headaches improve with manipulation.

The Role of the Chiropractor

The Chiropractor's Attitude with Patients, the Art of Adjustment, and a Mind-Body Approach

Someone once said that 50,000 chiropractors practice in the United States and 50,000 different ways of practicing chiropractic exist.[6] The author of this statement explained, "It is the attitude toward what the chiropractor does and how he/she delivers that adjustment to the patient. . . ." that creates successful chiropractic.

Having a positive attitude with patients, knowing the art of adjustment, and using a mind-body approach is good advice for the chiropractor who intends to treat headache. The prudence of this advice appears justified by the following two recent studies that examined the role of the chiropractor in healing.

Jaminson[7] examined the nature of the chiropractic model and found that use of verbal and nonverbal communication in chiropractic practice could be construed to create an environment conducive to healing. She specifically commented on the ability of the consultation to change the patient's perceptions and reduce anxiety and presented it as a substantial factor contributing to the potency of the chiropractic care. In addition, touch—whether diagnostic or therapeutic—emerged as a fundamental feature of chiropractic care.

Stude and Sweere[8] recommended a holistic approach to treat headache sufferers. In particular, they observed a severe headache sufferer who was unresponsive to previous cervical spine care. However, the patient responded favorably when chiropractic care included a more comprehensive evaluation and adjustments to regions of the lower spine not strictly associated with headache pain.

The Role of the Chiropractor as a Headache Diagnostician

Nearly every modern headache resource refers to the classification and diagnostic criteria for headache disorders, cranial neuralgias, and facial pain from the Headache Classification Committee of the International Headache Society[9] (Table 12-1). According to this arrangement, 13 major headache categories exist, with 162 headache types. For example, 17 types of migraine headache exist and 7 types of tension-type headaches exist. Presently, only 2 types of cervicogenic headache are recognized by this committee: cervical spine headache and retropharyngeal tendinitis headache. (Table 12-2 describes key differences between the clinical presentation of migraine and cervicogenic headaches.)

Fortunately, 94% of all headache episodes are caused by only three categories of headache: migraine, tension type, and cervicogenic. Migraine headache accounts for 16% with a point prevalence of 2.5%, tension-type headache accounts for 62% with a point prevalence of 10%, and cervicogenic headache accounts for 16% with a point prevalence of 2.5%.[10] Obviously, this makes the diagnostic challenge for the clinician far easier. (Box 12-1 describes the diagnostic criteria for cervicogenic headache.) The point prevalence of these headaches when added together (±15%) shows how common headache is in the adult population. Perhaps only the common cold has higher point prevalence.

Chiropractic management of patients with cervicogenic headache may encompass spinal adjustment, soft-tissue mobilization, and stretching techniques (Table 12-3). Long-term management includes addressing the postural component, pain-motor engrams, and imbalances in the upper

quarter, with attention to lifestyle, habits, and physical and emotional stress management.

Rebound Headache

Diagnosis of common headache may be difficult for the clinician due to the phenomenon of rebound headache, also called *analgesic headache* or *medication-induced headache*. Unlike other headache disorders, rebound headache is a newly recognized ailment. Rebound headache is a condition of daily or near-daily headache that develops in patients who have an underlying primary headache disorder, most commonly cervicogenic, migraine, or tension-type headaches.

Chiropractors are aware that headache patients may repeatedly take over-the-counter pain medication. Unfortunately, frequent use of these medica-

Table 12-1   *Quick-Reference Guide to Primary Headache*

Headache or Other Cranial Pains	Etiology
Cervicogenic headache	Mechanical joint pain, cervical spine
	Myofascial pain syndrome, cervical spine
	Articular disease, cervical spine
	Spondylosis and osteoarthritis
	Inflammatory arthritis
	Instability
Facial and nonheadache head pain	Temporomandibular joint articular disease
	Traumatic, degenerative, inflammatory, and infectious conditions
	Myofascial pain syndrome
	Cranial neuralgias and neuritis
	Arteritis and vascular disease
	Diseases of eye, ear, nose, throat, and teeth
Neurovascular headache	Migraine
	Cluster
	Toxic
	Rebound
	Hypertensive

Table 12-2   *Clinical Differences Between Migraine and Cervicogenic Headache*

	Migraine	Cervicogenic
Location	Unilateral tendency, infrequent sideshifting, origination frontally and spread posteriorly	Unilateral but possibly bilateral, particularly in occipital area, rarely sideshifting
Epiphenomena	Often severe photophobia, aura common	Photophobia uncommon, unilateral dimming of vision typical
Nausea or Vomiting	Nausea typical, vomiting uncommon	Mild nausea possible, vomiting rare
Frequency and Duration	Frequency varying usually only a few episodes per month with each episode lasting only 4 hours or so, possibly sustained (status migrainosus)	Frequent episodes, often daily, episodes possibly lasting in some degree for days
Mechanical Provocation	Atypical	Sustained neck posture, palpation, ipsilateral shoulder overuse
Vertebral Palpation	Variable local tenderness or restriction	Reproduction of headache from palpation, predictable restrictions from occiput to C3
Response to Adjustment	Variable, limited, possibly abort headache	Possibly abort headache, lasting relief reported

tions produces a new type of headache and causes an escalation of the headache symptoms. Daily or almost-daily (>2 to 3 times per week) use of even such over-the-counter medications as aspirin, acetaminophen, and ibuprofen, or more commonly a combination of sedatives and painkillers, is believed to interfere with the brain centers that regulate the flow of pain messages into the nervous system.

Everyone has a system in the brain to block pain. Burn-sufferers know that the pain may be very intense. However, after a short time, the pain starts to lessen. The body's natural pain-blocking system (the endogenous opiates such as endorphins) starts to relieve the pain. However, the daily use of painkillers seems to interfere with this process and can lead to rebound headache, also known as *medication-induced headache* or *analgesic headache*. In other words, medication use can change intermittent headaches into chronic and daily headaches.

Rebound headache generally has the following clinical characteristics:

- Chronic daily headache occurs for at least 6 months.
- Medication gives only transient or partial relief of the headache.
- Headache is present on waking.

- No other medical cause for the headache exists (e.g., hypertension, sinusitis).
- History of taking prescription or nonprescription pain relievers daily or almost every day is prevalent, contrary to directions on the package label.
- Overuse of medications causes the headache to rebound as the last dose wears off, leading to a cycle of taking more medication.

The following drugs are most often implicated in rebound headache:

- Acetaminophen or acetylsalicylic acid products
- Caffeine
- Narcotics
- Barbiturates
- Ergotamine products
- Nonsteroidal antiinflammatory drugs (NSAIDS)

The role of NSAIDS has not been clear, possibly because patients could only recently self-medicate with them. Although NSAIDS have been used as prophylactic agents in migraine headaches, frequent use of NSAIDS should be avoided in migraine patients until their role is more fully understood.

BOX 12-1

Diagnostic Criteria for Cervicogenic Headache

Major Signs and Symptoms

At least one of the following occurs:

Resistance to or limitation of passive neck movements

Changes in neck muscle contour, texture, tone, or response to active and passive stretching and contraction

Ipsilateral neck, shoulder, or arm pain of a rather vague nonradicular nature or occasional radicular arm pain

Pain triggered by neck movement or sustained awkward head positioning

Pain similar in distribution and character to spontaneously occurring pain elicited by pressure over the ipsilateral upper, posterior neck, or occiput area

Unilaterality of the headache without sideshift

Pain Characteristics

Precipitation or aggravation of headache, similar to the usually occurring one, precipitated by neck movements and/or sustained neck posture or awkward head positioning

Moderate-severe, nonthrobbing, and nonlancinating pain, usually starting in the neck

Varying duration, fluctuating, continuous

Pain localized to neck and occipital region, may project to forehead, orbital region, temples, vertex, or ears

Nonclustering pain episodes

Pain episodes varying in duration, possible fluctuating continuous pain

Other Important Criteria

Radiographic examination reveals at least one of the following:

Movement abnormalities in flexion/extension

Abnormal posture

Fractures, congenital abnormalities, bone tumors, rheumatoid arthritis, or other distinct pathology (not spondylosis or osteochondrosis)

Female predilection

Marginal or lack of effect from indomethacin, ergotamine, and sumatriptan

Minor, Rare, Nonobligatory Signs and Symptoms

Autonomic features:

Nausea

Vomiting

Dizziness

Phonophobia

Photophobia

Blurred vision on the eye ipsilateral to the headache

Difficulties in swallowing

Modified from Sjaastad O, Fredriksen TA, Pfaffenrath V: Cervicogenic headache: diagnostic criteria, *Headache* 38(6):442-445, 1998.

Table 12-3 *Source of Symptoms with Cervicogenic Headache*

Location of Complaint	Articulation Involved
Vertex	Occipitoatlantal
Frontal, periorbital, or temporal	Occipitoatlantal
Occipital and supraorbital or retroorbital	Atlantoaxial or C2-C3
Parietal	Occipitoatlantal or atlantoaxial
Neck pain and associated eye symptoms	C2-C3

Ominous Features in Headache Patients

The similarity of symptoms with benign headache in the early stage of a serious disease is common and is a source of potential confusion for the nonheadache specialist. For the purposes of this chapter, *ominous* refers to a condition that is not generally treatable with conservative measures or may lead to morbid outcomes. A complete discussion of this subject is not possible in this chapter, but the use of important guidelines should ensure the protection of the patient (Box 12-2).

BOX 12-2

Ominous Features in Headache Sufferers

The headache sufferer is considered to have an ominous clinical situation when the following occurs:

The headache fails to respond to care and continues to worsen.

The headache sufferer comes to the doctor with a new, sudden, and debilitating headache.

The headache continues and new problems emerge that do not fit the diagnostic profile of the headache.

The headache pain appears rapidly, rising to a peak within minutes and remains at that level.

The headache is aggressive and progresses and worsens with the appearance of constitutional symptoms and focal and/or nonfocal neurologic complaints.

The headache is uninterrupted and lasts longer than previous episodes, becoming more severe.

Some other worrisome findings include: recent head trauma, fever, loss of consciousness, altered consciousness, changes in vital signs, convulsions, aphasia, changes in mentation, emotional changes, headache awakening the patient from sleep, neck rigidity, unilateral blurring of vision.

Headache Models

Nearly as many headache models exist as headache researchers. Collecting, analyzing, and comparing all the headache models known to exist could take a long time. All the prevalent headache models cannot be discussed in this chapter; however, presenting the essential parts of the major theory used today, namely the unified headache model and the cervicogenic component to this model should be helpful in understanding the current investigations into this phenomenon.

The Unified Headache Model

In 1985, Featherstone[11] proposed that tension-type and migraine headaches do not exist as discrete pathophysiologic entities but form a contin-

uum. Then in 1994, Nelson[12] contributed to the chiropractic literature by adding cervicogenic headache to the continuum theory. In other words, the three most common headaches may share a common underlying mechanism. Essentially, this mechanism involves the trigeminocervical system, the cerebrovascular system, and the neurochemicals that maintain a gentle homeostatic control over these structures. Once disturbed, headache manifests and the greater the involvement of the cerebrovascular system, the more migraine-like the headache will be (Figure 12-2).

The continuum theory is not universally accepted, but its acceptance is increasing. Rasmussen's 1995 study[13] supports the idea that migraine and tension-type headaches are separate clinical entities. In his study, he suggested that migraine is primarily a constitutional disorder and tension-type headache is a more complex phenomenon influenced by several psychosocial factors, essentially leading to overload of the musculoskeletal and CNS homeostasis mechanisms. This model and similar ones are careful to note the obvious differences between the mechanism of onset of migraine versus tension-type headache and cervicogenic headache. A weakness or flaw in the physiologic mechanism of the CNS essentially triggers migraine. However, the critics of the continuum theory argue that no such flaw exists in the tension-type or cervicogenic headache sufferers. Instead, they believe these headaches are a result of overload and microtrauma. In other words, headache is the equivalent of a repetitive stress disorder for the CNS.

Cervicogenic Headache from a Somatovisceral Viewpoint

Cervicogenic headache is believed to be a common type of headache, perhaps more common than migraine. Sjaastad and others[14] introduced the term *cervicogenic headache* in 1983. Since then, more than 100 studies have been done on cervicogenic headache.[15] At one time, cervicogenic headache was thought to be a vascular headache, associated with vasoconstriction of the vertebral arteries and the sympathetic nervous system.[5] However, anatomic, physiologic, and clinical investigations have cast doubt on this idea.[16-19] Mechanisms other than sympathetic nervous involvement must be implicated in producing cervicogenic headache.

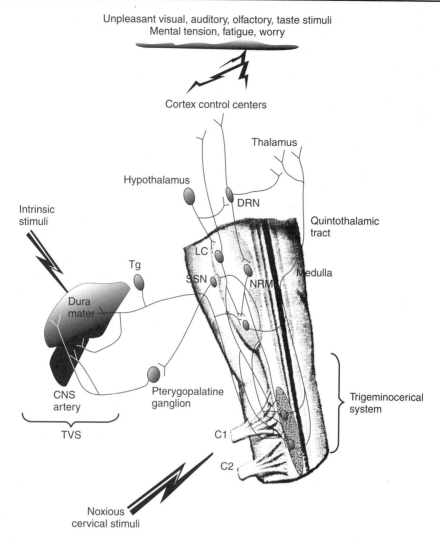

Figure 12-2 Input from C-fiber nociceptors triggers a maintained increase in the excitability of trigemino-vascular neurons that results in a phenomenon known as *central sensitization.* Based on the available evidence, a strong likelihood exists that headache, both tension-type and migraine, is associated with the induction of central sensitization in neurons of the spinal nucleus of the trigeminal pathway. Central sensitization is a form of neural plasticity responsible for generating hypersensitivity to normally nonpainful noxious stimuli, which results from changes in resting membrane potentials and activation of voltage-dependent ion channels in key central neurons.

Kerr[20] is credited with the discovery of the anatomic basis for cervicogenic headache, although he was unaware of the condition known by that name. Using animals, he uncovered an area at the junction of the brainstem and spinal cord called the *trigeminocervical nucleus* and demonstrated that an overlap of nociceptive (pain) cells from the upper three cervical nerves and ophthalmic division of the fifth cranial nerve occurred. Because of the close anatomic relationship of pain fibers from the cervical spine and

trigeminal system, pain impulses from the neck were proposed to transmit to the trigeminal system and were interpreted as headache. This phenomenon of referred headache from the upper cervical region has been termed the *Kerr principle.*[21] The basic underpinnings of the Kerr principle remain in the modern pathoanatomic explanation for cervicogenic headache.

Sources of cervicogenic headache include pain-sensitive tissues innervated by C1-C3 as these cervical nerves synapse with the trigeminocervical nuclei. These nerves innervate the joints and ligaments of the upper three cervical vertebrae, their associated anterior and posterior muscles, the sternocleidomastoid and trapezius muscles, the vertebral artery, and the dura mater of the posterior cranial fossa. Many different conditions of the cervical spine, including mechanical pain and joint and soft-tissue pathology, have been reported to cause cervicogenic headache (Box 12-3).

Although rare, pathologic causes of cervicogenic headache exist, including bony and soft-tissue anomalies of the craniovertebral junction, acquired craniovertebral lesions, and arthritic pathology of the upper cervical spine (Box 12-4). Trauma to the neck such as whiplash injury also is reported to cause cervicogenic headache. Balla and Iansek[22] studied 122 cases of acute whiplash and found that 75% developed headache, with 86% developing headache within the first week. Headache was reported in the occiput region (46%), generalized throughout the head (34%), and in areas other than the occiput region (20%).

The most common cause of chronic cervicogenic headache is believed to be mechanical pain (pain aggravated by movement but relieved by rest) from the muscles, ligaments, and joints of the upper cervical spine (Box 12-5). Vertebral restriction appears to contribute to the clinical syndrome of cervicogenic headache. Boquet and

others[23] thought that a combination of trigger points, hypertonicity of the ipsilateral trapezius muscle, and rotation of the C2 vertebra were associated with unilateral cervicogenic headache. Jaeger[24] reported similar findings such as trigger points, tenderness, and limited joint movement in the upper cervical spine ipsilateral to the headache in cervicogenic headache sufferers. She proposed that cervicogenic headache resulted from a combination of cervical joint dysfunction and myofascial pain.

Ng[25] examined 26 patients to test whether any radiographic relationship existed between the disposition of the upper three cervical vertebrae and occipital headache. X-rays of patients who suffered from occipital headache were compared with

---

BOX 12-4

Pathologic Causes of Cervicogenic Headache

Anomalies of craniovertebral junction
Basilar invagination
Congenital atlantoaxial dislocation
Occipitalization of atlas
Arnold-Chiari and Dandy-Walker malformation
Hydrocephalus and syringomyelia
Acquired lesions of craniovertebral junction
Meningiomas of foramen magnum
Neurofibromas and ependymomas
Multiple myeloma and metastatic tumor
Osteomyelitis, Pott's disease, and Paget's disease
Arthritis of the craniovertebral junction
Rheumatoid arthritis
Ankylosing spondylitis
Degenerative joint disease

BOX 12-3

Cervicogenic Headache Can Originate from these Tissues

Articulations
Occipitoatlas
C1-C2
C2-C3
C3-C4
Muscles
Prevertebral and postvertebral upper cervical muscles
Suboccipital musculature
Semispinalis capitus, longissimus capitus, and splenius capitus
Sternocleidomastoid and trapezius
Vertebral Artery
Posterior Cranial Fossa Dura Mater

BOX 12-5

Common Musculoskeletal Sources of Cervicogenic Headache

Upper cervical facet joints
Myofascial pain syndrome
Sprain or strain of the upper cervical spine
Suboccipital entrapment of the dura

x-rays of 25 asymptomatic patients concerning cervical curvature and anteroposterior, lateral, and rotational disposition of the upper cervical vertebrae. His results showed that the symptomatic group had a significantly greater degree of lateral inclination of C1 and C3, suggesting that a definite degree of association existed between abnormal upper cervical statics and occipital headache.

Fortunately, more agreement exists on the mechanism of headache than on the causes triggering the mechanism. Regarding the three categories of headache—migraine, tension-type, and cervicogenic—the trigeminal system is generally agreed to be the center of the headache mechanism. As noted earlier, the differences of opinion are in what disrupts the homeostasis of the trigeminal system that ultimately causes headache.

In 1992, Bogduk[26] proposed a neuroanatomic basis for cervicogenic headache through the convergence in the trigeminocervical nucleus between nociceptive afferents from the field of the trigeminal nerve and the receptive fields of the first three cervical nerves. The structures innervated by C1-C3 (muscles, joints, and ligaments of the upper three cervical segments, the dura mater of the spinal cord, the posterior cranial fossa, and the vertebral artery) may trigger the trigeminal system by repetitive noxious stimuli arising from the C1-C3 receptive fields.

In 1994, Darby and Cramer[27] further discussed the Bogduk-style pain generators and pain pathways of the head and neck, with a particular emphasis on the chiropractic approach to headache. They expanded the model to include the sensory innervation associated with autonomic fibers and displayed scientific evidence to identify the cervical region as a source of migraine. Essentially, using this model, they proposed that cervical arthritis, trauma, or other disease processes affecting the cervical spine may provide repetitive irritation of the nociceptive fibers running with the autonomic fibers of the cervical spinal nerves. Consequently, a vascular headache referred to as *cervical migraine* developed.

Specific Challenges to Effective Headache Management

The key to treating headache is not in the clinician's ability to recite the details of a particular headache theory; instead, successful headache management depends on the clinician's overall familiarity with the prevalent headache mechanisms. In other words, the chiropractor is responsible for maintaining familiarity with the subject of headache as it progresses in the clinical and scientific literature for several important reasons.

First, most headache sufferers want to know the reason they have headaches. In their quest for knowledge, they gather as much information as they can, sometimes to their detriment. In these cases, headache clinicians must have enough familiarity with whatever headache theory their patients are describing such that the doctors can communicate with patients and help them understand their problem better.

A case report from Olson[28] illustrates this point. The subject was a 56-year-old woman who sustained a whiplash-associated disorder caused by a motor vehicle accident. Eventually, she developed a chronic headache that was disabling and hindered her quality of life. For a year, she underwent a variety of diagnostic tests but medications and therapy were unsuccessful in relieving her complaints. Afterward, she expressed anger and frustration in not understanding the cause of her headache and did not want to endure additional therapy. The key to the successful outcome of her case arose through her doctors listening to her explain the ways she coped with and misunderstood her headache problem. With explanation, she realized that she needed to reduce her excessive cervical lordosis, a concept she was previously unable to associate with her headache complaint. After only a month of supine cervical traction and home exercise, she was finally able to reduce and control her headache.

Many headache sufferers also have absorbed a considerable amount of detailed but not necessarily cohesive information about their headaches from many visits to doctors, wanting to resolve their problems. These patients, when confronting headache doctors for the first time, often judge doctors' skills by their familiarity with the headache literature. This case is poignantly illustrated by a patient I saw, who obviously memorized relevant portions of volume one of Travell's and Simon's myofascial pain book. She firmly and correctly believed that doctors who were unfamiliar with the myofascial pain phenomenon were unlikely to be effective in headache management.

Headache management is greatly assisted by clinicians employing an appropriate headache model to use with the patient to foster common understanding. The lack of a common understanding undermines the entire process of headache treatment. More often than not, patient compliance with therapy gradually decreases, sometimes with the patient treating the headache with home medications. The medication is likely to lead to headache rebound phenomenon and with the worsening of the headache, the patient is further distanced from the chiropractor's headache treatment.

Further, clinicians must be alert for conflicting headache models because some patients are treated for their headaches by more than one doctor. The artful chiropractor manages to merge the conflicting models into a harmonious one.

For all its conflict and diversity, the headache literature is evolving, with excellent tips and tricks that greatly assist the chiropractor in treating headache. For example, Warner[29] reported a case involving a 42-year-old woman with a continuous, unilateral headache previously diagnosed as the rare type of headache known as *hemicrania continua*. Eventually, this headache ceased 3 weeks after she stopped taking analgesics on a frequent basis, thus prompting the notion that she was actually suffering from analgesic rebound headache.

The Present Challenge—Developing Evidence-Based Studies for Chiropractic Management of Headache

The basic problem is the fact that too few studies examining chiropractic and headache exist, with even fewer studies having significant scientific merit. Despite these deficiencies, some significant studies examining the role of chiropractic in headache management are worth mentioning, as are headache literature reviews and the works of the RAND organization[30] and Vernon.[31] These studies serve as a good framework for a review of the better chiropractic headache studies.

In 1982, Vernon[32] conducted an uncontrolled retrospective and prospective study on the role of manipulation in headache management. Unfortunately, the design limitations were such that the study could not provide a basis for testing the role of chiropractic intervention on headache. How-

ever, in this study, Vernon was the first to test a cohort of tension headache sufferers using a standardized outcome measure. This study was also limited by the fact that consistent diagnostic criteria for tension-type headache were not developed until 1988.

In 1983, Howe and others[33] compared manipulation with administration of azapropazone (Rheumox, an NSAID) in a randomized, controlled trial of 27 subjects. No significant difference was found between the groups on immediate assessment and after 3 weeks, but the small sample size detracted from the potential of this study. Droz's and Crot's 1985 retrospective study[34] on 332 occipital headache sufferers showed that 80% achieved a pain-free or almost pain-free status after eight to nine chiropractic treatments. Unfortunately, this study suffers from a significant number of biases that keep it from achieving scientific validity.

In 1987, Turk and Ratkolb[35] conducted a 6-month follow-up to the study of the effect of mobilization of the cervical spine in 100 chronic headache patients. Only 25 had no headache at 6 months, and 40 patients improved but still required medication. This study once held that manipulation might correct some underlying headache mechanism, but a significant number of design flaws prevent it from achieving scientific validity.

In 1990, Jensen and others[36] studied 23 patients with posttraumatic headache 1 year after head trauma using a prospective clinical controlled trial to discover whether specific manual therapy on the neck could reduce the headache. The study was completed by 19 patients.[19] Of these, 10 patients were treated twice with manual therapy and 9 were treated twice with cold packs on the neck over 2 weeks. Although a statistically significant change favoring manual therapy occurred, the study's design is questionable for many reasons, one being the fact that ice precipitates headache in some patients.[37]

In 1994, Whittingham and others[38] studied a particular type of manipulation. The objective of this pilot study was to investigate the effect of spinal manipulation for the relief of chronic headache of cervical origin, using a specific technique, *toggle recoil*, to treat the two upper cervical vertebrae. Unfortunately, the design of the study could not explain the speculation that four toggle recoil adjustments over a 2-week period improved headache. Because the results of this pilot study were not adequately controlled, they cannot be seen as proof supporting the clinical efficacy of manipulation for chronic headaches. As of yet, no follow-up to this pilot study has been reported.

In 1994, Mootz and others[39] conducted a small, prospective case series of a tension-type headache group of men for an 8-week treatment period, in which 16 treatments preceded by a no-treatment baseline period occurred. Unfortunately, the comparison between the baseline period and intervention period failed to achieve statistical significance. The McGill Pain Questionnaire did not appear to provide any useful information in assessing change in this sample. The findings of this study are limited by the small sample size.

In 1997, Nilsson and others[40] conducted a randomized, controlled trial with a blinded observer of a cohort of cervicogenic headache sufferers. Of these, 28 subjects received cervical manipulation twice a week for 3 weeks, and 25 subjects received low-level laser in the upper cervical region and deep friction massage including trigger points in the lower cervical and upper thoracic region twice a week for 3 weeks. The authors concluded that spinal manipulation had a significant positive effect in cases of cervicogenic headache. However, the manipulation group decreasing the use of analgesics by 36% and no change occurring in the soft-tissue group is important to point out. The spinal manipulation group also started with a range of daily analgesic use that was nearly twice as high as the soft-tissue group: 0 to 7.9 versus 0 to 4.4. Although the study has some scientific merit, the authors not addressing the potentially powerful role of improved headache outcomes because of a greater degree of abstinence from analgesics in the spinal manipulation group is important to point out.[41]

A few more chiropractic and manual medicine headache studies deserve mention. Although they lack scientific sophistication, they are memorable for their pioneering efforts.

Stodolny and Chmielewski[42] studied a small group of patients with cervical migraine managed with spinal manipulation. This study introduced the use of the Hautant test and the two-weight test, using bilateral scales to quantify asymmetry of weight-bearing, to assess disturbances of proprioception and symmetry of the perception of posture. Interestingly, the authors also proposed that vertebral restrictions of the upper cervical spine were important in the pathogenesis of cervical migraine and that their elimination significantly reduces the symptoms of cervical migraine.

Reports of resolution of chronic pediatric headache exist in the chiropractic literature. Hewitt[43] described a 13-year-old girl with a 1-year history of headache and neck pain for which he claimed to have basically cured after two chiropractic adjustments. Haney[44] reported on an 11-year-old girl with an 8-year history of headache with concomitant nausea, vomiting, dizziness, and foot pain, who responded well to 8 adjustments administered over 3 months. A similar case involving a male patient was presented by Cochran.[45]

A study by Stephens and Gorman[46] discussing pediatric headache resulting from vision problems is interesting. They described two pediatric patients who had constriction of the visual fields, one of whom suffered from chronic headache. The authors used computerized perimetry to document visual field improvement after spinal manipulation. After seven sessions of spinal manipulation to the neck and back of this 14-year-old girl, her visual fields and visual acuity returned to normal. The authors concluded that spinal manipulative therapy was responsible for the improved vision in these two cases.

In a study using Toftness technique, Gemmell and others[47] noted a 38-year-old woman with a 9-month history of severe biweekly basilar migraine headache accompanied by severe vertigo, tinnitus, nausea, vomiting, diarrhea, blurred vision, and numbness of the mouth, hands, and legs. After the eighth adjustment given in the second month of treatment, the patient was headache free.

Killinger[48] detailed the use of toggle-recoil technique for seven chronic headache sufferers. Although the clinical characteristics of the seven headache cases were poorly defined, the author described good-to-excellent relief of the patients' headaches.

Tuchin and others[49] described a patient with a history of migraine without aura who was treated for cervical spine dysfunction. During treatment, the patient showed a reduction in prevalence and intensity of headaches over a 4-month period. The authors addressed the fact that their analysis of the patient's outcome was complicated by the fact that whether the patient's headaches were common migraine or cervicogenic headache was not clear.

However, they provided an interesting discussion of a possible causative relationship between cervical spine dysfunction and common migraine. The authors also discussed the appropriateness of chiropractic treatment of chronic headache and migraine.

Wittingham and others[50] developed a pilot study examining the use of upper cervical spine toggle-recoil technique for the relief of chronic headache of cervical origin. Each of the 26 patients received four upper cervical toggle-recoil adjustments over a 2-week period. Their results indicated statistically significant outcomes ($p < 0.001$), including changes in headache frequency, duration, and severity in all but 2 of the patients. The overall duration of headaches decreased by 77%, the overall score for severity showed a 60% improvement in perceived pain, and the frequency of headache also improved by 62%.

Mootz and others[51] studied the effectiveness of diversified technique and soft-tissue therapy in the treatment of chronic episodic muscle tension–type headache in men. A total of 11 men between the ages of 18 and 40 years with a self-reported history of chronic headache for at least 6 months and an average of at least weekly headache episodes were recruited. Over 8 weeks, 16 outpatient sessions of chiropractic care were provided to each patient. Mean pretreatment-to-posttreatment headache frequency changed from 6.4 episodes per 2-week period to 3.1 per 2-week period, a statistically significant change ($p < 0.01$). Mean pretreatment-to-posttreatment headache duration changed from 6.7 hours per episode to 3.88 hours per episode, which was statistically significant ($p < 0.05$). Mean anchored pain-scale intensity ratings changed from 5.05 to 3.37 but was beyond statistical significance ($p = 0.059$). No significant changes occurred in any McGill Pain Questionnaire scores pretreatment and posttreatment. In this case series analysis of episodic tension headache in 10 men, typical chiropractic interventions of adjusting, muscle work, and moist heat significantly reduced self-reported frequency and duration of headache episodes after 12 treatments over an 8-week period.

Defranca and Levine[52] discussed a clinical condition known as *T4 syndrome*. The clinical features were nocturnal or early morning paresthesia, numbness, or a peculiar glovelike distribution of hand or forearm pain that may be associated with

headaches and upper back stiffness. In addition, no hard neurologic signs are present. Upper thoracic joint dysfunction, especially in the region of the T4 segment, appeared to be the major cause of the upper extremity symptoms and headaches. Manipulation of the dysfunctional upper thoracic segments may relieve these symptoms.

Anatomic and Physiologic Mechanisms

The concept that headache might originate from disorders in the neck is not new but the reason these headaches are initiated remains unclear. What follows is a brief portrayal of the mechanisms that could explain the initiation of headache from the cervical spine.

As discussed earlier, the branches of the first, second, and third cervical spinal nerves converge with the spinal nucleus of the trigeminal system. This convergence is presently seen as the neuroanatomic basis for headache triggered by the cervical spine. The finding of convergence between the trigeminal spinal nucleus and the upper cervical dorsal horn units is of considerable interest because it indicates a functional relationship of the trigeminal and cervical root systems. Errors in the homeostasis of this system may result from intrinsic faults in CNS neurotransmitter pathways, overload by chronic noxious stimuli, or both. Regardless, headache results and if the disruption in homeostasis is pervasive, headache epiphenomena occurs (e.g., aura, dizziness, nausea, paresthesias, blood vessel dilation, facial sweating, tinnitus).

Stimulation of the first and second cervical nerves has been shown to induce suboccipital, frontal, and supraorbital pain in human subjects.[53,54] The cervical facet joints produce headache with experimental noxious stimulation of these joints.[55,56] Each facet level appears to produce a clinically distinguishable characteristic pattern, and the corresponding zones of pain have been illustrated on pain charts (Figure 12-3). Upper cervical joint dysfunction or joint restriction is also thought to cause headache.[57]

Occipital neuralgia is popularly reported to result from compression of the greater occipital nerve by spasm of the trapezius muscle.[58] The anatomic and clinical evidence for this model has been strongly challenged.[59] Nevertheless, the diagnostic criteria for this form of headache have

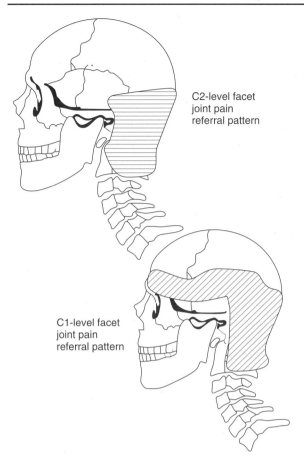

C2-level facet joint pain referral pattern

C1-level facet joint pain referral pattern

Figure 12-3 Headache pattern varies according to the level of origin in the cervical spine. (From Bogduk N, Marsland A: A cervical zygapophyseal joints as a source of neck pain, *Spine* 13:610-617, 1988.)

> ## BOX 12-6
>
> ### *Diagnostic Criteria for Occipital Neuralgia*
>
> **Primary Complaints or Findings**
> Neuralgic pain characterized as sharp, brief, and lancinating in the distribution of the relevant nerve
> Background pain of continuous aching component that may be present for days or weeks
> Paroxysmal jabbing pain in the distribution of the greater or lesser occipital nerves accompanied by diminished sensation or dysesthesia in the affected area
> **Secondary Complaints or Findings**
> Tearing of the eye
> Flushing of the face
> Occlusion of the ipsilateral nasal passage
> Tinnitus
> Visual blurring, retroorbital pain
> Vertigo and dizziness
> Nausea
> **Requisite Finding**
> Typical description of neuralgia pain, similar to the quality of trigeminal neuralgia
> Reproducible extracranial tenderness as the affected nerve is tender to palpation
> Tinel's sign over the affected nerve
> Resolution of pain through anesthetic block of the nerve

Modified from Kuhn WF, Juhn SC, Gilberstady H: Occipital neuralgias: clinical recognition of a complicated headache. A case series and literature review, *J Orofac Pain* 11(2):158-165, 1997.

---

been clearly identified (Box 12-6). Occipital neuralgia is now considered to be a true neuralgia like that of trigeminal neuralgia and may be induced by neuromata, scarring around the nerve, neural fibrosis, or densely adherent occipital lymph nodes.[60] The communication among the cervical nerve roots supplying the greater and lesser occipital nerves, the trigeminal system, and the acoustic and vestibular tracts may explain the visual, nasal, otic, and vestibular symptoms seen with this headache.

Noxious stimulation of suboccipital tissues such as muscles and ligaments has historically been reported to result in characteristic suboccipital and frontal headache.[61] Other cervicothoracic and cervicocranial muscles may be involved in the production of headache because they are susceptible to a variety of chronic low-level but repetitive

stresses that alter their functional status. This functional disturbance may cascade into abnormal stress of the suboccipital tissues.

Trigger points exist in the cervical musculature and are a source of head pain but not necessarily headache.[62] Some clinicians think that nociceptive impulses from posterior joint dysfunction reflexly increase the tension in certain neck muscles, leading to the formation of trigger points with referred pain to the head.[63]

Persistent contraction of the posterior neck muscles is commonly believed to be a source of neck pain and subsequent headache. The pathophysiology of this phenomenon, however, has been studied and the muscle contraction headache model is questionable.[64]

Arthritis of the cervical spine may be responsible for irritating or compressing the upper cervical roots and therefore may cause headache.[65] Bogduk and Marsland[66] demonstrated a headache mechanism produced by osteoarthritis of the C2-3 facet joint. By injection, they blocked the third occipital nerve that innervates this facet joint and mediates headache. A total of 7 out of 10 consecutive patients initiating treatment with suspected cervical headache were found to suffer from pain mediated by the third occipital nerve and stemming from the C2-3 facet joint.

Upper cervical joint dysfunction is consistently reported as a cause of headache. Joint dysfunction has been reported to occur in 70% to 90% of headache sufferers (Figure 12-4).[67,68] Senescence of the cervical spinal motion segment is manifested by changes in each anatomic component, although the pathoanatomic change that predominates varies. If sufficient compromise of local neural structures occurs, it will precipitate the onset of symptoms. The pattern of symptoms and any associated physical signs vary according to which structures are stimulated or compressed. Other less clearly understood patterns of local and referred symptoms may be mediated by the sinuvertebral nerves or the medial branches of the posterior ramus.[69]

Summary

Headache is mainly a somatovisceral phenomenon, mediated in part by disturbances arising in the cervical spine. The overlap between the upper cervical nerve roots and the trigeminal system, along with peripheral and central pain effects, figure heavily in the headache process. Because the muscles, ligaments, and joints of the cervical area are so richly supplied with sensory fibers, any change in the sensory input from them may overload the homeostatic mechanisms existing in the spinal cord, trigeminal system, and associated modulating centers.

Once the cervical area is disturbed, headache may ensue. The specific characteristics of the headache vary widely but ultimately determine the clinical diagnosis. Those headaches range from classic migraine to mixed headache to tension headache.

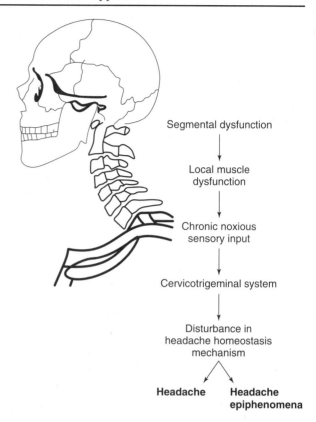

Segmental dysfunction

↓

Local muscle dysfunction

↓

Chronic noxious sensory input

↓

Cervicotrigeminal system

↓

Disturbance in headache homeostasis mechanism

↙   ↘

Headache   **Headache epiphenomena**

Figure 12-4 Cervical segmental dysfunction acts as part of an overall somatic dysfunction–noxious overload process. This may function as a potentiator of homeostatic disturbance, leading to headache and headache epiphenomena.

Strong visceral phenomena may arise from the cervical somatic structures, and the patient is diagnosed with cervical migraine. Cervical angina, resembling true angina pectoris but resulting from cervical spondylosis and nerve root compression, also has been reported.[70] Symptoms vary in severity and include neck pain and stiffness, occipital headache, and arm pain with sensory symptoms. All these visceral effects are believed to arise as epiphenomena of the primary disturbance in the headache homeostasis mechanism. The resultant disturbance in the trigeminovascular system is thought to mediate the epiphenomena seen with headache.

Although medications may be used to reset the homeostasis, the effect is often only temporary as the underlying etiology still remains. Hence the patient continues to suffer headache once the medications are withdrawn. Sometimes the medications used to resolve headache exacerbate it and cause rebound pain. Although not thoroughly

STUDY GUIDE

1. When was the earliest reported consideration given to extracranial sources of headache and by whom? What was said?
2. What are the origin and insertion of the RCMP muscle? When were the dural attachments discovered? Why might this be important in the etiology of headache?
3. In Boline's headache study, what was the major outcome difference between the group receiving chiropractic care and the group under allopathic care?
4. Discuss the findings in the Stude and Sweere headache study and their significance in terms of chiropractic analysis.
5. What is rebound headache? Name four common drugs often implicated. How would a clinician discover whether the patient is using any of these drugs?
6. When was the term *cervicogenic headache* first coined? Describe it in terms of referred pain.
7. What is the trigeminocervical nucleus and where is it located? What cervical nerves synapse with it?
8. Describe Nilsson's 1997 RCT involving cervicogenic headache sufferers.
9. Describe Tuchin's migraine case study and the factors complicating it. Are they important?
10. Explain the mechanism of occipital neuralgia. How might this appear during chiropractic analysis for the VSC?
11. Medication may appear to reset homeostasis. Why is the result usually temporary?

studied, manipulation of the cervical spine to treat headache may achieve its objective by affecting the homeostasis mechanism. If so, this explains many of the clinical observations noted in this chapter, thus providing clinicians with an evidenced-based approach to headache as a somatovisceral problem.

REFERENCES

1. Hack GD et al: Anatomic relation between the rectus capitis posterior minor muscle and the dura mater, *Spine* 20(23):2484-2486, 1995.
2. Rangnath M, Bartlett J, Palmer BJ: A man with a vision 1881-1961, *Int Rev Chiro* 35-37, 1995.
3. Marty G: Place of hysterectomy with adnexial preservation in the treatment of severe persistent catamenial migraine after age 45, *Bull Fed Soc Gynecol Obstet* 23(3):333-334, 1971.
4. Boline PD et al: Spinal manipulation vs. amitriptyline for the treatment of chronic tension-type headaches: a randomized clinical trial, *J Manipulative Physiol Ther* 18(3):148-154, 1995.
5. Zajecka J, Tracy KA, Mitchell S: Discontinuation symptoms after treatment with serotonin reuptake inhibitors: a literature review, *J Clin Psychiatry* 58(7):291-297, 1997.
6. Rousso A: The perfect technique, *Chiro Prod* 22-23, 1997.
7. Jamison JR: An interactive model of chiropractic practice: reconstructing clinical reality, *J Manipulative Physiol Ther* 20(6):382-388, 1997.
8. Stude DE, Sweere JJ: A holistic approach to severe headache symptoms in a patient unresponsive to regional manual therapy, *J Manipulative Physiol Ther* 19(3):202-207, 1996.
9. Headache Classification Committee of the International Headache Society: Classification and diagnostic criteria for headache disorders, cranial neuralgias and facial pain, *Cephalalgia* 7(Suppl 8):1-96, 1988.
10. Nilsson N: The prevalence of cervicogenic headache in a random population sample of 20-59 year olds, *Spine* 20(17):1884-1888, 1995.
11. Featherstone HJ: Migraine and muscle contraction headaches: a continuum, *Headache* 25(4):194-198, 1985.
12. Nelson CF: The tension headache, migraine headache continuum: a hypothesis, *J Manipulative Physiol Ther* 17(3):156-167, 1994.
13. Rasmussen BK: Epidemiology of headache, *Cephalalgia* 15(1):45-68, 1995.
14. Sjaastad O et al: "Cervicogenic" headache: an hypothesis, *Cephalalgia* 3(4):249-256, 1983.
15. As of August 1998. MEDLINE lists 89 articles. MANTIS lists 24 additional articles not found in the MEDLINE database.
16. Bogduk N, Lambert GA, Duckworth JW: The anatomy and physiology of the vertebral nerve in relation to cervical migraine, *Cephalalgia* 1:11-24, 1981.
17. Bovin G, Sjaastad O: Cervicogenic headache: responses to nitroglycerine, oxygen, ergotamine, and morphine, *Headache* 33:249-252, 1993.
18. Fredriksen TA: Cervicogenic headache: the forehead sweating pattern, *Cephalalgia* 8:203-209, 1998.
19. Fredriksen TA et al: Cervicogenic headache: pupillometric findings, *Cephalalgia* 8:93-103, 1998.

20. Kerr FL: A mechanism to account for frontal headache in cases of posterior fossa tumors, *J Neurosurg* 18:605-609, 1961.

21. Sjaastad O: The headache of challenge in our time: cervicogenic headache, *Funct Neurol* 5:155-158, 1990.

22. Balla J, Iansek R: Headache arising from the cervical spine. In Hopkins A, editor: *Headache—problems in diagnosis and management*, pp 243-267, London, 1988, Saunders.

23. Boquet J, Boismare F, Payenneville G: Lateralization of headache: possible role of an upper cervical trigger point, *Cephalalgia* 9:15-24, 1989.

24. Jaeger B: Are "cervicogenic" headaches due to myofascial pain and cervical spine dysfunction? *Cephalalgia* 9:157-164, 1989.

25. Ng S: Upper cervical vertebrae and occipital headache, *J Manipulative Physiol Ther* 3(3):137-141, 1980.

26. Bogduk N: The anatomical basis for cervicogenic headache, *J Manipulative Physiol Ther* 15(1):67-70, 1992.

27. Darby SA, Cramer GD: Pain generators and pain pathways of head and neck. In Curl DD, editor: *Chiropractic approach to head pain*, Baltimore, 1994, Williams & Wilkins.

28. Olson VL: Whiplash-associated chronic headache treated with home cervical traction, *Phys Ther* 77:417-424, 1997.

29. Warner JS: Analgesic rebound as a cause of hemicrania continua, *Neurology* 48(6):1540-1541, 1997.

30. Shekelle PG, Coulter I: Cervical spine manipulation: summary report of a systematic review of the literature and a multidisciplinary expert panel, *J Spinal Disord* 10(3):223-228, 1997.

31. Vernon HT: The effectiveness of chiropractic manipulation in the treatment of headache: an exploration in the literature, *J Manipulative Physiol Ther* 18(9):611-617, 1995.

32. Vernon H: Chiropractic manipulative therapy in the treatment of headaches: a retrospective and prospective study, *J Manipulative Physiol Ther* 5(3):109-112, 1982.

33. Howe DH, Newcombe RG, Wade MT: Manipulation of the cervical spine: a pilot study, *J R Coll Gen Pract* 33:564-579, 1983.

34. Droz J, Crot F: Occipital headaches, *Ann Swiss Chiro Assoc* 8:127-135, 1985.

35. Turk Z, Ratkolb O: Mobilization of the cervical spine in chronic headaches, *Man Med* 3(1):15-17, 1987.

36. Jensen OK, Nielsen FF, Vosmar L: An open study comparing manual therapy with the use of cold packs in the treatment of post-traumatic headache, *Cephalalgia* 10(5):241-250, 1990.

37. Robbins LD: Cryotherapy for headache, *Headache* 29(9):598-600, 1989.

38. Whittingham W, Ellis WB, Molyneux TP: The effect of manipulation (toggle recoil technique) for headaches with upper cervical joint dysfunction: a pilot study, *J Manipulative Physiol Ther* 17(6):369-375, 1994.

39. Mootz R, Dhami M, Hess J: Chiropractic treatment of chronic episodic tension type headache in male subjects: a case series analysis, *J Can Chiro Assoc* 38(3):152-159, 1994.

40. Nilsson N, Christensen HW, Hartvigsen J: The effect of spinal manipulation in the treatment of cervicogenic headache, *J Manipulative Physiol Ther* 20(5):326-330, 1997.

41. Rapoport A et al: Analgesic rebound headache in clinical practice: data from a physician survey, *Headache* 36(1):14-19, 1996.

42. Stodolny J, Chmielewski H: Manual therapy in the treatment of patients with cervical migraine, *J Man Med* 4:49-51, 1989.

43. Hewitt EG: Chiropractic care of a 13-year-old with headache and neck pain: a case report, *Proc Natl Conf Chiro Ped (ICA)* 90-98, 1993.

44. Haney VL: Chronic pediatric migraine-type headaches treated by long-term inderol prior to chiropractic care: a case report, *Proc Natl Conf Chiro Ped (ICA)* 132-140, 1993.

45. Cochran JA: Chiropractic treatment of childhood migraine headache: a case study, *Proc Natl Conf Chiro Ped (ICA)* 85-90, 1994.

46. Stephens D, Gorman F: The prospective treatment of visual perception deficit by chiropractic spinal manipulation: a report on two juvenile patients, *Chiro J Austral* 26:82-86, 1996.

47. Gemmell HA, Jacobson BH, Sutton L: Toftness spinal correction in the treatment of migraine: a case study, *Chiro Technique* 6(2):57-60, 1994.

48. Killinger LZ: A chiropractic case series of seven chronic headache patients, *Palmer J Res* 2(2):48-53, 1995.

49. Tuchin P, Brookes M, Swaffer T: A case study of chronic headaches, *Aust Chiro Osteopathy* 5(2):47-52, 1996.

50. Whittingham W, Ellis W, Molyneux T: The effects of manipulation (toggle recoil technique) for headaches with upper cervical joint dysfunction: a pilot study, *J Chiro* 17(6):369-375, 1994.

51. Mootz R, Dhami M, Hess J: Chiropractic treatment of chronic episodic tension type headache in male subjects: a case series analysis, *J Can Chiro Assoc* 38(3):152-159, 1994.

52. Defranca G, Levine L: The T4 syndrome, *J Manipulative Physiol Ther* 18(1):34-37, 1995.

53. Kerr FWL, Olafson RA: Trigeminal and cervical volleys, *Arch Neurol* 4:134-148, 1961.

54. Skillern PG: Great occipital-trigeminus syndrome as revealed by induction of block, *Arch Neurol Psychiatry* 72:335-340, 1954.

55. Kellgren JH: On the distribution of pain arising from deep somatic tissues with charts from segmental pain areas, *Clin Sci* 35-46, 1939.

56. Dwyer A, Aprill C, Bogduk N: Cervical zygapophyseal joint pain patterns: a study in normal volunteers, *Spine* 15:453-457, 1990.

57. Bogduk N: Headaches and cervical manipulation, *Med J Aust* 66:65-66, 1979.

58. Schultz M: Occipital neuralgia, *J Am Osteopath Assoc* 76:335-343, 1977.

59. Bogduk N: The anatomy of occipital neuralgia, *Clin Exp Neurol* 17164-17184, 1981.

60. Cox CL, Cocks GR: Occipital neuralgia, *J Med Assoc State Ala* 48(7):23-27, 1979.

61. Campbell DG, Parsons CM: Referred head pain and concomitants, *J Nerv Ment Dis* 99:544-551, 1944.
62. Travell JG, Simons DG: *Myofascial pain and dysfunction. The trigger point manual,* vol I, Baltimore, 1983, Williams & Wilkins.
63. Frolich R: Importance of muscular dysfunction in headaches, *Man Med* 26:113, 1988.
64. Pikoff H: Is the muscular model of headache still viable? A review of the conflicting data, *Headache* 24:186-198, 1984.
65. Edmeads J: Headaches and head pains associated with diseases of the cervical spine, *Med Clin North Am* 62:533-544, 1978.
66. Bogduk N, Marsland AJ: On the concept of third occipital headache, *Neurol Neurosurg Psychiatry* 49(7):775-780, 1986.
67. Boake HK: Cervical headache, *Can Fam Physician* 18:75-78, 1972.
68. Jirout J: Comments regarding the diagnosis and treatment of dysfunctions of the C2-C3 segment, *Man Med* 2:16-17, 1985.
69. Heller JG: The syndromes of degenerative cervical disease, *Orthop Clin North Am* 23(3):381-394, 1992.
70. Jacobs B: Cervical angina, *NY Sta J Med* 90(1):8-11, 1990.
71. Kuhn WF, Juhn SC, Gilberstady H: Occipital neuralgias: clinical recognition of a complicated headache. A case series and literature review, *J Orofac Pain* 11(2):158-165, 1997.
72. Bogduk N, Marsland A: The cervical zygapophyseal joints as a source of neck pain, *Spine* 13:610-617, 1988.

CHAPTER 13

Subluxation and the Special Senses

Charles S. Masarsky, DC • *Marion Todres-Masarsky, DC*

A small but growing body of clinical literature includes descriptions of disturbance of vision, hearing, and balance secondary to the vertebral subluxation complex (VSC). Most investigators in this arena hypothesize that these sensory effects are mediated through the influence of the VSC on the autonomic nervous system (ANS). For this reason, including a discussion of this topic in this textbook is appropriate.

Visual System

One controlled study by Briggs and Boone[1] on pupil diameter concerned the visual system. During a 4-day baseline period, 15 subjects had their pupils photographed using infrared film in a darkened room. Chiropractic analysis was performed during this same period, primarily based on heat-reading instrumentation and the Derefield-Thompson leg check procedure. A total of 8 subjects were found to have signs of cervical subluxation and 7 subjects did not. After adjustment of the subluxated subjects with toggle-recoil or diversified methods and light soft-tissue massage of the unsubluxated subjects, a fifth pupil measurement was performed. Although the subjects receiving massage demonstrated no postintervention change in pupillary diameter, change occurred in all the adjusted subjects—dilation in some and constriction in others. The authors suggested that cervical subluxation created imbalance in the tone of the sympathetic and parasympathetic innervation to the pupils. Therefore observation of pupillary diameter may have provided a noninvasive means for studying autonomic balance.

Gilman and Bergstrand[2] reported the case of a 75-year-old man with a 6-month history of total blindness after head trauma. After three upper cervical adjustments, he was able to tell the difference between light and darkness; after 11 adjustments administered over 3 months, he could distinguish colors and experienced a return of normal pupillary response; and after 5 months of care, he was able to read again.

Although spontaneous remission of posttraumatic blindness has been reported, it is rare after 6 months. The authors assumed that upper cervical VSC may have caused retinal vasospasm if sufficient irritation to the superior cervical sympathetic ganglia occurred that innervated most cranial blood vessels.

An impressive amount of ophthalmologic clinical research by Gorman and others,[3-6] published primarily in chiropractic research journals, featured automated static perimetry as a major outcome measure. In this technique, points of light of various intensities were projected at different spots on a hemispheric screen placed over a patient's head. The patient pressed a button each time a point of light was seen. Computerized mapping of the patient's visual field based on these responses identified perceptual defects not usually detected by less-sensitive techniques.

In the previously cited publications, Gorman and others[3-6] repeatedly noted improved perimetry results after general *pan-spinal* manipulation, usually performed after anesthetic was administered. Most results have been verified by an independent ophthalmologist. Patients have included adults and children, with traumatic and nontraumatic histories, mildly depressed visual sensitivity, and overt bilateral tunnel vision. Concomitant problems such as neck pain, headache, arm pain, dizziness, fatigue, and abdominal pain often resolved with the visual problems.

In more recent publications, Gorman and others[7] have presented cases in which no anesthetic was used. A 62-year-old man with monocular scotomata was managed with general cervical and thoracic manipulation under traction. Although complete resolution was often noted in previous cases with relatively few visits, this unanesthetized patient exhibited a partial but sharp improvement after each of 12 visits. The improvement in perimetry results abruptly plateaued each time. Gorman and others[7] referred to this as a *stepped* recovery because a graph of the results resembled stair steps. The step phenomenon appeared to be a feature of recovery in patients manipulated without anesthetic. Step phenomenon has been reported in other publications by Danny Stephens, DC, in which neither anesthetic nor traction were used.[8-10]

An almost universal finding in these patients was tenderness at the arch of the atlas. This tenderness generally cleared as visual competence was restored, which seemingly suggested a specific relationship between visual disturbance and upper cervical subluxation. Unfortunately, the Stephens-Gorman group has not reported a case in which specific upper cervical adjustments were used.

In the typical patient reported by Stephens[8-10] and Gorman and others[7], standard ophthalmoscopic examination failed to reveal any retinal problems. Unfortunately, this was misleading and caused many clinicians to resort to such diagnoses as *hysteric amblyopia, malingering,* and so on. Other researchers, particularly Gorman, have theorized that cervical dysfunction may disturb the sympathetic nerves surrounding the vertebral arteries, causing an electric disturbance to spread throughout the cranial arterial tree, resulting in hypoperfusion of the cerebrum in general and the visual centers in the occipital lobes in particular. This in turn could deprive cerebral neurons of enough oxygen to leave them electrically silent without causing cellular death. The idea that this hibernation-like state is possible in the nervous system has been well established since the early 1970s. The partial oxygen deprivation responsible for this state is called the *ischemic penumbra.* Much of the relevant literature in this area was recently reviewed by Terrett.[11]

The theory that visual dysfunction associated with the VSC actually reflected vertebrogenic brain dysfunction was reiterated in a paper by Carrick.[12] This study featured circumference measurement of maps of the left and right visual blind spot before and after chiropractic adjustment at C2. Although all people have a blind spot in each eye because of light insensitivity at the optic disk, enlargement of the blind spot is usually associated with problems in the visual cortex. Carrick[12] discovered that when C2 adjustment was delivered to the side of the larger map, symmetry and, by implication, cortical function increased. When the adjustment was delivered to the side of the smaller map, symmetry decreased.

Carrick[12] believed that various sensory modalities may affect each other at the central integration level, particularly at the thalamic level. If true, altered kinesthetic signals from a dysfunctional spinal motion segment could disrupt the central processing of visual signals. Successful adjustment of the subluxated segment would then be expected to improve kinesthetic and visual perception.

Kessinger and Boneva[13] reported visual acuity of subjects as measured by standard Snellen chart testing before receiving and 6 weeks after receiving upper cervical chiropractic care. The 67 subjects in this study were between the ages of 9 and 79. The most interesting finding was that the percentage of distance visual acuity (%DVA) increased among all subjects, including those with normal distance vision at the initial examination. For some reason, greater improvements in %DVA were noted in the right eyes of these subjects. Future studies should include data on handedness and eye dominance.

Alcantara and Parker[14] provided an instructive case study involving a 6-year-old boy with bilateral internal strabismus. The parents indicated that the patient's problem began to be noticeable at age 2. No other significant clinical history was noted, except for the child's umbilical cord being wrapped around his neck at birth. Analysis using Gonstead protocols revealed evidence of upper cervical, lower cervical, and sacral subluxations. Within 10 visits, based on optometric examination, the patient's internal strabismus was barely noticeable and his vision was measurably improved.

Visual dysfunction often accompanies headache. Chiropractic clinical literature associating some headaches with the VSC is accumulating (see Chapter 12).

Historic osteopathic and chiropractic research

also is important. Based on neuroanatomic considerations combined with long clinical experience, Homewood[15] stated that upper thoracic adjusting often benefits the eye and associated structures by normalizing sympathetic tone. Homewood[15] was in substantial agreement with pioneer osteopathic researcher Louisa Burns,[16-17] who advocated that upper thoracic and upper cervical dysfunctions should be ruled out in ocular disorders, based largely on the results of experimental animal research.

Last, D.D. Palmer suggested many correlations between spinal subluxations and disorders of the eye, including strabismus (T4), nystagmus (C3), and conjunctivitis (T6).[18]

Otovestibular Function

Otitis media is often accompanied by hearing loss that is either chronic or temporary. Hobbs and Rasmussen[19] described an adult case with a 30% to 60% conductive hearing loss verified by an otolaryngologist. Chiropractic adjustments included the cranial procedures of sacrooccipital technique, focusing on the right temporal bone. A follow-up hearing test after the fourth chiropractic adjustment indicated restoration of normal hearing. This recovery was stable at 2 years of follow-up.

Doyle and others[20] reported the case of a man with aerotitis media, a form of otitis media common in underwater divers and frequent airplane travelers. The patient's complaints at the first visit included a feeling of fullness in both ears, hearing loss, and tinnitus. A course of antihistamine treatment had failed to provide relief. Audiometry and tympanometry verified bilateral middle-ear dysfunction. On chiropractic analysis, signs of cervical subluxation clustered at C2 and C5. Diversified adjustments at these levels were performed twice per week for 5 weeks. After this regimen, audiometry and tympanometry results normalized and subjective complaints were resolved.

Heagy[21] presented a series of pediatric otitis media cases, one of which had 60% hearing loss in the left ear. All four patients had undergone unsuccessful antibiotic treatment and exhibited evidence of upper cervical subluxation on palpation and postural analysis. At the time of publication, all were free of otitis media signs and symptoms

without antibiotic or surgical intervention, based on parental reports, medical examinations, school attendance records, and in the one relevant case follow-up audiometry, for periods ranging from 5 months to 4 years.

The most common disturbance of vestibular function discussed in the chiropractic clinical literature is vertigo. Cote and others[22] reported three cases of cervicogenic vertigo in adults. In one case, dizziness, neck pain, and headache occurred after a woman was involved in an automobile accident. Deep digital pressure in the upper cervical spine reproduced the dizziness, which increased when she opened her mouth. This suggested upper cervical and temporomandibular joint involvement. Chiropractic adjustments focused on these two regions, and the patient was free of dizziness after 1 month of care. At 3 years of follow-up, the patient reported only one recurrence of vertigo that was resolved with a single chiropractic visit. The other two cases did not involve trauma, and both patients responded well to upper cervical adjusting.

A physical medicine group, Galm and others[23] reported on 50 vertigo patients with no remarkable findings of the ear, nose, and throat on neurologic examination. Of these patients, 31 demonstrated signs of upper cervical dysfunction. Response to high-velocity impulse manipulation was favorable for 24 of these 31 patients, with 5 of them reporting complete resolution of the vertigo.

A group of 31 patients with cervical migraine, or the symptom complex of headache, neck pain, and dizziness, was reported by manual medicine practitioners Stodolny and Chmielewski.[24] Assessment of each patient's equilibrium was performed before manual manipulation began. One test was interesting because of its similarity to certain chiropractic assessment procedures, called the *two-weight test*. (In this test, bilateral scales are used to measure the symmetry of weight bearing in the standing patient. The test is considered positive for possible disequilibrium if asymmetry of weight bearing exceeds 4 kg.) All 31 patients demonstrated evidence of atlantooccipital dysfunction, with some also demonstrating cervicothoracic dysfunction. Response to manipulation was favorable for the majority of the patients, based on symptomatic relief and improved symmetry in the two-weight test. No symptomatic exacerbation or complications were noted for any of these patients.

Virre and Baloh[25] reported a series of 13 cases of sudden hearing loss. Of these, 12 patients also suffered from vertigo. The clinical correlation of episodes of sudden deafness with migraine attacks, combined with the lack of history or clinical findings suggestive of viral infection, led the authors to speculate that the vasomotor instability associated with migraine can have profound effects on the vestibular and acoustic portions of the auditory nerve.

The effect of migraine on acoustic function was also evident in a study by Tuchin,[26] who described a series of four patients with migraine headache. Phonophobia was completely abolished for 2 of these patients after 2 months of chiropractic care.

Tinnitus, or *ringing in the ears,* can be distressing, sometimes leading to insomnia and even suicide. After an extensive review of the literature, Terrett[27] advised a trial of chiropractic care for tinnitus patients, with special emphasis on the cervical and upper thoracic spine. Blum[28] offered a case report of a woman shipping clerk who was exposed to a high-decibel noise in the loading dock area where she worked. She was unable to hear anything for approximately 30 minutes. As the day progressed, she began to experience ringing, hissing, buzzing, and warbling sounds. Treatment by an ear, nose, and throat medical specialist was not promising. When she first visited Dr. Blum's office, she was sleeping no more than 2 hours per night and would experience crying spells for 6 hours a day.

Chiropractic adjustments using sacrooccipital technique protocols for category II were instituted. (The category II protocols focus on a type of sacroiliac subluxation and correlates it with temporomandibular joint, cervical, and cranial dysfunction.) Relief was noted after the first visit. At the time the paper was written, the patient reported more than a 50% decrease in tinnitus intensity and improved sleep.

As anyone with an appreciation of chiropractic history knows, D.D. Palmer's first patient visited him with hearing loss. According to Palmer,[29] the following occurred:

> On Sept. 18, 1895, Harvey Lillard called upon me. He was so deaf for seventeen years that he could not hear the noises on the street. Mr. Lillard informed me that he was in a cramped position, and felt something give in his back. I replaced the displaced 4th dorsal vertebra by one move, which restored his hearing fully.

Unfortunately, this case description has been ridiculed by chiropractic detractors for more than a century. However, a similar case was reported by a medical author. In the previously cited tinnitus paper by Terrett,[27] a case by manual medicine practitioner John Bourdillon was reviewed. Bourdillon's patient was being treated for Meniere's disease, which include symptoms such as vertigo, tinnitus, and unilateral deafness. Only transient relief was obtained by cervical manipulation. When the T4-5 motion segment was addressed, the patient experienced ". . .dramatic and lasting relief of all the symptoms, including deafness."

The most frequently hypothesized mechanism for the association of T4 subluxation and hearing loss is that the preganglionic fibers from this level create a sympathetic disturbance in the superior cervical sympathetic ganglion. For many years this ganglion was considered the sole source of sympathetic fibers to the vasculature of the cochlea. In the early 1990s, sympathetic fibers from the stellate ganglion also were demonstrated to innervate the cochlear vasculature.[30] Obviously, the upper thoracic spine, including the T4 level, are responsible for preganglionic outflow to the stellate and superior cervical ganglion. Therefore although the explanation of Harvey Lillard regaining his hearing will never be known with certainty, our current understanding of the sympathetic innervation of the cochlear vasculature described earlier seems to suggest that a probable explanation exists.

STUDY GUIDE

1. Explain the possible significance of changes in pupillary diameter in terms of chiropractic analysis as discussed by Briggs and Boone.[1]
2. Which cervical ganglion innervates most cranial blood vessels? Discuss this in terms of the case study reported by Gilman and Bergstrand.[2]
3. What is the step phenomenon?
4. Describe ischemic penumbra.
5. Explain Carrick's findings associated with brain mapping.[12] How might this be useful to the clinician?
6. In the study by Kessinger and Boneva[13] which eye showed dominance? Why might this be important?
7. In the case study by Alcantara and Parker[14] regarding the 6-year-old boy with strabismus, what was a major item of significant clinical history? How might it be important?
8. According to Homewood[15] and Burns,[16,17] what spinal area other than the cervical is frequently involved in ocular disorders?
9. Why might the VSC make a person vulnerable to otitis media? Discuss this in terms of the studies cited.
10. What is cervicogenic vertigo? How might this be related to the VSC?
11. What symptom of the VSC appeared along with hearing loss in the papers by Virre and Baloh[25] and Tuchin?[26] What neurologic mechanism was suggested?
12. Where was the primary subluxation in the tinnitus case reported by Blum?[28]
13. Regarding the Harvey Lillard case, where did D.D. Palmer[29] report finding the subluxation? Explain a possible mechanism by which this might have caused hearing loss.

REFERENCES

1. Briggs L, Boone WR: Effects of a chiropractic adjustment on changes in pupillary diameter: a model for evaluating somatovisceral response, *J Manipulative Physiol Ther* 11:181, 1988.
2. Gilman G, Bergstrand J: Visual recovery following chiropractic intervention, *Chiropr: J Res Chiropr Clin Invest* 6:61, 1990.
3. Gorman RF: Monocular visual loss after closed head trauma: immediate resolution associated with spinal manipulation, *J Manipulative Physiol Ther* 16:308, 1993.
4. Gorman RF: Automated static perimetry in chiropractic, *J Manipulative Physiol Ther* 16:481, 1993.
5. Gorman RF et al: Case report: spinal strain and visual perception deficit, *Chiro J Austral* 24:131, 1994.
6. Gorman RF: The treatment of presumptive optic nerve ischemia by spinal manipulation, *J Manipulative Physiol Ther* 18:172, 1995.
7. Gorman RF: Monocular scotomata and spinal manipulation: the step phenomenon, *J Manipulative Physiol Ther* 19:344, 1996.
8. Stephens D, Gorman RF: The association between visual incompetence and spinal derangement: an instructive case history, *J Manipulative Physiol Ther* 20:343, 1997.
9. Stephens D, Gorman RF, Bilton D: The step phenomenon in the recovery of vision with spinal manipulation: a report on two 13-year-olds treated together, *J Manipulative Physiol Ther* 20:628, 1997.
10. Stephens D et al: Treatment of visual field loss by spinal manipulation: a report on 17 patients, *J Neuromusculoskel Syst* 6:53, 1998.
11. Terrett AGJ: Cerebral dysfunction: a theory to explain some of the effects of chiropractic manipulation, *Chiro Technique* 5:168, 1993.
12. Carrick FR: Changes in brain function after manipulation of the cervical spine, *J Manipulative Physiol Ther* 20:529, 1997.
13. Kessinger R, Boneva D: Changes in visual acuity in patients receiving upper cervical specific chiropractic care, *J Vertebr Sublux Res* 2(1):43, 1998.
14. Alcantara J, Parker JA: Management of a patient with bilateral esotrophia and subluxations, *J Manipulative Physiol Ther,* 1999 (in press).
15. Homewood AE: *The neurodynamics of the vertebral subluxation,* p 251, St. Petersburg, Fla, 1977, Valkyrie Press.
16. Burns L: Eyes and vertebral lesions, *J Am Osteopath Assoc* 40:487, 1941.
17. Burns L: Study of certain structures concerned in pupillary reactions following second thoracic lesions, *J Am Osteopath Assoc* 36:409, 1937.
18. Palmer DD: *The science, art and philosophy of chiropractic,* p 925, Portland, Ore, 1910, Portland Printing House.
19. Hobbs DA, Rasmussen SA: Chronic otitis media: a case report, *ACA J Chiro* 28:67, 1991.
20. Doyle EP, Dreifus LI, Dreifus GL: Aerotitis media: a case report, *Chiropr Sports Med* 9:89, 1995.
21. Heagy DT: The effect of the correction of the vertebral subluxation on chronic otitis media in children, *Chiro Pediatr* 2(2):6, 1996.

22. Cote P, Mior SA, Fitz-Ritson D: Cervicogenic vertigo: a report of three cases, *J Can Chiro Assoc* 35:89, 1991.
23. Galm R, Rittmeister M, Schmitt E: Vertigo in patients with cervical spine dysfunction, *Eur Spine J* 7:55, 1998.
24. Stodolny J, Chmielewski H: Manual therapy in the treatment of patients with cervical migraine, *J Man Med* 4:49, 1989.
25. Virre ES, Baloh RW: Migraine as a cause of sudden hearing loss, *Headache* 36:24, 1996.
26. Tuchin PJ: A case series of migraine changes following a manipulative therapy trial, *Aust J Chiro Osteopath* 6(3):85, 1997.
27. Terrett AGJ: Tinnitus, the cervical spine, and spinal manipulative therapy, *Chiro Technique* 1:41, 1989.
28. Blum CL: Spinal/cranial manipulative therapy and tinnitus: a case history, *Chiro Technique* 10:163, 1998.
29. Palmer DD: *The science, art and philosophy of chiropractic*, p 137, Portland, Ore, 1910, Portland Printing House.
30. Ren T et al: Effects of stellate ganglion stimulation on bilateral cochlear blood flow, *Ann Otol Rhinol Laryngol* 102:378, 1993.

CHAPTER 14

Endocrine Disorders

Anthony Rosner, PhD

Initially, the way in which the endocrine system and chiropractic are related may not seem obvious. Many more traditional approaches to chiropractic have focused on the biomechanical aspects of musculoskeletal pain.[1] However, as Herzog suggested, three primary mechanisms exist that have been associated with the beneficial effects of spinal manipulation for neck and back pain. Reflexogenic and neurophysiologic sequelae and the aforementioned biomechanical consequences should be considered.[2] The neurophysiologic elements, in turn, involve two distinct domains: neurologic and hormonal. Again, much of chiropractic's rationale has been historically framed in neurologic terms with relatively little attention paid to its hormonal counterparts. This chapter seeks to address this imbalance by focusing on the underrepresented hormonal element with attention to the following three areas:

1. The way pain is associated with the endocrine system and the implications in the relief of pain through spinal manipulation
2. The way stress is associated with the endocrine system and the way its detrimental effects on health may be relieved by spinal manipulation
3. A description of specific endocrine disorders and their responses to spinal manipulation

Effects on Pain and Immunologic Activity

The endocrine system can be called into play by two distinct mechanisms for pain and its alleviation. The first relates to the actual production of pain, its enhancement and attenuation, and the appearance of biochemical endproducts that have hormonal activity. The second takes into account the role of stress in producing what may be considered the psychoneuroendocrine response, which has tremendous bearing on the onset of many diseases and disorders.

Localized Production of Pain and Its Modulation

The reason an action potential is created and transmitted through the neuronal axon is beyond the scope of this discussion; however, a typical neurotransmitter for C and Aδ fibers, acetylcholine, must successfully cross the synaptic cleft and bind to a receptor on the opposite side to renew the cycle of nerve transmission through the length of the neighboring neuron.

An oversupply of acetylcholine can cause overstimulation or even paralysis in the neurons downstream from the binding sites. Normally, this untoward circumstance is prevented by the continuous breakdown of acetylcholine by the enzyme cholinesterase, leading to the uptake of fragments of the original neurotransmitter and its resynthesis into fresh acetylcholine in the axonal region of the original neuron (Figure 14-1).

Other neurotransmitters may be expected to follow a similar mechanism. One such entity is the peripatetic peptide Substance P, the first peptide to have been proposed as a neurotransmitter, which is found in the gut, salivary glands, and most areas of the central nervous system (CNS).[3] The release of specific substance P receptors in the synaptic cleft[4] is modulated by opioid peptides known as *enkephalins*[5] (Figure 14-2).

Release of a cocktail of mediators that are primarily algesic follows nociceptive stimulation, originating from such inflammatory centers as mast cells, macrophages, and lymphocytes. Included in this mix of pain stimulators is Substance P and products of the arachidonic acid pathway such as the prostaglandins and leukotrienes (Figure 14-3).[6] Any or all of these chemicals act to sensitize nociceptors, lowering their thresholds to

further stimulation, such that normally benign stimuli then become perceived as pain. This is the basis of peripheral sensitization. Cells in the dorsal horn of the spinal cord become sensitized by repeated nerve stimulation in a process known as *windup,* leading to central sensitization.[7] The fact that prostaglandins are produced by this mechanism and then exert their effects on distant

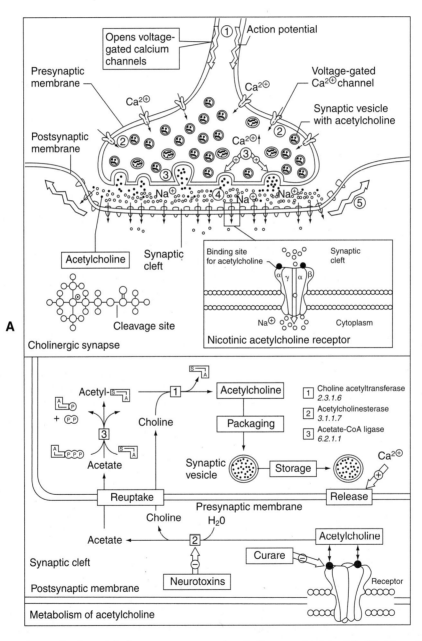

Figure 14-1 A, Role of acetylcholine as a neurotransmitter in the synaptic cleft. (Modified from Koolman J, Rohm KH: *Color atlas of biochemistry,* p 321, New York, 1996, Thieme.)

sites qualifies them as hormones. Later in this chapter, the consequences of prostaglandin production and the way they might be limited by spinal manipulation are discussed and become clear.

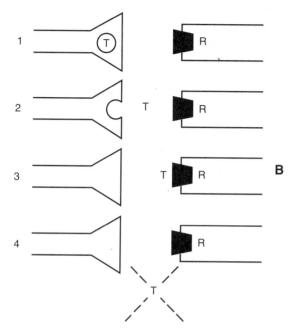

Figure 14-1 B, Role and metabolism of neurotransmitter in the synaptic cleft. (Modified from Koolman J, Rohm KH: *Color atlas of biochemistry*, p 321, New York, Thieme.)

The Role of Psychoneuroendocrine Stress Responses

The conscious experience of pain may be shaped by mental, emotional, and sensory mechanisms and by the primary stimulus.[8] This has given rise to the biopsychosocial concept of illness rather than disease, a model that has been proposed to be effective in clinical practice[9] and has become the centerpiece in the newer concepts of back pain.[10] The psychologic and psychosocial influences on the course of human disease have led to the science of psychoneuroimmunology (PNI), used to describe the communication system between mind and body first popularized through the work of Benson[11] and ultimately by Ader.[12] Much research showed that through a complex system of feedback loops and interactions, a close communication among the CNS, the immune system, and hormones by means of the hypothalamic-pituitary-adrenal (HPA) axis existed[13] (Figure 14-4).

Stress and the Production of Hormones Relationships among stress, the HPA axis, and chiropractic have been elegantly and exhaustively presented by Morgan.[13] The biochemistry of stress first became a topic of interest from the investigations of Hans Seyle, the "father of stress," who in 1936

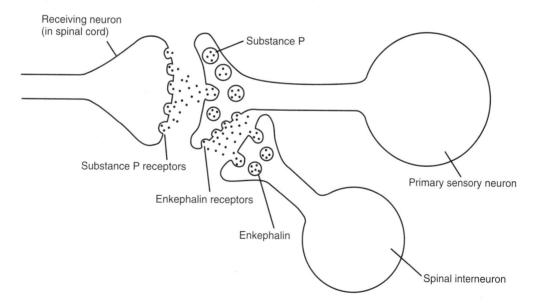

Figure 14-2 Proposed gating mechanism at the first synaptic relay in the spinal cord, regulating transmission of pain information from the peripheral pain receptor to the brain. (Modified from Iversen LL: The chemistry of the brain, *Sci Am* 241(3):134-149, 1979.)

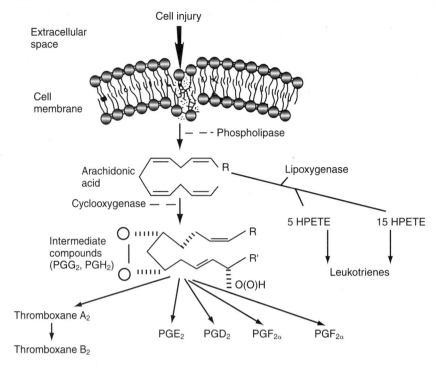

Figure 14-3 Sequence of chemical events following cell injury at the site of pain in the peripheral nervous system, leading to the synthesis of prostaglandins and other products from arachidonic acid. (Modified from Raj RP: *Pain medicine: a comprehensive review,* p 13, St Louis, 1996, Mosby.)

proposed the following four stages of the stress reaction[14,15]:

1. Alarm reaction, with sympathoadrenomedullary output
2. Stage of resistance, with activation of the HPA axis
3. Stage of adrenal hypertrophy, gastric ulceration, and thymic and lymphoid shrinkage, known as the *general adaptation syndrome*
4. Exhaustion and death

The biochemical basis of stress begins when distinct chemical entities, including the neuropeptides and neurohormones, function as neurologic transmitters of stress. Even before the development of an endocrine system, neuropeptides appear to have evolved from microbes as a primary means of intercellular communication.[16] The end result is the complex pathway shown in Figure 14-5, the most important aspect of which is the secretion of corticosteroids, in particular, glucocorticoids, including cortisol, from the adrenal cortex in response to adrenocorticoid

(ACTH) secretion from the anterior lobe of the pituitary. Glucocorticoids subsequently exert a variety of effects on cardiovascular, muscle, and immunologic activity, many of which are detrimental. The connection between increased cortisol levels and stressful events has been well documented.[17,18]

Probably the best known component of this pathway is the sympathetic system, which is responsible for producing the adaptive "fight or flight" response to stress through the production of epinephrine and norepinephrine from the adrenal medulla and sympathetic nerve terminals. In chronic stress, increased catecholamine secretion is observed. One of the net effects of this function is to raise blood pressure by a mechanism involving the production of renin, which in turn increases the levels of angiotensin that subsequently induces aldosterone secretion. The latter acts on the kidney to produce sodium retention, which leads to the secondary retention of water, expansion of extracellular fluids, vasoconstriction, and ultimate increase in blood pressure.[19]

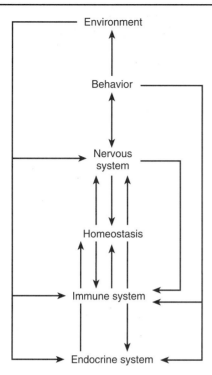

Figure 14-4 Interaction of stress with various body systems. (Modified from Morgan LG: Psychoneuroimmunology, the placebo effect and chiropractic, *J Manipulative Physiol Ther* 21(7):484-491, 1998.)

Numerous control mechanisms complicate matters, including the following[16]:

1. Regulation of ACTH by corticotropin-releasing hormone (CRH) from the hypothalamus
2. Presence of glucocorticoid receptors in the limbic system and hypothalamus to modulate the production of glucocorticoids in response to either environmental or emotional stimuli
3. Existence of other positive and negative feedback loops that regulate CRH levels

Stress and Aberrations of Immunologic Activity Numerous observations have suggested that stress plays a major role in promoting a variety of disorders, some of which are life threatening.

Infectious Disease
1. Although acute short-term stress plus exercise may enhance leukocyte and natural killer cell function, chronic stress often displays the opposite effect. This is borne out in individuals who are recently widowed or unemployed.[20]
2. Individuals under high stress experience higher infection rates to all five cold viruses tested.[21,22]
3. Herpes infections become more active in student nurses and college students experiencing immunosuppression from stress or colds.[22]
4. CD4 counts in HIV-infected men decline faster in individuals suffering from depression.[23]

Heart Disease
1. In response to stress, vascular epithelial cells may express heat shock proteins that could then trigger a cascade, leading to atherosclerotic lesions, accelerated by high serum cholesterol levels.[24]
2. Chronic stress may promote cardiovascular reactivity, resulting in increased cortisol and NK cell cytotoxicity, posing a particular risk for the elderly.[23,25]

Gastrointestinal Dysfunction
1. Irritable bowel syndrome, diarrhea, colitis, and abdominal pain have been long and closely associated with stress and may result from alteration of the permeability of the gastric mucosa affecting fluid and electrolyte absorption rates.[25]
2. Gastric alterations have been implicated in explaining increased allergic reactions by allowing previously restricted macromolecules to enter the bloodstream.[26]

Insulin-Dependent Diabetes Mellitus
1. The mechanism of insulin-dependent diabetes mellitus involves the destruction of islet cells of the pancreas, presumably from an autoimmune process.
2. Animal models display elevated rates of insulin-dependent diabetes mellitus development after exposure to chronic stress.[13]

Systemic Lupus Erythrematosus
1. An autoimmune disorder has long been implicated as the cause of systemic lupus erythrematosus.
2. Systemic lupus erythematosus is believed to provide the strongest evidence linking the

effect of psychologic factors to the immune system.[27]

Low-Back Pain and Major Depression
1. Adults aged 20 to 39 with elevated indicators of allergic reactions (asthma, hay fever, pet allergies, or allergy-shot reactions) are much more likely to report low-back pain and to be diagnosed with major depression.[28]
2. Proinflammatory cytokines activate the HPA axis in response to various threats to homeostasis.[29]
3. Glucocorticoids released as a response to this activation quench the immune and inflammatory responses.[30,31]

Although all aspects of these relationships have yet to be explained, endocrine and neurologic signals clearly trigger reactions in the immune system. Recent observations from Turnbull[29,30] also show that the peptide mediators (interleukins IL-1 and IL-6 and tumor necrosis factor alpha) not only regulate local immune and inflammatory responses but also stimulate many CNS-mediated responses through the HPA axis. The production of immune complexes also promotes the release of prostaglandin E_2, which promotes the eventual synthesis of immunosuppressive cytokines.[32]

Chiropractic and the Relief of Stress

Hormones play a major if not dominant role in communications between the central nervous and immune systems. Chiropractics' effort in health management to control stress-related hormones is discussed next. Chiropractic should become aware of this from at least two perspectives.

1. Two major studies[33,34] published in leading medical journals within the past year have been incorrectly interpreted to indicate that chiropractic is ineffective for treating the respective conditions under study simply because cavitations, as indicators of high-velocity thrusting and commonly regarded by some as the gold standard of chiropractic,[35] did not show any association with improvements. Rather, the control treatments, involving deep-friction massage and perhaps trigger-point therapy,[34] have been referred to as *mimic* or *sham treatments*,[33] and entailed considerable contact with the patient and cannot be simply disregarded as irrelevant.
2. EMG responses to SMT have been reported to occur regularly with latencies too short to involve the central recruitment of muscles.[2,36] They are more likely of reflex origin and coincide with the timings of spinal adjustments achieved with instruments, in which cavitations are expected to be absent.[37] The reflex responses observed may in fact be largely responsible for the reduction of pain and decrease of muscle hypertonicity observed after SMT,[2,36] skirting the idea that the beneficial effects of chiropractic are achieved through the audible release.

In pointing out the inaccuracy of the one-dimensional stereotype of chiropractic as the cracking of joints, these findings underscore the importance of low-force techniques and the management of stress—whether achieved through contact, relaxation techniques, biofeedback, other forms of mind-body medicine, exercise, or any combination. In blinded clinical trials, 30% to 40% of patients have been observed to experience significant relief from a placebo.[38] In nonblinded clinical trials that must necessarily be employed to evaluate manual medicine, only larger placebo effects involving greater numbers of patients can be anticipated. Kaptchuk[35] argued, "the chiropractic approach to healing relies on the opposite of double-blindedness; it enlists the full participation and awareness of both" (physician and patient). It fills a major gap in established medicine by enabling the physician to validate the patient's pain experience.[35] In terms of reduction of overall stress, a recent randomized clinical trial found that spinal manipulation significantly decreased the intensity of emotional arousal reported by phobic college students.[39] Spinal manipulation, consistent with the calming effect of stress reduction, may also reduce salivary cortisol levels over several weeks.[40] This, in turn, might be expected to affect blood pressure.

The chiropractor is involved with a broad spectrum of health issues, including primary care[41,42] and maintenance.[42-44] In this manner, the reduction of stress and its deleterious effects discussed previously could be achieved.

Chiropractic and the Relief of Pain

In terms of outcomes, recent evidence regarding the effectiveness of chiropractic in reducing pain from low-back pain, headache, and some somatovisceral disorders has been reviewed.[34,45-50] In terms of mechanisms, this discussion focuses on the levels of two metabolites responding to spinal manipulation: beta-endorphins or enkephalins and prostaglandins.

Beta-Endorphins or Enkephalins

Beta-endorphins or enkephalins have been proposed to display a gating, palliative effect at the first synaptic relay in the spinal cord, limiting the transmission of pain information from the peripheral pain receptor to the brain (see Figure 14-2).[51] Described in 1972 by Pert,[52] these molecules represented a class of opioid peptides that bound to specific receptors and displayed marked analgesic

effects.[53,54] For the next decade a variety of therapeutic modalities were appearing to exert their pain-relieving effects at least partly because of their capacities to induce increases in endorphin levels.[55-60] Thus a great impetus to explore the relationships between spinal manipulation and beta-endorphin levels existed that has regrettably been the subject of only a few studies presenting conflicting results.

Unlike the remainder of the studies summarized in Table 14-1, the research by Vernon[61] revealed approximately an 8% increase in the level of plasma endorphins 5 minutes after a single rotary manipulation in asymptomatic men aged 23 on average. Of all the studies reviewed,[61-64] only Vernon[61] synchronized his observations within 3 hours, in which the known diurnal variations of beta-endorphins in the human are at 80% of their maximum values and in a period of decline.[60] The two effects are as follows:

1. Assurance that increases observed during the experimental period could not be attributed to natural cyclic variations
2. Limitations of increases observed to a ceiling

Table 14-1 *Summary of Trials Measuring Beta-Endorphin Levels Involving Chiropractic Intervention*

Author	Design	Branches	Number of Subjects	Presenting Condition	Outcomes	Change	Time Intervals
Vernon[61]	RCT	Control	27 men	Asymptomatic	BP	None	−20 min to
		Sham		Asymptomatic	HR	None	+40 min at
		SMT		Asymptomatic	ANX	#	5 min intervals
					BE	+	
Christian[62]	RCT	Sham	40 men	Asymptomatic	BP	None	Baseline
		SMT		Asymptomatic	HR	None	+5 min
		Sham		C/T pain*	BE	None	+30 min
		SMT		C/T pain*	ACTH	None	
					Cortisol	#	
Luisetto[63]	Pros SMT	SMT	11 women	Neck and arm pain	BE	None	Pretreatment and posttreatment
					CT	−	
Richardson[64]	RCT	Control	31 men and women	?	BE	None	−60 min
		SMT		?			posttreatment +60 min

Pros SMT, Prospective study of *SMT* patients; *SMT,* Spinal manipulative therapy; *RCT,* Randomized controlled trial; *BP,* Blood pressure; *HR,* Heart rate (pulse); *ANX,* Anxiety; *BE,* Plasma beta-endorphin; *CT,* Plasma calcitonin; *ACTH,* Adrenocorticotropic hormone; **,* Cervical and thoracic pain; *#,* Decrease seen in all experimental groups.

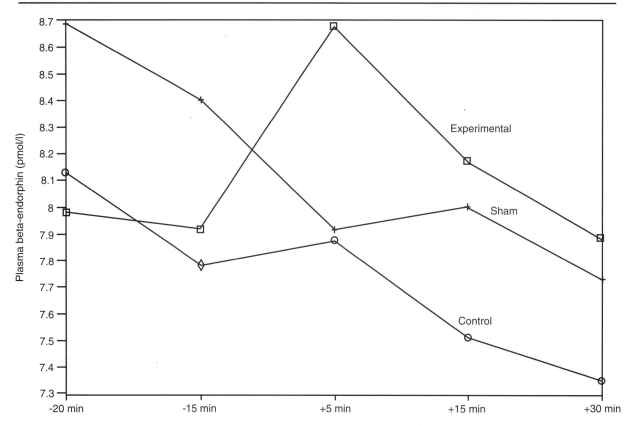

Figure 14-5 Mean beta-endorphin levels before and after spinal manipulation. (Modified from Vernon HT et al: Spinal manipulation and beta-endorphin: a controlled study of the effect of a spinal manipulation on plasma beta-endorphin levels in normal males, *J Manipulative Physiol Ther* 9(2):115-123, 1986.)

Other design differences between the trials reviewed in the table include the following:

1. With chiropractic techniques being unspecified[62,63] or of the osteopathic, long-lever variety,[64] only the Vernon investigation[61] likely involved rotary maneuvers.
2. The presence of gender and age differences in the patients recruited in the trials other than the Vernon study[61] may have presented confounding elements, obscuring the outcomes measured.
3. Vernon's study[61] was the only one to employ two measurements taken within 20 minutes at baseline and closely spaced postintervention measurements at 5-minute intervals, which would be expected to more closely match the rapid postintervention physiologic events reported by Herzog[2] and are more indicative of the short half-life of plasma beta-endorphin[65] (Figure 14-5).

4. The precision of the RIA beta-endorphin assay used by Christian[62] was reported to have a between-assay variation of 11% to 13%, exceeding and threatening to invalidate the 8% variation reported by Vernon[61] if the same analytical technique was used in the two investigations.
5. With few exceptions, beta-endorphin levels reported by Christian[62] were below the detection limit.

In summary, the hypothesis that spinal manipulation increases beta-endorphin levels, in turn providing a mechanism by which it leads to the reduction of pain, apparently remains largely untested. The variations within and among subject groups and of measurement times make combining the observations of Table 14-1 into a consistent pattern virtually impossible. As in most research, they raise further questions and future investigative efforts need to be refined.

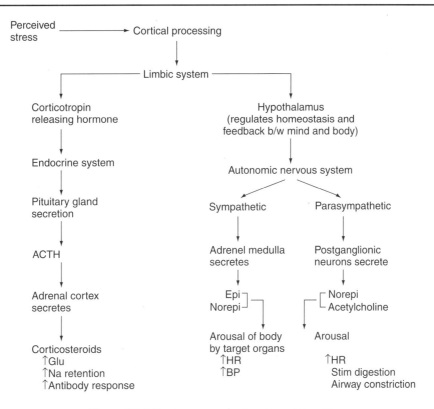

Figure 14-6 Psychoneuroendocrine stress responses.

However, the following two observations are notable:

1. Effects (anxiety in the Vernon trial[61] and cortisol levels in the Christian study[62]) sometimes pertained to all experimental groups, raising questions concerning the placebo effect and the presence of appropriate sham measures.
2. The average decrease in cortisol levels and the lack of corresponding changes of the average levels of ACTH in the Christian investigation[62] might suggest that the pathway was not operative (Figure 14-6); however, a closer examination of the individual patient values indicates that many data points were actually missing, severely compromising any systematic analysis.[62] Larger patient groups with a more robust statistical analysis are needed in any repeated investigation.

Prostaglandins

The link between prostaglandins and pain is best exemplified by primary dysmenorrhea (PD), the painful menstruation in the absence of organic pelvic pathologic change that has been reported to occur in up to half of all women of childbearing age and resulting in 600 million lost working hours at the cost of $2 billion annually.[66] In this condition, increased production and release of two endometrial fractions of prostaglandins (PGE_2 and PGF_{2a}) during menstrual sloughing of the endometrium triggers a corresponding escalation of uterine smooth muscle contraction plus vasospasm of the uterine arterioles, leading to ischemia and the cramping sensation of dysmenorrhea.[66-68] The implication of prostaglandins in causing PD is made even more pronounced by the fact that relief from PD is achieved through the use of nonsteroidal antiinflammatory (NSAIDS) drugs such as ibuprofen, naproxen, and mefanamic acid, which all exert their effects by inhibiting the activities of the enzymes in the cyclooxygenase pathway leading to the synthesis of prostaglandins (see Figure 14-3). NSAIDs appear to be effective in reducing pain in 70% to 85% of women diagnosed with PD.[66] Furthermore, oral contraceptives also are effective in treating PD[66,69] and reduce the levels of PGs in menstrual fluid.[70]

This information, together with the results from several case and anecdotal studies,[71-75] and one small clinical trial with a control group[76] suggest that spinal manipulation reduced the pain reported from PD and prompted Brennan to begin her investigations at the National College of Chiropractic in the early 1990s. Her attempt was to correlate the clinical effects observed after manipulation with actual prostaglandin levels and resulted in a pilot study[77] and a full-scale clinical trial.[78]

In the pilot study, Brennan and others[77] recruited a total of 45 women and subjected them to either side-posture manipulation (in the spinal region bounded by T10 and L5-S1 and associated with the neural connections to the uterus[71,75]) or a sham procedure of lower force, measuring pain using a visual analog scale and Menstrual Distress Questionnaire, 15 minutes before and 60 minutes after treatment. These measurements were combined with venipunctures at corresponding times to measure a PGF_{2a} metabolite ($KDPGF_{2a}$) thought to be the most appropriate analyte for the parent compound because of its longer half-life, stability during collection, and higher plasma concentrations. The actual assay for the PG metabolite was accomplished by a radioimmunoassay procedure.

In the women who had abdominal and back pain and menstrual distress, their scores declined in both groups after treatment, with the manipulated group displaying nearly twice the effect in all three criteria, easily reaching statistical signifi-

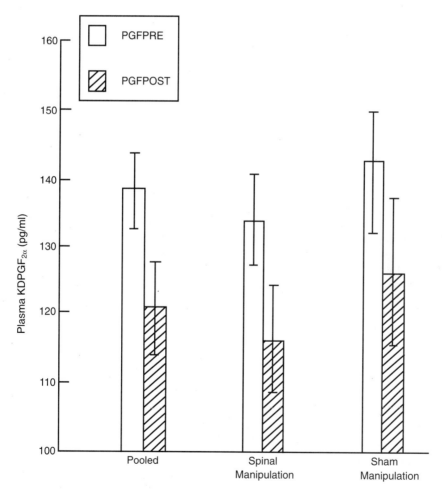

Figure 14-7 Prostaglandin metabolite levels and spinal manipulation. Pretreatment and posttreatment group means (±SE) for plasma levels of $KDPGF_{2a}$ in spinal-manipulated ($n = 20$), sham-manipulated ($n = 19$) and pooled ($n = 39$) subjects. (Modified from Kokjohn K et al: The effect of spinal manipulation on pain and prostaglandin levels in women with primary dysmenorrhea, *J Manipulative Physiol Ther* 15(5):279-285, 1992.)

cance. The corresponding KDGPF$_{2a}$ levels declined by nearly 50% after the interventions; however, in this instance, differences between sham and manipulated groups did not reach statistical significance (Figure 14-7). A considerable placebo effect is evident, observed in a previous trial of PD that employed either medications or a placebo.[79] The sham procedure appears to remain poorly defined as suggested earlier; active elements within the protocol have produced partial declines in pain and distress scores and in PG metabolite levels. As suggested by the authors, increased leuketriene levels resulting from increased lipoxygenase activity (see Figure 14-3)[66] is also possible and may contribute to the pain experienced in PD. In the more recent full-scale trial, similar results were observed, only this time the differences in VAS scores between the sham and manipulated groups were statistically insignificant.[78]

PG levels may indeed be reflective of the pain experienced in PD; however, to what extent reflection occurs is uncertain. Major difficulties in defining the active elements of spinal manipulation continue to occur, as shown by the positive results obtained with the sham procedures used.

Specific Endocrine Disorders and Responses to Spinal Manipulation

From the foregoing discussions, little doubt exists that the human endocrine and nervous systems are extensively interconnected. With the nervous system being placed at the conceptual centerpiece of chiropractic,[80] the link between chiropractic adjustments and the endocrine system should be apparent. Unfortunately, a lack of research attempting to explore the management of endocrine disorders by chiropractic exists. Only the following five areas, some including only isolated case reports for support, can be currently considered.

Primary Dysmenorrhea

The uterus has been postulated to be involved in the cramping associated with PD and the effect is likely to be in part caused by prostaglandins.[66-68] For these reasons, this clinical condition may be considered to be an endocrine disorder, the effects of which appear to be alleviated by spinal manip-

ulation[77,78,81-84] and by medication.[78] With the designs and effects of clinical trials having just been presented,[77,78] brief considerations of the uncontrolled case studies preceded Brennan's research[77] remains.

The first encouraging case study documented the improvement reported by a fraction of the 5 patients treated by Arnold-Frochet.[72] Pain diaries were subsequently used by a single patient during 3 months of treatment by manipulation and soft-tissue therapy and revealed significant reductions of the intensities and number of episodes of pain during therapy.[73] Finally, osteopathic manipulative treatment was shown to decrease the EMG activity of the lumbar spinae erector muscles and abolish spontaneous EMG activity in addition to the reports of 12 patients of diminished low-back pain and menstrual cramping.[81]

Premenstrual Syndrome

Closely related to but not similar to dysmenorrhea is premenstrual syndrome, which has up to 150 symptoms including breast tenderness, abdominal cramps, low back pain, headaches, joint pain, and psychologic and behavioral effects including irritability, mood changes, depression, food craving, insomnia, and loss of libido.[82] Unlike dysmenorrhea, the etiology of this condition has been more difficult to describe or define.

Numerous case studies have supported the possibility that spinal manipulative therapy may be effective in alleviating this condition. The earliest report by Hubbs[83] revealed a significant decrease in intensity and duration of back pain and premenstrual symptoms 2 months after adjustment.[83] Other case reports followed,[84] including the use of the PMT-Cator disc, a more objective scale throughout the menstrual cycle[85] that revealed a palliative effect of SMT,[86] and a case series.[87]

The case series conducted by Walsh[87] involved 8 patients, 5 of whom showed statistically significant reduction in PMS symptom scores during the treatment compared with the pretreatment phase. After SMT, 2 subjects reported that their symptoms had stayed reduced after treatment and the remaining 3 subjects found that their symptoms had returned to baseline levels.[87]

These moderately encouraging observations led to a randomized clinical trial involving 45 subjects who were divided into two groups, one receiving chiropractic adjustments for 3 cycles, then a sham treatment for 3 additional cycles after a 1-cycle hiatus as a wash-out, and the other receiving the sham and manipulative treatments in the reverse order. The sham treatment consisted of the use of an Activator instrument at the lowest setting, and adjustments entailed drop-piece, manual, and soft-tissue therapies. With 25 patients having completed the study, both groups showed significant decreases of their outcome scores with no significant differences observed between the treatment groups.[88] As is the case for many but not all clinical trials involving chiropractic, the effects of the sham procedure approximated those resulting from the manipulative technique identified as the presumably active component of therapy.

Aldosterone and Hypertension

The links of chiropractic management to the autonomic nervous system and reducing anxiety have led to conflicting observations regarding the effect of chiropractic procedures on blood pressure. Two clinical trials, one using the Activator[89] and the other using a cervical chair procedure,[90] yielded statistically significant lowerings of systolic and diastolic readings, with the decreases averaging 2 to 3 mm Hg. A more recent pilot study suggested a modest decrease in diastolic blood pressure after adjustments.[91]

Because of the strong rationale for linking serum aldosterone levels with blood pressure (see Primary Dysmenorrhea), one would immediately ask whether the concentrations of this particular hormone are responsive to spinal manipulations. Such an investigation occurred, using either Gonstead or States contacts. Out of 9 patients tested, a statistically and clinically significant aldosterone decrease of 50% was observed in patients treated within the first 10 days of the study; however, hormone concentrations rebounded to pretreatment levels within 4 days after the final treatment. The authors in this study, who did not present actual data, observed that, as in the previous studies,[89,91] a modest decrease of blood pressure could be observed immediately after the adjustment; however, these reductions were not maintained during the study.[92] Further studies with larger patient cohorts, including a time-frame of

sodium retention, are necessary to provide details for this putative model, depicting the possible management of hypertension by chiropractic manipulation. In particular, data are needed that would answer the following:

1. How many adjustments are needed and which variety would produce maximal lowering of blood pressure?
2. How enduring would these effects be postintervention?

Diabetes Mellitus

The damaging effects of glucose in diabetic patients may be mitigated by therapies used to elicit autonomic reflexes that favor homeostasis. Reducing stress, in particular, would be expected to reduce the incidence and magnitude of glucose spikes resulting from gluconeogenesis. An attractive candidate for such a therapy is chiropractic intervention.

Only the most preliminary evidence involving individual case studies tentatively supports this hypothesis. One investigation involving two patients undergoing a neurovascular dynamic technique[93] indicated that such common complications as the deterioration of vision or the development of foot ulcers did not occur in these individuals.[94] In the remaining study, glucose and glycosylated hemoglobin levels in a diabetic patient were observed to return to near normal levels after chiropractic adjustments.[95] Obviously, the therapies involved have not been shown to be directly responsible for these favorable outcomes. In the absence of substantial alternative data the direct management of insulin levels by medical means remains the intervention of choice for managing diabetes mellitus.

Perimenopausal Hot Flashes

The intense vasodilations in the skin associated with menopause, known as *hot flashes,* have been proposed to be associated with vasomotor tone. Proposing that vertebral subluxations could be a factor for producing hot flashes, Weber and Masarsky[97] reported that a 90% decrease in the frequency of hot flashes was recorded from clinical records and a single perimenopausal patient's diary after intervention with cervical and upper thoracic adjusting. The superior cervical sympathetic ganglion, supplying sympathetic innervation to the blood vessels of the hypothalamus and pituitary,[96] becomes a critical neuroendocrine junction that acts as the primary locus of control of events of the menstrual cycle. The authors suggested that this entity could be adversely affected by the dysfunctional spinal units corrected by manipulation.[97]

Far more research addressing these metabolic and other hormonal imbalances is mandatory if a connection between chiropractic care and endocrine function is to be documented and theorized. The history of documentation supporting the beneficial role of chiropractic in the management of low-back pain[44,48,49] and headache[46,49] need only be observed to realize that such an objective may be within reach.

STUDY GUIDE

1. Name two ways the endocrine system is related to pain and its control.
2. Does substance P stimulate or depress pain?
3. Name three biopsychosocial mechanisms that may be related to the conscious experience of pain and the primary stimulus.
4. Who was Hans Selye? Relate his four stages of reaction to stress to possible results of the VSC. Where is the earliest mention of the effects of the psyche regarding chiropractic located?
5. Describe the role of the "fight or flight" mechanism in terms of endocrine function.
6. Describe the incidence of viral infection in individuals suffering from high levels of stress. How is the CD4 count in HIV-positive individuals affected by depression? Do any benefits occur through chiropractic intervention?
7. How do glucocorticoids affect the immune inflammatory response? Describe a possible pathway to this reaction that could be initiated by the VSC.
8. What part of the nervous system is affected by the HPA axis? What is the HPA axis?
9. Can an adjustment that does not create cavitation produce changes on an EMG? How?
10. Discuss Kaptchuk's argument[35] regarding the usefullness of double-blind studies in terms of chiropractic research. What is another field of science in which double blinding may not be possible or prudent?
11. Discuss the study on salivary cortisol levels and spinal manipulation. What would be the next step in this study?
12. Name two metabolites with levels possibly affected by chiropractic care. Describe their role in the relief of pain.
13. Describe the Brennan study[77] on primary dysmenorrhea.
14. Natural biologic events may be accompanied by unnecessary negative symptoms; therefore describe and discuss the Masarsky and Weber[97] paper on hot flashes.

REFERENCES

1. Triano J: Interaction of spinal biomechanics and physiology. In Haldeman S, editor: *Principles and practice of chiropractic,* ed 2, Norwalk, Conn, 1992, Appleton & Lange.
2. Herzog W, Scheele D, Conway PJ: Electromyographic responses of back and limb muscles associated with spinal manipulative therapy, *Spine* 24(2):146-153, 1999.
3. von Euler US, Pernow B: *Substance P,* New York, 1977, Raven Press.
4. Emson PC: Peptides as neurotransmitter candidates in the CNS, *Prog Neurobiol* 13:61-116, 1979.
5. Jessell TM, Iversen LL: Opiate analgesics inhibit substance P release from rat trigeminal nucleus, *Nature* 268(5620):549-551, 1977.
6. Raj RP: *Pain medicine: a comprehensive review,* p 13, St Louis, 1996, Mosby.
7. Woolf CJ: Evidence for a central component of post-injury pain hypersensitivity, *Nature* 306(5944):686-688, 1983.
8. Melzack R, Casey KL: Sensory, motivational and central control determinations of pain. In Kenshalo DR, editor: *The skin senses,* Springfield, Ill, 1968, Charles C Thomas.
9. Waddell G: A new clinical model for the treatment of low-back pain, *Spine* 12(7):632-644, 1987.
10. Waddell G: *The back pain revolution,* New York, 1998, Churchill Livingstone.
11. Benson H, Greenwood MM, Klemchuk H: The relaxation response: psychophysiologic aspects and clinical applications, *Int J Psychiatry Med* 6(1):87-98, 1975.
12. Ader R, Cohen H, Felten D: Psychneuroimmunology: interactions between the nervous system and the immune system, *Lancet* 345:99-103, 1995.

13. Morgan LG: Psychoneuroimmunology, the placebo effect and chiropractic, *J Manipulative Physiol Ther* 21(7):484-491, 1998.
14. Seyle H: Stress and duress, *Comp Ther* 1:9-13, 1975.
15. Johnson E et al: Mechanisms of stress: a dynamic overview of hormonal and behavioral homeostasis, *Neurosc Biobehav Rev* 16:115-130, 1992.
16. Vishwanath R: The psychoneuroimmunological system: a recently evolved networking organ system, *Med Hypotheses* 47:265-268, 1996.
17. Bassett JR, Marshall PM, Spillane R: The physiological measurement of acute stress (public speaking) in bank employees, *Int J Psychophysiol* 5(4):265-273, 1987.
18. Kirschbaum C, Hellhammer DH: Salivary control in psychobiological research: an overview, *Neuropsychobiology* 22(3):150-169, 1989.
19. Laragh JH et al: The renin axis and vasoconstriction volume analysis for understanding and treating renovascular and renal hypertension, *Am J Med* 58(1):4-13, 1975.
20. Waddell G et al: Chronic low-back pain, psychologic distress, and illness behavior, *Spine* 9(2):209-213, 1984.
21. Walker L: Psychological assessment and intervention: Future prospects for women with breast cancer, *Semin Surg Oncol* 12:76-83, 1996.
22. Schedlowski M, Schmidt M: Stress and the immune system, *Naturwissenschaften* 83:214-220, 1996.
23. Cohen S, Tyrrell D, Smith A: Psychological stress and susceptibility to the common cold, *New England J Med* 325(9):606-612, 1991.
24. Avina-Zubieta J, Paez F, Galindo-Rodriguez G: Rheumatic manifestations of neurological and psychiatric diseases, *Curr Opin Rheumatol* 9:51-55, 1997.
25. Berin M, Perdue M: Effect of psychoneural factors on intestinal epithelial function, *Can J Gastroenterol* 11:353-357, 1997.
26. Schmidt MA, Smith LH, Sehnert KW: *Beyond antibiotics,* Berkeley, Calif, 1993, North Atlantic Books.
27. Ader R, Cohen N: Psychoneuroimmunology: conditioning and stress, *Ann Rev Psychol* 44:53-85, 1993.
28. Hurwitz EL, Morgenstern H: *The effects of asthma, hay fever, and other allergies on major depression and low-back pain,* Manchester, United Kingdom, Oct 2-3, 1998, Proceedings of the Third International Forum for Primary Care Research on Low Back Pain.
29. Turnbull AV, Rivier C: Regulation of the HPA axis by cytokines, *Brain Behav Immun* 9(4):253-275, 1995.
30. Buckingham JC et al: Activation of the HPA axis by immune insults: roles and interactions of cytokines, eicosanoids, glucocorticoids, *Pharmacol Biochem Behav* 54(1):285-298, 1996.
31. Myers FH, Jawetz E, Goldfien A: *Basic and clinical pharmacology,* ed 4, pp 341-351, Los Altos, Calif, 1978, Lange Medical Publications.
32. Faist E, Schinkel C, Zimmer S: Update on the mechanisms of immune suppression of injury and immune modulation, *World J Surg* 20:454-459, 1996.
33. Balon J et al: A comparison of active and simulated chiropractic manipulation as adjunctive treatment for childhood asthma, *New England J Med* 339(15):1013-1020, 1998.
34. Bove G, Nilsson N: Spinal manipulation in the treatment of episodic tension-type headache, *JAMA* 280(18):1576-1579, 1998.
35. Kaptchuk TJ, Eisenberg DM: Chiropractic: origins, controversies, and contributions, *Arch Intern Med* 158:2215-2224, 1998.
36. Herzog W, Conway P, Scheele D: *Reflex responses associated with spinal manipulation,* pp 105-107, Vancouver, British Columbia, July 16-19, 1998, Proceedings of 1988 International Conference on Spinal Manipulation.
37. Fuhr AW, Smith DB: Accuracy of piezoelectric accelerometers measuring displacement of a spinal adjusting instrument, *J Manipulative Physiol Ther* 9(1):15-21, 1986.
38. Brown W: The placebo effect, *Sci Am* 278:90-95, 1998.
39. Peterson KB: The effects of spinal manipulation on the intensity of emotional arousal in phobic subjects exposed to a threat stimulus: a randomized, controlled, double-blind clinical trial, *J Manipulative Physiol Ther* 20(9):602-606, 1997.
40. Tuchin PJ: The effect of chiropractic spinal manipulation on salivary cortisol levels, *J Austral Chiropr Osteopath* 7(2):86-92, 1998.
41. Bowers LJ, Mootz RD: The nature of primary care: the chiropractor's role, *Top Clin Chiro* 2(1):66-84, 1995.
42. Hawk C, Dusio ME: A survey of 492 U.S. chiropractors on primary care and prevention-related issues, *J Manipulative Physiol Ther* 18(2):57-64, 1995.
43. Jamison JR: Preventive chiropractic and the chiropractic management of visceral conditions: is the cost to chiropractic acceptance justified by the benefit to health care? *Chiro J Austral* 21(3):95-101, 1991.
44. Haldeman S, Chapman-Smith D, Peterson DM: *Guidelines for chiropractic quality assurance and practice parameters,* Gaithersburg, Md, 1993, Proceedings of the Mercy Center Concensus Conference, Aspen.
45. Nelson C et al: The efficacy of spinal manipulation, amiltriptyline, and the combination of both therapies for the prophylaxis of migraine headache, *J Manipulative Physiol Ther* 21(8):511-519, 1998.
46. Hurwitz EL et al: Manipulation and mobilization of the cervical spine, *Spine* 21(15):1746-1760, 1996.
47. Rosner AL: *The role of subluxation in chiropractic,* Arlington, Va, 1997, Foundation for Chiropractic Education and Research.
48. Bigos S et al: *Acute low-back pain problems in adults,* No 14, Clinical Practice Guideline, Rockville, Md, 1994, Agency for Health Care and Policy Research Publication 95-0642.
49. Rosner A: Musculoskeletal research. In Redwood DC, editor: *Ontemporary chiropractic,* pp 163-187, New York, 1996, Churchill Livingstone.
50. Masarsky C, Todres-Masarsky M: *Somatovisceral aspects of chiropractic: an evidence-based approach,* New York, Churchill Livingstone (in press).
51. Iversen LL: The chemistry of the brain, *Sci Am* 241(3):134-149, 1979.
52. Pert C: *Molecules of emotion,* p 368, New York, 1979, Scribner.
53. Hughes J et al: Identification of two related pentapeptides from the brain with potent opiate agonist activity, *Nature* 258:577-579, 1975.

54. Li CH, Chung D, Doncen BA: Isolation, characterization and opiate activity of beta-endorphin from human pituitary glands, *Biochem Biophys Res Commun* 72:1542, 1976.

55. Pomeranz B, Chiu D: Naloxone blockade of acupuncture analgesia: endorphin implicated, *Life Sci* 9:1757-1762, 1976.

56. Harber VJ, Sutton JR: Endorphins and exercise, *Sports Med* 1:154-171, 1984.

57. Szczudik A, Lypka A: Plasma immunoreactive beta-endorphin and enkephalin concentration in healthy subjects before and after electroacupuncture, *Acupunct Electrother Res* 8:127-137, 1983.

58. Malizia E, Andrencci G, Paolucci D: Electoacupuncture and peripheral beta-endorphin and ACTH levels, *Lancet* 2:535-536, 1979.

59. Hughes GS et al: Response of plasma beta-endorphins to transcutaneous electrical nerve stimulation in healthy subjects, *Phys Ther* 64(7):1062-1066, 1984.

60. Elkiss M, Ingall JRF, Dooley J: Pilot study on the effects of transcutaneous electrical nerve stimulation on the level of plasma beta-endorphin, *J Am Osteopath Assoc* 84:144-147, 1984.

61. Vernon HT et al: Spinal manipulation and beta-endorphin: a controlled study of the effect of a spinal manipulation on plasma beta-endorphin levels in normal males, *J Manipulative Physiol Ther* 9(2):115-123, 1986.

62. Christian GF et al: Immunoreactive ACTH, beta-endorphin, and cortisol levels in plasma following spinal manipulative therapy, *Spine* 13(12):1411-1417, 1988.

63. Luisetto G et al: Plasma levels of beta-endorphin and calcitonin levels before and after manipulative therapy of patients with cervical arthrosis and Barr's syndrome. In Mazarelli JP, editor: *Chiropractic interprofessional research*, pp 47-52, Torino, Italy, 1982, Edizioni Minerva Medica.

64. Richardson DL et al: The effect of osteopathic manipulative treatment on endogenous opiate concentrations, *J Am Osteopath Assoc* 84:127, 1984 (abstract).

65. Strand F: *Physiology: a systems approach*, New York, 1983, Collier Macmillan.

66. Dawood MY: Dysmenorrhea, *Clin Obstet Gynecol* 33:168-178, 1990.

67. Pickles PR: Prostaglandins and dysmenorrhea, *Acta Obstet Gynecol Scand Suppl* 87:7-12, 1979.

68. Rosenwaks Z, Seegar-Jones G: Menstrual pain: its origin and pathogenesis *J Reprod Med* 25:207-212, 1980.

69. Chan WY, Dawood MY, Fuchs F: Prostaglandins in primary dysmenorrhea. Comparison of prophylactic and nonprophylactic treatment with Ibuprofen and the use of oral contraceptives, *Am J Med* 70:535-540, 1981.

70. Hauksson A et al: The influence of a combined oral contraceptive on uterine activity and reactivity to agonists in primary dysmenorrhea, *Acta Obstet Gynecol Scand Suppl* 69:31-34, 1989.

71. Hitchcock ME: The manipulative approach to the management of primary dysmenorrhea, *J Am Osteopath Assoc* 75:97-100, 1976.

72. Arnold-Frochot S: Investigation of the effect of chiropractic adjustments on a specific gynecological symptom: dysmenorrhea, *J Aust Chiro Assoc* 10(1):6-10, 14-16, 1981.

73. Liebl NA, Butler LM: A chiropractic approach to the treatment of dysmenorrhea, *J Manipulative Physiol Ther* 13(3):101-106, 1990.

74. Radler M: Dysmenorrhea: chiropractic application, *Am Chiro* :29-32, 1984.

75. Wiles M: Gynecology and obstetrics in chiropractic, *Gynecol Obstet* 24:163-166, 1980.

76. Thomason PR et al: Effectiveness of spinal manipulative therapy in treatment of primary dysmenorrhea: a pilot study, *J Manipulative Physiol Ther* 2(3):140-145, 1979.

77. Kokjohn K et al: The effect of spinal manipulation on pain and prostaglandin levels in women with primary dysmenorrhea, *J Manipulative Physiol Ther* 15(5):279-285, 1992.

78. Hondras M, Brennan PC: The effect of spinal manipulation on pain and prostaglandin levels in women with primary dysmenorrhea: a randomized, full-scale clinical trial, *Pain*, 81:105-114, 1999.

79. Fedele L et al: Dynamics and significance of placebo response in primary dysmenorrhea, *Pain* 36:43-47, 1989.

80. Palmer DD: *The chiropractor*, Los Angeles, 1914, Beacon Light Printing.

81. Boesler D et al: Efficacy of high-velocity low-amplitude manipulative technique in subjects with low-back pain during menstrual cramping, *J Am Ostepath Assoc* 93(2):203-214, 1993.

82. Sveinsdottin H, Reame N: Symptom patterns of women with PMS complaints, *J Adv Nurs* 16(6):689-700, 1991.

83. Hubbs EC: Vertebral subluxation and premenstrual tension syndrome: a case study, *Res Forum* 2:100-102, 1986.

84. Smith VC, Rogers SR: Premenstrual and postmenstrual syndrome, its characteristics and chiropractic care, *Am Chiro* 14(3):4-6, 1992.

85. Magos AL, Studd JWW: A simple method for the diagnosis of PMS by use of a self-assessment disk, *Am J Obstet Gynecol* 158:1024-1028, 1988.

86. Stude DE: The management of symptoms associated with premenstrual syndrome, *J Manipulative Physiol Ther* 14(3):209-215, 1991.

87. Walsh MJ, Chandraraj S, Polus BI: The efficacy of chiropractic therapy on premenstrual syndrome: a case series study, *Chiro J Austral* 24(4):122-126, 1994.

88. Walsh MJ, Polus B: *A randomised placebo controlled clinical trial on the efficacy of chiropractic therapy on premenstrual syndrome*, pp 92-95, Vancouver, British Columbia, July 16-19, 1998, Proceedings of the International Conference on Spinal Manipulation.

89. Yates RG et al: Effects of chiropractic treatment on blood pressure and anxiety: a randomized, controlled trial, *J Manipulative Physiol Ther* 11(6):484-488, 1988.

90. *Palmer Technique Manual*, Davenport, Iowa, 1980, Palmer College of Chiropractic.

91. McKnight ME, DeBoer KF: Preliminary study of blood pressure changes in normotensive subjects undergoing chiropractic care, *J Manipulative Physiol Ther* 11(4):261-266, 1988.

92. Wagnon RJ, Sandefur RM, Ratliff CR: Serum aldosterone changes after specific chiropractic manipulation, *Am J Chiropr Med* 1(2):66-70, 1988.

93. Bennett TJ: *Dynamics of correction of abnormal function*, Sierra Madre, Calif, 1977, Ralph J. Morris.

94. Nelson WA: Diabetes mellitus: two case reports, *Chiro Technique* 1(2):37-40, 1989.

95. Kfoury PW: Chiropractic and holistic management of type II diabetes mellitus, *Dig Chiropr Econ* 37(4):37-40, 1995.

96. Adams RD, Victor M: *Principles of neurology,* ed 4, p 435, New York, 1989, McGraw-Hill.

97. Weber M, Masarsky CS: Cervicothoracic subluxation and hot flashes in a perimenopausal subject: a time-series case report, *J Vertebr Sublux Res* 1(2):33-38, 1996.

CHAPTER 15

Somatovisceral Involvement in the Pediatric Patient

Marion Todres-Masarsky, DC • *Charles S. Masarsky, DC* • *Claudia A. Anrig, DC* • *Steven T. Tanaka, DC* • *Joel Alcantara, DC*

Although the first recorded chiropractic adjustment of a child (B.J.'s son, D. David Palmer, by his grandfather, D.D. Palmer) occurred in 1906, earlier instances may have gone unreported.[1] The first chiropractic textbook about pediatrics was published by Craven[2] in 1924. The publisher was the Palmer School of Chiropractic, and the book was part of the "Green Book" series.

Medical Prejudice

Despite this long history of responsible professional care, significant sectors of the medical profession and the insurance industry have vehemently opposed chiropractic care for children until now. In her foreword of a recent chiropractic pediatric textbook, medical pediatrician Helen Rodriguez-Trias[3] stated that she was indoctrinated to totally reject chiropractic during her medical education. Unfortunately, medical opposition to chiropractic care for children combined with insurance industry refusal to include such care in their health plans often influences parents to exclude chiropractic from their children's health care.

One of the flash points for this opposition has been chiropractic care for children with visceral involvements. A 1994 condemnation of chiropractic care for children with otitis media, tonsillitis, and colic by medical pediatricians in Canada was cited by York University faculty members who did not want to be affiliated with the Canadian Memorial Chiropractic College.[4] The controversy surrounding chiropractic pediatrics and chiropractic care for infants and children with visceral in-

volvements requires a concise review in this chapter, even though much of the material has already been discussed in previous chapters.

In the appendix at the end of this chapter, a general description of the neurologic examination of the pediatric patient is provided. The approach to the patient with somatovisceral and neurologic complaints has too often been exclusionary (e.g., at any sign of underlying pathology or neurologic delay the patient was supposed to be "referred out" for allopathic care). With appropriate attention to neurologic and chiropractic findings, chiropractic must not abdicate responsibility to the patient without first giving careful consideration to the possible health benefits available through chiropractic care in conjunction with any appropriate medical comanagement. This must be achieved through a careful, attentive case history and examination.

Otitis Media and Chiropractic

Although chiropractic care for children with otitis media was specifically criticized as unscientific in the previously mentioned statement by the Canadian pediatricians, the scientific case for such intervention has been growing. (Some of the relevant literature is discussed in Chapter 13 and in the immune system section in Chapter 16.[5-10]) Two additional reports on children with otitis media are by Peet[11] and by Fallon and Vallone.[12]

Peet[11] described a 5-year-old boy who suffered from otitis media with effusion every 3 to 6 weeks, despite numerous courses of antibiotics. Postural analysis revealed abnormal carriage of the head and thorax. Palpation of the upper cervical spine revealed grossly asymmetric tone of the suboccipital muscles and malposition consistent with upper cervical subluxation as demonstrated on x-ray.

In accordance with Chiropractic Biophysics protocols (CBP), upper cervical adjustments were delivered with the patient placed in the mirror image of his postural distortions. Based on his mother's account and otoscopic examination, improvement was evident 2 days after the first adjustment. A total of 10 more visits were scheduled over the next 4 weeks. Follow-up x-rays taken at that point indicated substantial reduction in upper cervical malposition, with improvements also noted in posture and suboccipital muscle tone. Visit frequency was reduced to once per week for 6 weeks, then once every 3 weeks for 6 months. During a total of 6 months of chiropractic care the child had only one middle ear infection with mild effusion, compared with approximately monthly episodes during the 2 years before chiropractic care.

Vallone and Fallon[12] presented the results of a survey of 33 doctors of chiropractic enrolled in a postgraduate course in chiropractic pediatrics. Methods used by at least 75% of the respondents were considered to represent consensus. Spinal adjustments, manual lymphatic drainage of the cervical musculature, and removal of potential allergens from the diet (particularly wheat and dairy products) were recommended to manage the pediatric otitis media patient.

The immune system section in Chapter 16 also reviews additional pediatric research not directly related to otitis media.[13-15]

Colic and Other Issues

Chiropractic care for infants with colic was also denounced as unscientific in the recent statement by Canadian pediatricians. However, some of chiropractic's more interesting clinical research has occurred in this area.[16-20] (Most of the research pertaining to infantile colic was reviewed in Chapter 9.)

Chapter 11 discussed many chiropractic research papers concerning pediatric asthma and studies including adults and children.[21-28]

Chapter 13 reviewed a number of studies linking the VSC to visual deficit.[29-32]

Subluxation and the Pediatric Bladder

The body of research connecting the VSC to pediatric bladder dysfunction is gradually increasing in the chiropractic literature. Although some chiropractic research on one aspect of this relationship—pediatric nocturnal enuresis was cited briefly in Chapter 8, additional commentary is warranted. The etiology of primary nocturnal enuresis (bedwetting not related to infection or genitourinary pathology) is generally unknown. Medical intervention often entails courses of antidepressant treatments or other drug therapies.

One asthma paper cited previously also involved nocturnal enuresis.[23] Other well-described cases of nocturnal enuresis improvement under chiropractic care have been presented by Gemmell and Jacobson[33] and Blomerth.[34]

Two controlled studies involving pediatric nocturnal enuresis also exist. Leboef and others[35] presented a study in which the bedwetting children served as their own controls. Baselines were established by monitoring the children for 2 to 4 weeks before the chiropractic adjustments were administered. Based on parental reports, no significant difference was found between the baseline and intervention periods. These researchers did not report which spinal levels were adjusted, and no subluxation-based outcome measures were described, which was a serious methodologic flaw.

A contrasting view was provided in a recent study by Reed and others.[36] After a 2-week baseline period the children were divided into two groups, with one group receiving sham adjustments administered with an Activator instrument set on 0 tension and the other group receiving actual adjustments, generally in the upper cervical and sacroiliac areas.[36] The group receiving actual adjustments experienced a statistically significant 17.9% decrease in the frequency of wet nights, compared with a slight increase in wet-night frequency among the group receiving sham adjustments.

An instructive case was published by Borregard,[37] in which a 13-year-old boy had an initial complaint of bilateral knee pain. During physical examination the doctor could not identify any local knee dysfunction. Incidental mention of a history of recurrent urinary tract infections and bladder incontinence was made during the intake interview. The incontinence resulted from a reduced perception of bladder filling; by the time the patient was aware of bladder fullness, he could not get to the bathroom in time. This is known as *neurogenic bladder.*

The only remarkable x-ray finding was spina bifida occulta at S1. Borregard[37] administered adjustments to L3-4 and both sacroiliac motion segments. Knee pain was gone within 1 week. Urinary incontinence was resolved within 2 weeks, concurrent with the clearing of signs of lumbar and sacroiliac VSC. An exacerbation 4 months later was resolved with a single adjustment.

The case of a 12-year-old girl with pain in the lower back and left flank with concomitant daytime incontinence was reported by Stude and others.[38] A pediatrician and a urologist, who evaluated the patient, were unsuccessful in producing a definitive diagnosis. Findings on static and motion palpation and x-ray were consistent with the VSC involving L3-4 and the left sacroiliac motion segments. A combination of diversified adjusting and dietary modifications for 3 weeks, or 9 visits, produced a 50% reduction in the low back pain and flank pain. Some reduction in daytime urinary incontinence also ensued. No further progress occurred for the next 3 months.

At 3 months, periarticular pain on digital pressure was noted during an examination of the sacrococcygeal joint. The patient then recalled a slip-and-fall injury to that area just before the appearance of urinary incontinence. After adding minimal-force intrarectal adjusting of the coccyx to her care in 4 visits the patient reported her first days without pain and leakage. No recurrences of either the musculoskeletal or urinary symptoms have developed during 4 years of follow-up.

Vallone[39] reported the case of a 7-year-old girl with recurrent urinary tract infection.[39] The results of previous allopathic and homeopathic interventions had been disappointing. About 2 years before she visited the doctor the patient injured her thoracolumbar junction while attempting a gymnastic maneuver on her bed. No apparent history of urinary tract infection before this incident existed.

Motion palpation revealed evidence of the VSC at T7, L2, and S2. Diversified adjustments to these segments, combined with myofascial work for the pelvic floor muscles, were administered twice a week for 3 weeks. At the end of this regimen the patient was free of urinary tract infection signs

and symptoms and free of the VSC based on follow-up motion palpation. An exacerbation followed while she was playing with her older brother 2 weeks later. The same levels were found to be subluxated, and her pain resolved with one adjustment. At 9 weeks of follow-up, no recurrence occurred.

Subluxation and the Pediatric Central Nervous System

Much chiropractic literature concerning central nervous system disorders involves pediatric cases. This may be because of the vulnerability of the developing pediatric central nervous system.[40] For instance the primitive reflexes of the neonate such as the Babinski response do not disappear until approximately ages 6 to 24 months. Myelination is not complete in the spinal cord and cerebrum until approximately 2 years of age. A number of brain structures, including the reticular formation, commissural neurons, and intercortical association areas are not fully mature until after age 10. This immature state of development may render children more vulnerable than adults to VSC-related central nervous system dysfunction. For this reason, clinical research in this arena is of great interest.

Giesen and others[41] presented a time-series study of 7 hyperactive children. During a placebo period these patients were given sham adjustments with an Activator instrument placed on 0 tension, and parents kept a diary of each child's activity level. Electodermal testing provided a measure of sympathetic arousal, and a motion recorder disguised as a wristwatch was used to measure activity levels during a simulated homework assignment.

After the placebo period, Gonstead, Palmer upper cervical or diversified adjustments were administered at various levels once a week, depending on examination results and doctor-patient comfort. Improvement was noted for all measures and for all 7 patients, from the placebo phase to the end of the treatment phase. This improvement was statistically significant, despite the small number of patients.

In addition to this prospective case series a number of promising case reports have been presented. Phillips[42] reported abatement of hyperactivity symptoms in a 10-year-old boy after 11 chiropractic visits, in which diversified spinal adjusting was combined with Upledger craniosacral therapy. After 5½ relatively symptom-free months, based on parental and school reports, the boy suffered 2 falls, at least one of which involved minor head trauma. An increase of hyperactivity symptoms followed, which was resolved by a single adjustment.

Thomas and Wood[43] reported the case of a 13-year-old girl who spent most of the day staring into space while avoiding eye contact.[43] On the rare occasions when she spoke, she would utter only one word at a time. Detailed examination and treatment for 9 years before initial chiropractic treatment included visits to the Mayo Clinic and the National Institutes of Health, producing no improvement. After 3 upper cervical adjustments over 4 days, based on National Upper Cervical Chiropractic Association (NUCCA) protocols, the patient began to make eye contact and to speak in complete sentences. Unfortunately, the patient only responded to NUCCA adjustments, and no practitioner knowledgeable of this technique was available where the family lived. Return visits to the NUCCA practitioner on at least 2 subsequent occasions resulted in transient improvements.

Much biomechanic and neurologic individuality exists among people. As a result, certain patients only respond to a singular form of adjusting and fail to respond to others. Apparently, the patient described by Thomas and Wood is in this category.

Arme[44] reported the case of a 7-year-old boy who exhibited memory loss, inability to concentrate, and general agitation after a motor vehicle accident. A medical specialist diagnosed attention deficit disorder. Treatment with Ritalin was somewhat successful. Upper and midcervical adjusting using Thompson protocols was initiated at 4 months posttrauma. During the course of chiropractic management the Ritalin dose was reduced by the attending medical doctor. At 17 weeks of care the Ritalin was withdrawn, and the patient's behavior appeared normal to the medical doctor, the school system, and his mother. Unfortunately, his mother discontinued chiropractic care for her son after legal settlement. When Arme's report was published the patient was taking Ritalin as a result of returned attention deficit disorder symptoms.

Araghi[45] reported the case of a 5-year-old girl with the inability to talk (oral apraxia). Magnetic resonance imaging of the brain, electroencephalography, chromosome evaluation, and hearing tests were all unremarkable. After 3 years of intensive speech therapy the patient had acquired some sign language skills and the ability to pronounce 4 letters of the alphabet. The night after her first adjustment (at C1, with the Gonstead technique used) the patient spoke her first word; while signing for apple juice, she said, "Apple." After 1 year of care, she was able to speak in 3-word sentences. Although she has below normal language skills expected for her age, this speech is quite an improvement.

Manuele and Fysh[46] reported the case of a 7-year-old girl with acquired verbal aphasia. Before the age of 18 months this patient's language development had been normal. Approximately 6 weeks after vaccination for diphtheria, pertussis, tetanus, measles, mumps, and rubella, her vocabulary suddenly diminished to 2 words. After more than 5 years of speech therapy, her vocabulary had only increased to 4 words. After 7 chiropractic adjustments focused on the C1-2 and temporal-sphenoidal motion segments for approximately 7 weeks the patient's vocabulary had increased to approximately 60 words. Although establishing a definite causal relationship between the aphasia and the vaccination is not possible, postvaccination complications have been reported with latencies of 12 weeks or more.[47]

Peet[48] reported the case of an 8-year-old boy diagnosed with attention deficit disorder at the age of 3 years, medicated with Ritalin and Prozac since the age of 5. These medications provided only partial improvement. After 6 weeks of chiropractic care focused on the upper cervical region, using Chiropractic Biophysics protocols, the patient was medication free for 3 weeks, and school reports indicated improvement in cognition skills, task concentration, emotion control, and decreased aggressiveness.

Seizure disorders are among the most dramatic central nervous system manifestations. Goodman[49] described a 5-year-old girl with a 9-month history of grand mal seizures. At the first visit the patient had not experienced a seizure-free day in 6½ months and could barely talk or stand. Upper cervical specific adjustments were administered daily for 3 days. After a transient increase in seizure frequency, she was seizure-free for 4 weeks.

When the author's study was published the patient was reported to be functioning as a normal 7-year-old. She now attends regular classes at school, requires no medication, and is almost entirely free of seizures (when she has a seizure, they are petit mal). She is examined for signs of upper cervical subluxation every 2 to 3 months.

Hyman[50] reported the case of a 5-year-old boy with a 3-year history of petit mal seizures. The patient would spend 4 to 5 seconds motionless, with a blank stare 4 to 6 times every hour. After 2 months of chiropractic care focused on the upper cervical region, seizure frequency had been reduced to no more than one per day, and the attending medical doctor had gradually eliminated medication.

Hospers[51] presented a series of 5 cases (4 of which were children), with complaints including seizures, hyperactivity, and inability to concentrate. The major outcome measure used in the study was computerized electroencephalography (CEEG), or *brain mapping.* In this procedure a computer software program analyzes brain activity measured from scalp electrodes. The display is a diagram of the brain, with the percentage of various types of brain-waves written or color-coded over the various lobes. Previous research has identified normal values for each brainwave type (alpha, beta, delta, theta) from each cerebral lobe for various age groups. After 4 patients received Life Upper Cervical adjustments and 1 patient received category II pelvic blocking based on Sacrooccipital Technique protocols, all 5 patients demonstrated improved CEEG results, with concomitant symptomatic relief.

Woo reported[52] a case of myelopathy in an 11-year-old boy. The myelopathy was related to an injury sustained during practice of the flopping high jump, in which the athlete lands on the neck and upper back. If the landing is off center, severe lateral flexion forces are introduced into the cervicothoracic spine. Despite 3 months of hospitalization and steroid therapy the patient continued to deteriorate. At his initial visit the patient had lost bladder and bowel control, was unable to stand, and suffered from iatrogenic Cushing's disease. After 2 months of adjustments at the C7-T1 motion segment the patient was able to walk with crutches. At 9 years of follow-up, he could run, needed no crutches, and had no bladder or bowel complaints.

Sleep Disturbance

Although sleep disturbance is often handled as a secondary issue in chiropractic research concerning infantile colic and other disorders, little has been published regarding sleep disorders as clinical problems.

Rome[53] described· a 12-month-old boy who would wake up 7 to 8 times each night. This disturbed sleep was not secondary to urinary urgency or any other apparent cause. After the first adjustment of the C1-2 and T8-9 motion segments, with gentle fingertip pressure, the child slept soundly for 7 hours. At 6 months of follow-up the mother described her son as a healthy toddler with normal sleeping habits.

The Kentuckiana Experience

Barnes[54] reported 2 cases of special needs children. One was a 9-year-old girl with spastic cerebral palsy. This patient came to the doctor in a brace prescribed by her medical orthopedist to correct internal rotation of both hips. Adjustments were administered twice per week. At 7 months the orthopedist reviewed follow-up x-rays of the patient and indicated that the "spontaneous remission" permitted brace removal and release from further orthopedic treatment.

Barnes' second case[54] was a 16-year-old boy with high-functioning autism and a 2-year history of voluntary bowel control failure, with at least one encopresis incident per day. After 13 sessions of spinal and cranial adjusting over 5½ months the patient was able to resume after-school activities because he had no recurrences in 2 months. At 7 months of follow-up, no further encopresis episodes were reported.

The cases described by Barnes,[54] were patients of the Kentuckiana Children's Center in Louisville, Kentucky. Kentuckiana has been providing nonprofit chiropractic care to children with learning disabilities, cerebral palsy, autism, seizure disorders, and other central nervous system manifestations since 1957. Chiropractic adjustments are part of a multidisciplinary program that includes nutritional therapy, counseling, special education, visual and speech therapy, Doman-Delacato patterning, and dental and medical care.

Unfortunately, no indexed journals were avail-

Table 15-1   *Apgar Scoring*

Score	Color	Heart Rate	Reflex Irritability	Muscle Tone	Respiratory Effort
0 points	Blue, pale	Absent	No response	Flacid	Absent
1 point	Blue extremities, pink body	Less than 100	Grimacing	Minimal flexion of extremities	Weak, irregular
2 points	Pink	Greater than 100	Sneezing or coughing	Flexion of extremities	Crying, good effort

able for chiropractic publication when Kentuckiana was created, and clinician researchers such as Barnes[54] have only recently been able to have some of the center's work published. However, Kentuckiana is still a unique model of effective, long-standing interdisciplinary cooperation in a clinically challenging environment.

Summary

Although most pediatric chiropractic care is not published in the research literature a significant portion of the existing clinical literature concerns nonmusculoskeletal conditions and complaints. A recent survey at a chiropractic college teaching clinic confirmed that pediatric patients were common and their complaints often included ear infection, sinus trouble, allergies, bedwetting, and respiratory and gastrointestinal problems.[55]

Although no responsible doctor of chiropractic would claim that the VSC correction is the only health care children need the available research literature strongly supports a significant role for chiropractic care in the pediatric population. Interprofessional cooperation in this area will hopefully become more common. The blanket condemnation of chiropractic care for infants and children that continues from major sectors of the medical profession and the insurance industry contradicts a growing body of evidence.

Appendix: Neurologic Examination of the Pediatric Patient

The examination of the pediatric patient, as with all patients, begins with a thorough case history, after which the clinician progresses to a combination of established neurologic, orthopedic, and chiropractic tests (although in most cases the child was previously examined by a medical pediatrician and therefore some tests are duplications). Any positive findings are reason to perform more specifically directed tests. Careful observation of infants or toddlers should occur because they cannot verbalize their fears, discomforts, or disabilities. The clinician must also consider the patient's age because the pediatric nervous system is not fully developed, and whether a test or reflex is positive or negative, normal or abnormal, depends on the child's development stage.[56]

The neonate is assessed immediately after birth to determine the integrity of the autonomic nervous system based on the patient's Apgar score, named after Virginia Apgar, who developed the system in 1953 (Table 15-1).[57] At 1 minute a total score of 3 to 4 indicates severe (physical) depression, a score of 5 to 6 indicates mild depression, and a score of 7 to 10 is normal. The test is repeated at 5 minutes and, if necessary, at 10 minutes. Neurologic examination involves the cardinal testing of sensory, motor, and deep tendon reflexes after careful visual inspection of the patient, noting posture, symmetry of the upper and lower extremities, spontaneous movement, facial expression, and eye movement. Postural finding of cervical hyperextension may indicate severe brainstem or meningeal irritation. The thumb curled under flexed fingers (cerebral thumb) may indicate cerebral abnormalities.

Examination of tone in extraspinal and paraspinal muscles and of the newborn's resistance to passive movement or gravity should occur. All tests should be done bilaterally. Static palpation of the spine should occur to evaluate rigidity, unusual alignment, or hypermobility. Motion palpation of the pediatric spine should ensue to study individual vertebral units from the cervical spine to the sacrum to assess aberrant motion and joint

Table 15-2 *Primitive Automatisms*

Protocol	Normal Finding
Rooting Response	
Corner of newborn's mouth touched	Head turns ipsilaterally, mouth grasps examiner's finger
Plantar Grasp	
Newborn's foot plantar flexed, with hip and knee flexion	Plantar flexion of toes over examiner's hand occurs
Palmar Grasp	
Finger placed on newborn's hand from ulnar side	Fingers grasp examiner's finger
Moro's Reflex	
Newborn held supine, with body and head supported, head allowed to drop	Symmetrical abduction of upper extremities, extension of fingers, adduction of arms, with loud cry occurs
Galant's Reflex	
Paravertebral musculature stroked 2-3 cm from midline, from shoulder to buttocks	Lateral curvature of trunk toward stimulated side occurs
Stepping Response	
Infant's soles placed on a surface	Infant extends knee and hip simultaneously

Table 15-3 *Infant's Development Milestones*

Activity	Age (Months)
Sitting up unaided	4-5
Rolling over	3-5
Crawling	5-7
Creeping	6-9
Walking*	11-14

Modified from Fallon J: Chiropractic pediatrics. In Redwood D, editor: *Contemporary Chiropractic,* p 284, New York, 1997, Churchill Livingstone.

*Language development appears around the same time as walking, with the child initiating one recognizable word between ages 10 and 14 months.[60,61]

play, in all pertinent directions, for each spinal level and pelvic landmark.

Sensory examination may be traditionally done by applying gentle pressure to the palms and soles of the newborn, but the infant's response is too variable to consider such testing reliable.

An infant's alertness may be assessed by observing for hyperirritability or lethargy, in which reflex testing may be performed. Responses should be brisk but may vary according to the age of the patient and the development of the corticospinal tracts. A Babinski response of fanned, extended toes, with flexion of the big toe, is normal in the infant and the young child, sometimes up to the age of 24 months. The same response in an older patient would indicate an upper motor–neuron lesion.

Cranial nerves can be tested in the infant by observing spontaneous ocular motions and making note of any ptosis. The facial nerve may be assessed by observing the child's face while the child is crying and smiling. Obviously, an older child can follow more specific directions or imitate the examiner's expressions. Sucking, swallowing, and gag reflexes, which are survival skills for the infant, demonstrate the competence of cranial nerves V, VII, IX, X, and XII. The acoustic blink test is accurate for checking hearing acuity in the infant. More specific testing of all cranial nerves is more easily done as the child matures.

Automatisms are primitive reflexes and may be present at birth, depending on development of the patient. They usually disappear by the age of 6 months.[58] Some more important automatisms include the rooting response, plantar and palmar grasp, Moro's reflex, Galant's reflex, and stepping response (Table 15-2).

Observation is an extremely important tool when clinicians examine infants. The clinician should watch the patient's actions while the parent gives the history. If possible the clinician should watch the infant at play. Special note of the child's ability to crawl, walk, or sit upright should be taken. (Table 15-3) Balance, sitting and standing, should be monitored and facial expressions and eye movements should be observed.

When the clinician observes the preschooler, speech patterns, motor development, and hyperactivity or hypoactivity should be noticed. Testing can be enhanced by using toys, eye contact, and gestures to get and hold attention. The slightly older child should also be observed for appropriate social skills development and learning ability. When a child has reached adolescence the examination is similar to the adult.

STUDY GUIDE

1. What year did the first reported chiropractic pediatric adjustment occur? What other important event in chiropractic history occurred in that year? What are the connections? When was the first chiropractic pediatric textbook published?
2. Why did York University faculty members not want to be affiliated with Canadian Memorial Chiropractic College? Where did the faculty members obtain the information on which this opinion was based?
3. In Borregard's case,[37] what was the connection between the patient's complaint and the patient's bladder problem? How was the secondary problem discovered?
4. What is a frequent etiologic factor in many pediatric complaints, either somatovisceral or musculoskeletal?
5. Describe the existing chiropractic studies on pediatric attention deficit hyperactivity disorder.
6. When did the patient in Manuele's and Fysh's study[46] of acquired verbal aphasia become symptomatic? Connect this with D.D. Palmer's three causes of subluxation and with the information on stress and neuroimmunology in Chapter 14.
7. Describe the potential frequency of seizures in some pediatric cases. Why does this happen?
8. What does CEEG or brain mapping measure? How is this useful in chiropractic research and particularly in pediatric research?
9. Describe the clinical setting at the Kentuckiana Children's Center. Considering the information that comes from this setting, why have these cases only recently been written about and published?

REFERENCES

1. Palmer DD: *The Science, art and philosophy of chiropractic,* p 579, Portland, Ore, 1910, Portland Printing House.
2. Craven JH: *Chiropractic hygiene and pediatrics,* Davenport, Iowa, 1924, Palmer School of Chiropractic.
3. Rodriguez-Trias H: Foreword. In Anrig CA, Plaugher G, editors: *Pediatric chiropractic,* p vii, Baltimore, 1998, Williams & Wilkins.
4. Johnson T: Angry scientists fight university's attempt to affiliate with chiropractic college, *Can Med Assoc J* 160(1):99, 1999.
5. Phillips NJ: Vertebral subluxation and otitis media: a case study, *Chiropr: J Res Chiropr Clin Invest* 8:38, 1992.
6. Thill L et al: The response of a patient with otitis media to chiropractic care, *Life Work* 3:23, 1995.
7. Froehle RM: Ear infection: a retrospective study examining improvement from chiropractic care and analyzing for influencing factors, *J Manipulative Physiol Ther* 19:169, 1996.
8. Fysh PN: Chronic recurrent otitis media: case series of five patients with recommendations for case management, *J Clin Chiropr Ped* 1:66, 1996.
9. Heagy DT: The effect of the correction of the vertebral subluxation on chronic otitis media in children, *Chiro Pediatr* 2(2):6, 1996.
10. Fallon JM: The role of the chiropractic adjustment in the care and treatment of 332 children with otitis media, *J Clin Chiropr Ped* 2:167, 1997.
11. Peet JB: Case study: chiropractic results with a child with recurring otitis media accompanied by effusion, *Chiro Pediatr* 2:8, 1996.
12. Vallone S, Fallon JM: Treatment protocols for the chiropractic care of common pediatric conditions: otitis media and asthma, *J Clin Chiropr Ped* 2:113, 1997.
13. Van Breda WM, Van Breda JM: A comparative study of the health status of children raised under the health care models of chiropractic and allopathic medicine, *Chiropr: J Res Chiropr Clin Invest* 5:101, 1993.
14. Rose-Aymon S et al: The relationship between intensity of chiropractic care and incidence of childhood diseases, *Chiropr: J Res Chiropr Clin Invest* 1:70, 1989.
15. Araghi HJ: Juvenile myasthenia gravis: a case study in chiropractic management. In: *Proceedings of the national conference on pediatrics and chiropractic,* p 122, Arlington, Va, 1993, International Chiropractors Association.
16. Klougart N, Nilsson N, Jacobsen J: Infantile colic treated by chiropractors: a prospective study of 316 cases, *J Manipulative Physiol Ther* 12:281, 1989.
17. Pluhar GR, Schobert PD: Vertebral subluxation and colic: a case study, *Chiropr: J Res Chiropr Clin Invest* 7:75, 1991.
18. Hyman CA: Chiropractic adjustments and infantile colic: a case study. In: *Proceedings of the national conference on chiropractic and pediatrics,* p 65, Arlington, Va, 1994, International Chiropractors Association.
19. Fallon JP, Lok BJ: Assessing the efficacy of chiropractic care in pediatric cases of pyloric stenosis. In: *Proceedings of the national conference on chiropractic and pediatrics,* p 72, Arlington, Va, 1994, International Chiropractors Association.
20. Killinger LZ, Azad A: Chiropractic care of infantile colic: a case study, *J Clin Chiropr Ped* 3:203, 1998.
21. Hviid C: A comparison of the effect of chiropractic treatment on respiratory function in patients with respiratory distress symptoms and patients without, *Bull Eur Chiropr Union* 26:17, 1978.
22. Nilsson N, Christiansen B: Prognostic factors in bronchial asthma in chiropractic practice, *Chiro J Austral* 18:85, 1988.

23. Bachman TR, Lantz CA: Management of pediatric asthma and enuresis with probable traumatic etiology. In: *Proceedings of the national conference on chiropractic pediatrics,* p 14, Arlington, Va, 1991, International Chiropractors Association.

24. Lines DH: A wholistic approach to the treatment of bronchial asthma in a chiropractic practice, *Chiro J Austral* 23:4, 1993.

25. Peet JB, Marko SK, Piekarcyk W: Chiropractic response in the pediatric patient with asthma: a pilot study, *Chiro Pediatr* 1:9, 1995.

26. Graham RL, Pistolese RA: An impairment rating analysis of asthmatic children under chiropractic care, *J Vertebr Sublux Res* 1(4):41, 1997.

27. Peet JB: Case study: eight year old female with chronic asthma, *Chiro Pediatr* 3:9, 1997.

28. Balon J et al: A comparison of active and simulated chiropractic manipulation as adjunctive treatment for childhood asthma, *New England J Med* 339:1013, 1998.

29. Stephens D, Gorman F: The prospective treatment of visual perception deficit by chiropractic spinal manipulation: a report on two juvenile patients, *Chiro J Austral* 26:82, 1996.

30. Stephens D, Gorman F: The association between visual incompetence and spinal derangement: an instructive case history, *J Manipulative Physiol Ther* 20:343, 1997.

31. Stephens D, Gorman F, Bilton D: The step phenomenon in the recovery of vision with spinal manipulation: a report on two 13-year-olds treated together, *J Manipulative Physiol Ther* 20:628, 1997.

32. Kessinger R, Boneva D: Changes in visual acuity in patients receiving upper cervical specific chiropractic care, *J Vertebr Sublux Res* 2(1):43, 1998.

33. Gemmell HA, Jacobson BH: Chiropractic management of enuresis: a time-series descriptive design, *J Manipulative Physiol Ther* 12:386, 1989.

34. Blomerth PR: Functional nocturnal enuresis, *J Manipulative Physiol Ther* 17:335, 1994.

35. Leboeuf C et al: Chiropractic care of children with nocturnal enuresis: a prospective study, *J Manipulative Physiol Ther* 14:110, 1991.

36. Reed WR et al: Chiropractic management of primary nocturnal enuresis, *J Manipulative Physiol Ther* 17:156, 1994.

37. Borregard PE: Neurogenic bladder and spina bifida occulta: a case report, *J Manipulative Physiol Ther* 10:122, 1987.

38. Stude DE, Bergmann TF, Finer BA: A conservative approach for a patient with traumatically induced urinary incontinence, *J Manipulative Physiol Ther* 21:363, 1998.

39. Vallone SA: Chiropractic management of a 7-year-old female with recurrent urinary tract infections, *Chiro Technique* 10:113, 1998.

40. Tanaka ST, Martin CJ, Thibodeau P: Clinical neurology. In Anrig CA, Plaugher G, editors: *Pediatric chiropractic,* p 479, Baltimore, 1998, Williams & Wilkins.

41. Giesen JM, Center DB, Leach RA: An evaluation of chiropractic manipulation as a treatment of hyperactivity in children, *J Manipulative Physiol Ther* 12:353, 1989.

42. Phillips CF: Case study: the effect of utilizing spinal manipulation and craniosacral therapy as the treatment approach for attention deficit-hyperactivity disorder. In: *Proceedings of the national conference on chiropractic and pediatrics,* p 57, Arlington, Va, 1991, International Chiropractors Association.

43. Thomas MD, Wood J: Upper cervical adjustments may improve mental function, *J Man Med* 6:215, 1992.

44. Arme J: Effects of biomechanical insult correction on attention deficit disorder, *J Chiro Case Rep* 1(1):6, 1993.

45. Araghi HG: Oral apraxia: a case study in chiropractic management. In: *Proceedings of the national conference on chiropractic and pediatrics,* p 34, Arlington, Va, 1994, International Chiropractors Association.

46. Manuele JD, Fysh PN: Acquired verbal aphasia in a 7-year-old female: case report, *J Clin Chiropr Ped* 1:89, 1996.

47. Mitchell LA et al: Chronic rubella vaccine-associated arthropathy, *Arch Intern Med* 153:2268, 1993.

48. Peet JB: Adjusting the hyperactive/ADD pediatric patient, *Chiro Pediatr* 2(4):12, 1997.

49. Goodman R: Cessation of seizure disorder: correction of the atlas subluxation complex. In: *Proceedings of the national conference on chiropractic and pediatrics,* p 46, Arlington, Va, 1991, International Chiropractors Association.

50. Hyman CA: Chiropractic adjustments and the reduction of petit mal seizures in a five-year-old male: a case study, *J Clin Chiropr Ped* 1:28, 1996.

51. Hospers LA: EEG and CEEG studies before and after upper cervical or SOT category II adjustment in children after head trauma, in epilepsy, and in "hyperactivity". In: *Proceedings of the national conference on chiropractic and pediatrics,* p 84, Arlington, Va, 1992, International Chiropractors Association.

52. Woo CC: Post-traumatic myelopathy following flopping high jump: a pilot case of spinal manipulation, *J Manipulative Physiol Ther* 16:336, 1993.

53. Rome PL: Case report: the effect of a chiropractic spinal adjustment on toddler sleep pattern and behavior, *Chiro J Austral* 26:11, 1996.

54. Barnes T: Chiropractic management of the special needs child, *Top Clin Chiropr* 4(4):9, 1997.

55. Nyiendo J, Olsen E: Visit characteristics of 217 children attending a chiropractic college teaching clinic, *J Manipulative Physiol Ther* 11:78, 1988.

56. Tanaka ST, Martin CJ, Thibodeau P: Clinical neurology. In Anrig C, Plaugher G, editors: *Pediatric chiropractic,* pp 522-525, Baltimore, 1998, Williams & Wilkins.

57. Forrester J, Anrig C: The prenatal and perinatal period. In Anrig C, Plaugher G, editors: *Pediatric chiropractic,* pp 127-128, Baltimore, 1998, Williams & Wilkins.

58. Fallon J: Chiropractic pediatrics. In Redwood D, editor: *Contemporary chiropractic,* p 281, New York, 1997, Churchill Livingstone.

59. Fallon J: Chiropractic pediatrics. In Redwood D, editor: *Contemporary chiropractic,* p 284, New York, 1997, Churchill Livingstone.

60. Wall H, Gottlieb M, McGhee S: Growth and development. In Hughes JG, editor: *Synopsis of pediatrics,* p 25, St Louis, 1980, Mosby.

61. Tanaka S, Martin CJ, Thibodeau P: Clinical neurology. In Anrig C, Plaugher G, editors: *Pediatric chiropractic,* p 538, Baltimore, 1998, Williams & Wilkins.

CHAPTER 16

The Somatovisceral Interface: Further Evidence

Marion Todres-Masarsky, DC • *Charles S. Masarsky, DC* • *Everett Langhans, DC*

Subluxation and the Immune System

With the increase in antibiotic-resistant strains of pathogenic microbes, nonpharmaceutical strategies for boosting the competence of the immune system are attracting unprecedented attention in the scientific press and the general media. Therefore chiropractic researchers are beginning to address the possibility that decreased immunocompetence may be a feature of subluxation and the vertebral subluxation complex (VSC).

Although otitis media sometimes involves sterile effusion, it is often linked to viral or bacterial infections of the middle ear. Many chiropractic studies have indicated a favorable clinical response by otitis media patients to chiropractic care, many of whom had clear infectious involvement.[1-7] Whether the results in these cases represent enhancement of general immunocompetence, local improvement in tissue tone, including improved drainage through the eustachian tubes and enhanced lymphatic drainage from the ears, or a combination is not yet clear.

Van Breda and Van Breda[8] surveyed parents, who were either medical doctors or doctors of chiropractic, regarding various aspects of their children's health histories. The children whose parents were doctors of chiropractic were typically adjusted once per week or more, and the children whose parents were medical doctors were not adjusted. At least one bout of otitis media was reported among 80% of the medical children versus 31% of the chiropractic children. (Some of the medical doctors commented that otitis media was a universal childhood experience; therefore the question on otitis media was invalid.) At least one bout of tonsillitis was reported among 42% of the medical children versus 27% of the chiropractic children. The differ-

ence between the groups was statistically significant for both conditions.

Rose-Aymon and others[9] presented a survey involving pediatric patients receiving chiropractic care. Although a small sample size precluded assessment of statistical significance, the pilot data suggested an inverse relationship between the frequency of chiropractic adjustments and the incidence of chickenpox, mumps, measles, and German measles.

Thomas and Wilkinson[10] published a case study of a woman with frank spina bifida from T11 to L2. She suffered from many problems, including long-standing, recurrent bladder infections despite a daily regimen of antibiotics. After receiving chiropractic care (a variety of techniques for 5 years), her infections became less frequent. When the authors' report was published the patient had been infection-free for more than 1 year without antibiotics.

Araghi[11] presented the case of a 2-year-old girl with myasthenia gravis. Myasthenia gravis is now widely viewed as an autoimmune condition, in which acetylcholine receptors at the myoneuronal junction are attacked by the patient's white blood cells. After 5 months of steady deterioration despite medical attention the patient began to respond after a single Gonstead adjustment at the upper cervical and sacroiliac levels.

A second case involving myasthenia gravis was described by Alcantara and others.[12] A 63-year-old man came to the chiropractor with multiple complaints, including swelling of the tongue, dysphagia, nausea, digestive problems, weakness in the eye muscles, dyspnea, myopia, diplopia, and headaches. In addition, he experienced difficulty in ambulation resulting from loss of balance and coordination. Contact-specific, high-velocity, and low-amplitude adjustments were applied to sub-luxation sites. As a result, myasthenia gravis is no longer debilitating to the patient; he is medication-free and lives normally.

The possibility that autoimmune disorders may respond to chiropractic care was further reinforced by a case of psoriasis presented by Behrendt.[13] The patient was a 52-year-old man who had not experienced a nonmedicated remission from psoriatic skin lesions in approximately 6 years before visiting the doctor. The patient was adjusted according to Network Chiropractic Analysis protocols. Although the adjustments varied with each visit, C2, C5, the sacrum, and the coccyx were the most frequently adjusted levels. When the authors' report was published, psoriatic skin lesions covering the body had been maintained at 1% or less without oral medication, compared with 5% with medication, and as much as 20% nonmedicated before chiropractic care.

A number of clinical and experimental studies have recently appeared that include laboratory data as outcome measures. In a review of uncontrolled pilot investigations, Allen[14] described studies indicating increased serum immunoglobulin levels and increased lymphocyte counts after chiropractic adjustments. This review also offered an instructive summary of work by Brennan's research team.[17]

Lee and Jenson[15] presented the case of a patient with liver cancer (hepatocellular carcinoma). When the patient's most recent bout of liver cancer was confirmed by CT scan and alpha-fetal protein levels, he declined medical intervention but requested that his health maintenance organization continue monitoring his progress. The only intervention was upper cervical analysis and adjustment. Alpha-fetal protein levels were normalized within 6 months of beginning intensive chiropractic care, with remission confirmed on CT scan after 8 months. The patient is reportedly well at 3 years postremission.

A small but potentially groundbreaking clinical study was offered in 1994 by Selano and others.[16] A total of 10 human immunodeficiency virus-(HIV) positive patients were randomly assigned to 2 groups. The experimental group received upper cervical adjustments according to Grostic protocols, and the control group received sham adjustments, with the Grostic instrument trigger depressed and no impulse delivered to the atlas

vertebra. The study lasted 6 months, with no record of visit frequency noted.

The most interesting outcome measure in this study was the CD4 count at the beginning and end of the study because a decline in the white blood cell level is an essential immunodeficiency measure in HIV-positive patients. In the control group, CD4 count declined by a mean of 7.96%. In the experimental group, CD4 count increased by a mean of 48%. Despite the small number of subjects in this study the results approached statistical significance, making further chiropractic research on this subject possible.

Brennan's research team[17] is the most widely published group in chiropractic neuroimmunology. In a 1991 study, they injected a nontoxic sealant into the posterior facet joints of 4 dogs at various thoracic and lumbar levels, in an attempt to mimic the VSC through surgical joint fixation. A total of 4 other dogs underwent sham surgery, in which the sealant was injected near the facet joints, at a location not causing fixation. White blood cell functional activity was measured in both groups during postsurgical recovery.

Although functional activity levels of lymphocytes and polymorphonuclear neutrophils were depressed in both groups, the dogs that had sham surgery recovered normal white blood cell function more rapidly than the dogs with spinal joint fixation. These results support the hypothesis that immunosuppression can result from the VSC.

In another study by Brennan and others[18] using human volunteers, thoracic manipulation (diversified maneuvers at levels indicated by motion palpation), sham manipulation (light-force thrust with no audible or palpable joint release), and soft-tissue manipulation (light massage at the gluteal area) groups were compared. Blood was drawn before and after these interventions. Polymorphonuclear neutrophils and monocytes demonstrated increased functional activity after thoracic manipulation but not after sham or soft-tissue manipulation.

The difference between groups was statistically significant. Polymorphonuclear neutrophils are phagocytic white blood cells. Monocytes are also phagocytic and are involved in the process that activates lymphocytes to produce antibodies when nonself proteins are present. The functional activity of these cells was measured through a process called *chemiluminescence,* or light emission by white blood cells in the presence of certain reagents. The amount of light emission is proportional to the rate of metabolic activity during phagocytosis.

A second component of this study explored the role of a particular neurotransmitter (substance P) in communication between the spine and white blood cells. Unfortunately, the results were inconclusive.

Brennan's team[18] is the first chiropractic research group to seriously explore molecular communication pathways between the nervous system and the immune system. Before their investigations, receptors for a variety of neurotransmitters had been identified on certain populations of white blood cells. Some white blood cells apparently also secrete neurotransmitters, establishing a possible molecular infrastructure for two-way communication between neurons and white blood cells. Fidelibus[19] presented an interesting review of this research.

Broadly, white blood cells can seemingly act as mobile neurons with defensive capabilities. The theoretic and applied aspects of this new understanding should be beneficial for future chiropractic researchers.

Adductor-Type Spasmodic Dysphonia

Adductor-type spasmodic dysphonia (ASD) is a rare, puzzling speech disorder of unknown etiology. A person afflicted with ASD experiences a choking sensation whenever conscious speech is attempted resulting from glottis closure by hyperadduction of the vocal folds. This strain-strangle phonation could be aptly described as "choking on one's own words." Once the condition plateaus, spontaneous recovery is rare.

Treatment ranges from relatively gentle interventions such as speech therapy and psychotherapy to more invasive measures such as botulinum injection or surgery. These invasive measures generally focus on the recurrent laryngeal nerve, the vagus branch that innervates the vocal folds.

Wood[20] described a 46-year-old man who experienced a minor head cold accompanied by hoarseness. Although the other head cold symptoms disappeared, the hoarseness progressed for 4 to 8 weeks, until the patient was unable to talk. Consultations with numerous specialists at two teaching hospitals revealed no frank pathology of the vocal apparatus and a diagnosis of ASD of hysteric origin. Psychotherapy was therefore recommended. At the time of presentation the patient had suffered from ASD symptoms for 6 months.

The patient related in writing that upper cervical stiffness and suboccipital headache had appeared concurrently with the voice problem. Examination revealed hypomobility and tenderness at the C1-2 motion segment, and x-ray examination revealed malposition at that level. Wood explained to the patient that the upper cervical problem could be a source of irritation to one of the nerves controlling the vocal apparatus (the vagus), simultaneously causing the neck stiffness and headache. A 2-week clinical trial of diversified adjusting was recommended.

Complete resolution of the headaches, neck stiffness, and ASD symptoms ensued within 2 weeks (5 visits). A partial exacerbation occurred several months later and was resolved within 4 visits. At 4 years of follow-up, no further episode was noted.

Reflex Sympathetic Dystrophy

Reflex sympathetic dystrophy (RSD) is a condition not fully understood, characterized by vasoconstriction (sometimes reaching cyanosis) and pain after an injury. The pain is usually not proportionate to the severity of the original injury, and spontaneous resolution is rare. Medical treatment often involves anesthetic injection into the sympathetic ganglion or ganglia innervating the involved area, in an effort to reverse the sympathetic hyperactivity characteristic of RSD.

Ellis and Ebrall[21] described the case of a 13-year-old girl with lower extremity RSD. After jumping to the ground from a height of 10 feet, the patient stated that her left foot hurt, felt cold, and sometimes became blue and white. Initial medical evaluation produced a diagnosis of "posttraumatic injury of ligamentous dislocation with possible reflex sympathetic dystrophy." After 9 weeks of unsuccessful physical therapy, the diagnosis was changed to "injury to the left foot with conversion reaction," (conversion reaction indicates psychogenic symptoms) and psychotherapy was recommended. At the first doctor visit the patient required crutches to walk.

Chiropractic examination revealed dysfunction at the L5-S1 and left sacroiliac motion segments, along with fixation involving the left talus. The involved motion segments were adjusted using the Gonstead technique, and a home program of passive stretching was initiated. The patient reported substantial relief after 3 weeks of care. After 3½ months the patient was able to ambulate without crutches, and at 5½ months the patient was able to play basketball.

A case of upper extremity RSD was reported by Langweiler and Febbo.[22] About 4 weeks before the first doctor visit a 24-year-old woman began experiencing stiffness in the upper thoracic spine. Within 12 days, severe burning pain, numbness, sweating, and swelling were noted in her right arm and hand. After several medical examinations, RSD was diagnosed, and injection of anesthetic into the stellate ganglion was recommended. The patient opted for a trial of chiropractic care before considering this more invasive intervention.

Motion palpation revealed hypomobility at the T3-4 and C5-6 motion segments. Diversified adjustments were administered 3 times per week for 6 weeks, with electroacupuncture as adjunctive therapy. At the end of this period, subjective improvement was accompanied by better pinch and grip strength. After 8 more weeks of chiropractic care, the patient was referred to a rehabilitation center for concurrent work hardening. When the authors' case report was published the patient returned to full-time work as a data entry processor for 1 year with no apparent difficulties.

Myoclonic Seizures

Most people have experienced the normal myoclonic jerk when going to sleep. In myoclonic seizures, similar jerk-like, involuntary phasic contractions of muscles or groups of muscles occur in rapid succession, often while the patient is awake.

Woo[23] reported the case of a 24-year-old woman who suffered from myoclonic seizures of the inner thigh and abdominal musculature. These seizures occurred day and night for 17 years, after a diving injury, in which the patient's lower back was hyperextended when she dove into the water. The violence of the abdominal contractions was occasionally intense enough to cause the patient to regurgitate her meals. Previous electroencephalo-graphic examination was negative, making any classic type of epilepsy unlikely. Antiseizure medications were not successful in controlling this patient's seizures.

Thoracolumbar VSC was indicated by palpation. The seizures became less frequent after a single adjustment at the thoracolumbar junction. When the author's journal article was published the patient was seizure-free for 3 months.

Duff[24] reported the case of a 30-year-old woman who was awakened during sleep with migraine, slurred speech, vomiting, pain behind the right eye, blurred vision, and mild myoclonic seizures. Extensive medical evaluation included blood work, x-rays, and electroencephalography, computerized tomography, and magnetic resonance imaging examinations. All of the test results were negative, and a diagnosis of myoclonic seizures of unknown etiology was determined.

When the patient returned to the chiropractic office 18 months later, she was experiencing 30 to 40 myoclonic seizures a day, despite taking antiseizure medication. A history of multiple sports injuries to the cervical spine was noted, as were myoclonic jerks provoked during cervical range of motion testing. X-ray examination and thermocouple instrument scanning for paraspinal temperature asymmetry indicated the presence of upper cervical VSC.

The day after the first upper cervical adjustment using toggle recoil protocols the patient had only 2 myoclonic seizures. By the third day, she had no seizures, and a progress examination indicated a reduction in paravertebral temperature asymmetry. An exacerbation after a fall 2 days later was resolved with a single adjustment. At 2 years of follow-up, the patient remained seizure free.

Multiple Sclerosis

The etiology of multiple sclerosis is uncertain. Although the visualization of sclerotic demyelination lesions in the central nervous system through magnetic resonance imaging techniques has improved the assessment of this condition, diagnoses remains difficult. Typical signs and symptoms include motor weakness, numbness, ataxia, blurred vision, and positive L'Hermittes sign (electric-like pain spreading down the body into the extremities on passive head flexion).[25]

Patients with multiple sclerosis typically experience many series of apparently spontaneous worsening symptoms and remission. These unpredictable cycles make assessing the role of the VSC in aggravation and the chiropractic adjustment in remission of multiple sclerosis difficult. Nevertheless, chiropractic literature on this topic is currently being written.

Gonstead maintained that loss or reversal of the normal lordotic cervical curve could cause a patient with multiple sclerosis to be more vulnerable to irritations because of adverse tension on the spinal cord.[26] The author recommended that close attention be given to restoration of this curve.

In the literature review by Roberts and others,[27] they briefly described a 35-year-old man with a medical diagnosis of multiple sclerosis. The patient apparently responded well to unspecified cervical and upper thoracic adjusting.

Stude and Mick[28] presented the case of a 32-year-old man with a medical diagnosis of multiple sclerosis based on clinical signs and supported by magnetic resonance imaging findings. The patient's symptoms included fatigue, diplopia, gait imbalance, eye twitching, general muscular weakness, and enuresis at the first chiropractic visit. Deep tendon reflexes were hyperactive in the lower extremities, with the Achilles reflex demonstrating mild clonus. Thoracolumbar and lumbosacral VSC were identified through motion palpation and x-ray examination. Minutes after diversified adjusting at these levels, the patient reported that all symptoms had subsided. The patient visited the doctor 2 more times for the next 3 weeks, and then he discontinued the visits for several months. The patient denied any return of symptoms during the hiatus from care.

Kirby[29] reported the case of a 24-year-old woman who received a diagnosis of multiple sclerosis from a medical neurologist 3 months before her first chiropractic visit.[29] Diagnosis was based on physical examination and magnetic resonance imaging findings. The results of treatment with steroidal therapy and a low-fat diet were not promising.

At the initial examination, she was suffering from fatigue, depression, blurred vision, and numbness and tingling in all four extremities. Decreased sensation was noted in the L1-S2 dermatomes, and L'Hermittes' test results were positive. Palpation and x-ray examination findings were consistent with upper cervical VSC.

Upper cervical instrument adjusting was administered 14 times for 120 days. The patient was monitored for an additional 80 days after the final adjustment. By the end of the 200 days the extremity numbness had substantially improved, and L'Hermittes' test produced less intense pain. Energy levels, emotional well being, and general health, as measured by the Rand SF-36 health survey, also improved considerably (see Chapter 6).

Killinger and Azad[30] reported four retrospective cases from the recently rediscovered clinical records of the B.J. Palmer Chiropractic Clinic between 1948-1953. In those years, diagnosis was based on history and neurologic signs because magnetic resonance imaging was not available. Because today's formal pencil-and-paper instruments were also not available, outcomes pertaining to quality of life were taken from patient diaries and correspondence.

An illustrative case involved a 51-year-old woman with a medical diagnosis of multiple sclerosis discerned at 9 years before her initial examination. Lack of coordination in her legs, along with numbness in the left foot, required cane use for walking. Numbness in both hands prevented her from easily grasping objects and from writing. She suffered from insomnia and was unable to work for 3 months. About 3 days after her first upper cervical adjustment, using HIO protocols, the patient reported that the numbness in her left foot was gone, ambulation had improved, her ability to grasp and manipulate objects had progressed so that she could now easily write in her diary, and her sleep quality was much improved. About 9 months later, she returned to her full-time job as a night nursing supervisor.

Emotional and Behavioral Disorders

One of the classic tenets of chiropractic is that emotional stressors can create or worsen the VSC and vice versa. During the first half of the twentieth century, this principle was taken so seriously that chiropractic psychiatric hospitals were created. The most well-known facility was Clear View Sanitarium in Davenport, Iowa (1926-1961). At Clear View, patients were evaluated by medical doctors and psychologists, but chiropractic adjustments were the only intervention used. Although journal publication was not available for chiropractic clinician-researchers in those years, some of the clinical work performed at Clear View, along with theoretic commentary, was published in a book edited by Schwartz.[31]

Koren and Rosenwinkel[32] correlated spinal x-ray findings with personality profiles, measured by a well-established pencil-and-paper instrument, the Minnesota Multiphasic Personality Inventory (MMPI). X-rays from 40 patients in a private chiropractic practice were evaluated according to the protocols of Spinal Stressology. Atlas angle (deviation of the atlas plane line from the horizontal plane) was significantly correlated with three MMPI scales: hypochondriasis (the tendency to somatize emotional problems), hysteria (the tendency to dramatize and overrespond to stimuli), and paranoia (the tendency to feel persecuted).

Spinal length correlated considerably with the masculinity-femininity scale, which measures identity with sexual stereotypes. The thoracic apex (the distance from the center of the body of the most posterior vertebra and a vertical line drawn from the most anterior point on the tip of the second sacral tubercle) correlated with hypomania (depression and low energy) but only in the standing position.

Several chiropractic cases involving anxiety disorders were published during the 1990s. Sullivan[33] reported the case of a 42-year-old woman with a 1-year history of severe anxiety attacks. The first attack occurred shortly after a motor vehicle accident. This patient also suffered from agoraphobia, nightmares, dizziness, insomnia, tachycardia, memory loss, inability to concentrate, and urinary bladder urgency. The findings of motion palpation, x-ray examination, and surface electromyography (SEMG) clustered at the C5-6, T5-6, and L5-S1 motion segments.

For 2 months the patient was seen 3 times per week for chiropractic adjustments using Gonstead protocols and once per week for counseling and biofeedback training. At the end of 2 months the patient reported a sharp reduction in anxiety, along with complete resolution of agoraphobia, bladder urgency, insomnia, and dizziness. After 4 more months of care, anxiety was completely resolved, concurrent with improvement in the motion palpation and SEMG findings.

Potthoff and others[34] reported the case of a 52-year-old woman with a long-standing anxiety dis-

order. At the time of her initial examination, panic attacks were occurring several times per week, characterized by cardiac palpitations and a feeling of doom. Each attack would last several hours. Over the years, a variety of antidepressants and tranquilizers were prescribed; at the first doctor visit, she was taking antianxiety medication and receiving counseling and relaxation training. These measures were of little apparent benefit.

Motion palpation findings clustered at the upper and midcervical, upper and midthoracic, and right sacroiliac areas. The patient was instructed to come to the office for an adjustment at the onset of a panic attack. Response to diversified adjusting was generally rapid and dramatic. During one of her panic attacks the patient's blood pressure would typically be approximately 182/102 mmHg and pulse rate would be 120 bpm. About 4 minutes after the adjustment the patient's blood pressure would drop to 140/80 mmHg and the pulse rate would slow to 76 bpm. This was accompanied by subjective dispersal of the anxiety state.

Initially the patient would visit about 4 times per week, sometimes taking 2 visits on the same day. The attacks gradually became less frequent. When the authors' report was published the patient had been free of panic attacks for more than 2 months—the longest period in many years. This was accomplished even with decreased medication dose (at her medical doctor's request).

Peterson[35] presented a small but interesting controlled clinical trial involving anxiety. A total of 18 volunteers with long-standing phobic reactions to spiders, snakes, mice, or other insects or animals were divided into experimental and control groups. After viewing a color photograph of the fear-inducing creature (phobogenic stimulus) for 20 seconds the volunteers indicated their anxiety levels on a visual analog scale (VAS), and their pulse rates were measured.

After this initial phobogenic exposure, control subjects were given a sham adjustment, using an Activator instrument set on 0 tension. The experimental subjects were adjusted at T1, T5, and T8, while contemplating their phobia (the procedure called for in Neuroemotional Technique). Afterwards, another 20-second phobogenic exposure occurred and a second set of VAS and pulse rates were measured.

The experimental subjects demonstrated a statistically significant improvement in VAS scores and the control subjects did not. Pulse rates did not change significantly for either group.

Tourette's syndrome is a peculiar condition of unknown etiology, characterized by motor tics and uncontrolled vocalizations. The vocalizations may include sniffing, grunting, barking, and sudden utterances of obscenities. In severe cases these bizarre symptoms make a normal life virtually impossible for the patient. Medical management is often unsuccessful.

Trotta[36] presented the case of a 31-year-old man with Tourette's syndrome, which was originally diagnosed at 4 years of age. His symptoms primarily consisted of uncontrollable sniffing and grunting, with increased severity at night and during stress. These symptoms were worsening 6 years before his initial examination, despite medical intervention.

X-ray analysis, thermographic scan, and the supine leg check indicated the presence of upper cervical VSC. A total of 8 adjustments, using Life Upper Cervical protocols, were administered for 12 weeks. In most cases a reduction in symptoms was noted immediately after the adjustment. According to the Stress Audit Profile (a pencil-and-paper instrument that monitors patient stress levels), significant reduction in stress levels occurred almost immediately and remained lower than at the time of the first visit throughout the 12 weeks of chiropractic care. Unfortunately, long-term follow-up care was not possible because the patient discontinued care.

Many of the behavioral disorder studies involved pediatric patients (see Chapter 15).[35-43]

Coma

Probably the most spectacular case in the chiropractic literature was described by Plaugher and others.[44] A 21-year-old man was comatose for more than 1 year after a motor vehicle accident. After 3 modified Gonstead upper cervical adjustments the patient woke up with a concomitant return of normal levels of pulse rate and blood pressure. Adjustments were later performed at L5-S1 and various levels of the thoracic spine. At the time of the authors' published work the patient was able to walk with the help of crutches.

Dermatologic Disorders and the VSC

Chronic dermatologic disorders offer convenient opportunities to study the somatovisceral interface. Changes in these disorders are readily triggered by alterations in cutaneous vasomotor tone, glandular activity, stress physiology, and immune responses. Visual inspection and photography offer noninvasive and cost-effective outcome measures.

Unfortunately the chiropractic literature on dermatologic conditions is scant. A case involving psoriasis in the immune system section was previously discussed.[13] Lacunza and others[45] reported the case of a 16-month-old girl with eczema lesions covering her entire body except the diaper area. This lesion distribution was present for 10 months before her initial examination. The patient was also constipated during this period. Homeopathic medication, dietary changes, and previous chiropractic care had failed to provide relief.

A total of 2 adjustments were administered according to Alphabiotic protocols (an upper cervical technique, in which the supine patient is placed on an incline table) for 4 days. At 4 days the severity and distribution of the eczema lesions were reduced by approximately 50%. After 7 more adjustments administered over approximately 3 weeks the eczema was barely noticeable and bowel movements were occurring daily. Unfortunately, long-term follow-up was not possible because of transportation difficulties.

A biomedical team led by Tait[46] reported a series of brachioradial pruritis (BRP) cases. BRP usually involves itching over the lateral elbow, although the posterior shoulder and interscapular area can be involved. Symptoms can be unilateral or bilateral. Patients are often examined with no visible rash in the involved area. Although topical medication and avoidance of sun exposure provide relief for some patients, treatment fails for the majority of people and the etiology remains obscure.

Tait and others[46] are dermatologists who became aware of several instances in which BRP was apparently relieved after manipulation by orthopedists trained in manual medicine. The manipulative technique was described by Cyriax; it involves a general cervical rotary move, with the head turned away from the symptomatic side. Of 14 patients surveyed, relief was reported to last from 2 days in one case to apparent permanent resolution in another after manipulative therapy.

Chiropractic Care and Wellness

In some studies an effort occurs to analyze the effects of the VSC correction on general health and wellness. Instruments such as the RAND SF-36 (SF-36) and the Global Well-Being Scale (GWBS) were discussed in Chapter 6. These instruments were used by Owens and others[47] in a multisite research project. Patients from 10 different upper cervical practices completed the SF-36 and GWBS at specified intervals in their care. Statistically significant improvements in SF-36 scales related to physical and emotional health and vitality were noted from the first visit to maximal chiropractic improvement. These improvements were accompanied by reduction in radiographic signs of upper cervical subluxation and improvement in GWBS scores. These results are preliminary in an on-going planned investigation.

The SF-36 was also used as a major outcome measure in an investigation of Bio-Energetic Synchronization Technique (BEST) by Morter and Schuster.[48] The SF-36 was administered before care and 4 days after a BEST adjustment; statistically significant improvements were noted. This improvement was accompanied by change in fasting salivary pH, which is believed to reflect autonomic balance. Unfortunately, normal values have not yet been established for fasting salivary pH, making this aspect of the study difficult to interpret. However, Morter and Schuster[48] reportedly plan similar follow-up studies.

Blanks and others[49] developed a new pencil-and-paper instrument to assess wellness and quality of life in an investigation of Network chiropractic care. Based on responses from 2818 patients of Network practitioners, statistically significant improvement in wellness and quality of life was noted, comparing current status with status "before Network." This new instrument is still being developed and validated; therefore the reported results must be considered preliminary.

Athletes are a potentially valuable group of subjects for study because they are relatively healthy people who constantly stress their bodies to achieve maximal performance. Therefore their response to chiropractic care is one way the adjust-

ment improves general wellness in asymptomatic people. Although cases involving athletic injuries are somewhat common in the chiropractic literature, the study of the well athlete under chiropractic care is in the preliminary stage.

Lauro and Mouch[50] studied 50 athletes involved in a variety of activities, including football, volleyball, track, cross-country running, weight lifting, body building, rugby, and aerobic dancing. A total of 11 tests were used to measure various aspects of athletic ability, including agility, balance, kinesthetic perception, power, and reaction time. After initial testing the experimental group received a chiropractic analysis, which included Gonstead and Palmer upper cervical x-ray marking, thermoscribe pattern analysis, Derefield leg check, static palpation, and motion palpation. Adjustment techniques included toggle-recoil, Gonstead, diversified, and Thompson. Technique and visit frequency were determined on an individual basis, and the control group was not adjusted.

After 6 weeks the control group exhibited statistically significant improvement in 2 of the 11 tests, and the experimental group exhibited statistically significant improvement in 8 tests.

The results of the Nelson hand reaction test were interesting—a measure of the speed of reaction with the hand in response to a visual stimulus occurs. After 6 weeks the control group exhibited less than 1% improvement in this test, and the experimental group exhibited more than 18% improvement.

A smaller but more focused study on athletic ability in patients under chiropractic care was conducted by Schwartzbauer and others.[51] A total of 21 players on a men's college baseball team were randomly assigned to control (observation only) or experimental (upper cervical chiropractic care) groups. Statistically significant improvements were noted at 14 weeks in long jump distance and muscle strength in the experimental group but not the control group. The experimental group also exhibited statistically significant improvement in capillary counts, and the control group did not. Capillary counts were made by viewing the nailbed of the right and left middle fingers through a microscope at 60× magnification. The number of capillaries visible in one microscopic field of view was recorded. As microcirculation to the fingers improved, capillary count increased.

Summary

Studies involving general health and wellness are instrumental in chiropractic research. The results of such research may help to confirm what has been informally observed by many clinicians— that the VSC is a general depressor of well-being and therefore may be considered a global risk factor for future illness and injury in the asymptomatic patient. In this arena the chiropractic adjustment is not only viewed as a treatment for specific injuries and disorders but is also regarded as a supportive general health measure.

STUDY GUIDE

1. What are three possible mechanisms by which chiropractic adjustments are specifically beneficial in improving the health of patients with otitis media?

2. Define myasthenia gravis. Why should some benefit through chiropractic be expected for people with this condition?

3. Why are research projects using correctly presented laboratory work so useful in supporting the evidence of chiropractic adjustments as the primary vehicle of improvement in many of the cases?

4. What is chemoluminescence?

5. Why do some white blood cells function as mobile neurons?

6. What is adductor-type spasmodic dysphonia? What is the current treatment of choice for ASD? How could the chiropractic adjustment be capable of relieving the problem using, in part, the same pathway as the treatment of choice without exposing the patient to further trauma.

7. What is reflex sympathetic dystrophy? What is a conversion reaction? Chiropractors treat many patients whose medical testing does not reveal pathology and who will appear emotionally stable, yet have an obvious problem. Can pain make a rational person appear less emotionally stable? Write a brief paragraph about an imaginary patient who has been medically diagnosed with a conversion reaction after injury, explaining the findings and which mechanism should be used to help regain the patient's health. Exchange paragraphs with a colleague and critique each other's explanation. Look for accuracy and easy comprehension.

8. In Duff's study[24] of a patient with myoclonic seizures, the findings in the EEG, CAT scan, and MRI were negative, yet the patient had a clear problem. Why did none of the above sophisticated tests show the source of that problem?

9. Name four symptoms of MS that can be discovered through routine history and examination. Explain these symptoms in terms of the condition of the patient's nervous system. What did Gonstead say about MS?

10. Many health professionals think MS is becoming more prevalent. Although some of this may be because of the invention of the MRI, which allows the plaques that are characteristic of the condition to be seen, what are some other aspects of modern life that may contribute to MS. For each of the possible contributing factors, discuss a way in which removing nerve interference may directly effect the patient.

11. What kind of professionals were on the team at Clear View Sanitarium? How was patient care divided among them?

12. Describe and compare the two cases that were concerned with the relief of anxiety attacks.

13. Why are dermatologic disorders such convenient opportunities to study the somatovisceral interface? Name three aspects of general physiology that when altered can change these disorders quickly.

14. According to Selano and others[16] what was the relationship of the CD4 counts of the subjects being adjusted to that of the controls?

15. Name two instruments that can be used to study changes in general health and wellness in the chiropractic patient.

16. Why are athletes such valuable research subjects for wellness studies?

17. What is the Nelson hand reaction test and what does it measure? Describe the results of the Nelson hand reaction test in Lauro's and Mouch's study.[50]

18. Why is capillary count a useful measure of general wellness?

REFERENCES

1. Hobbs DA, Rasmussen SA: Chronic otitis media: a case report, *ACA J Chiro* 28:67, 1991.
2. Phillips NJ: Vertebral subluxation and otitis media: a case study, *Chiropr: J Res Chiropr Clin Invest* 8:38, 1992.
3. Thill L et al: The response of a patient with otitis media to chiropractic care, *Life Work* 3:23, 1995.
4. Froehle RM: Ear infection: a retrospective study examining improvement from chiropractic care and analyzing for influencing factors, *J Manipulative Physiol Ther* 19:169, 1996.
5. Fysh PN: Chronic recurrent otitis media: case series of five patients with recommendations for case management, *J Clin Chiropr Ped* 1:66, 1996.
6. Heagy DT: The effect of the correction of the vertebral subluxation on chronic otitis media in children, *Chiro Ped* 2(2):6, 1996.
7. Fallon JM: The role of the chiropractic adjustment in the care and treatment of 332 children with otitis media, *J Clin Chiropr Ped* 2:167, 1997.
8. Van Breda WM, Van Breda JM: A comparative study of the health status of children raised under the health care models of chiropractic and allopathic medicine, *Chiropr: J Res Chiropr Clin Invest* 5:101, 1993.
9. Rose-Aymon S et al: The relationship between intensity of chiropractic care and incidence of childhood diseases, *Chiropr: J Res Chiropr Clin Invest* 1:70, 1989.
10. Thomas RJ, Wilkinson M: Chiropractic care in adult spina bifida: a case report, *Chiro Technique* 2:191, 1990.
11. Araghi HJ: Juvenile myasthenia gravis: a case study in chiropractic management. In: *Proceedings of the national conference on pediatrics and chiropractic*, p 122, Arlington, Va, 1993, International Chiropractors Association.
12. Alcantara J et al: Chiropractic management of a patient with myasthenia gravis and vertebral subluxations, *J Manipulative Physiol Ther* 22:333, 1999.
13. Behrendt M: Reduction of psoriasis in a patient under network spinal analysis care: a case report, *J Vertebr Sublux Res* 2(4):196, 1998.
14. Allen JM: The effects of chiropractic on the immune system: a review of the literature, *Chiro J Austral* 23:132, 1993.
15. Lee G, Jenson CD: Remission of hepatocellular carcinoma in a patient under chiropractic care: a case report, *J Vertebr Sublux Res* 2(3):125, 1998.
16. Selano JL et al: The effects of specific upper cervical adjustments on the CD4 counts of HIV positive patients, *Chiro Res J* 3:32, 1994.
17. Brennan PC et al: Immunologic correlates of reduced spinal mobility: preliminary observations in a dog model. In Wolk S, editor: *Proceedings of the 1991 international conference on spinal manipulation*, p 118, Arlington, Va, 1991, Foundation for Chiropractic Education and Research.
18. Brennan PC et al: Enhanced phagocytic cell respiratory burst induced by spinal manipulation: potential role of substance P, *J Manipulative Physiol Ther* 14:399, 1991.
19. Fidelibus JC: An overview of neuroimmunomodulation and a possible correlation with musculoskeletal system function, *J Manipulative Physiol Ther* 12:289, 1989.
20. Wood KW: Case report: resolution of spasmodic dysphonia (focal laryngeal dystonia) via chiropractic manipulative management, *J Manipulative Physiol Ther* 14:376, 1991.
21. Ellis WB, Eball PS: The resolution of chronic inversion and plantarflexion of the foot: a pediatric case study, *Chiro Technique* 3:55, 1991.
22. Langweiler MJ, Febbo TA: Reflex sympathetic dystrophy syndrome: a case report, *J Neuromusculoskel Syst* 1:69, 1993.
23. Woo CC: Traumatic spinal myoclonus, *J Manipulative Physiol Ther* 12:478, 1989.
24. Duff BA: Documented chiropractic results on a case diagnosed as myoclonic seizures, *Chiropr: J Res Chiropr Clin Invest* 8:56, 1992.
25. Balduc HA: Neurological system. In Lawrence DJ, editor: *Fundamentals of chiropractic diagnosis and management*, p 112, Baltimore, 1990, Williams & Wilkins.
26. Plaugher G et al: Spinal management for the patient with a visceral concomitant. In Plaugher G, editor: *Textbook of chiropractic: a specific biomechanical approach*, p 374, Baltimore, 1993, Williams & Wilkins.
27. Roberts JW, Sturgeon JS, Thomas RJ: Multiple sclerosis and early diagnosis: a literature review, *ACA J Chiro* 27:75, 1990.
28. Stude DE, Mick T: Clinical presentation of a patient with multiple sclerosis and response to manual chiropractic adjustive therapies, *J Manipulative Physiol Ther* 16:595, 1993.
29. Kirby SL: A case study: the effects of chiropractic on multiple sclerosis, *Chiro Res J* 3:7, 1994.
30. Killinger LZ, Azad A: Multiple sclerosis patients under chiropractic care: a retrospective study, *Palmer J Res* 2:96, 1997.
31. Schwartz HS: *Mental health and chiropractic*, New York, 1973, Sessions Publishers.
32. Koren T, Rosenwinkel E: Spinal patterns as predictors of personality profiles: a pilot study, *Int J Psychosom* 39:10, 1992.
33. Sullivan EC: The chiropractic management of anxiety: a case report, *ACA J Chiro* 29:29, 1992.
34. Potthoff S, Penwell B, Wolf J: Panic attacks and the chiropractic adjustment: a case report, *ACA J Chiro* 30:26, 1993.
35. Peterson KB: The effects of spinal manipulation on the intensity of emotional arousal in phobic subjects exposed to a threat stimulus: a randomized, controlled, double-blind clinical trial, *J Manipulative Physiol Ther* 20:602, 1997.
36. Trotta N: The response of an adult tourette patient to life upper cervical adjustments, *Chiro Res J* 1:43, 1989.
37. Giesen JM, Center DB, Leach RA: An evaluation of chiropractic manipulation as a treatment of hyperactivity in children, *J Manipulative Physiol Ther* 12:353, 1989.
38. Phillips CF: Case study: the effect of utilizing spinal manipulation and craniosacral therapy as the treatment approach for attention deficit-hyperactivity disorder. In: *Proceedings of the national conference on chiropractic and pediatrics*, p 57, Arlington, Va, 1991, International Chiropractors Association.
39. Thomas MD, Wood J: Upper cervical adjustments may improve mental function, *J Man Med* 6:215, 1992.

40. Arme J: Effects of biomechanical insult correction on attention deficit disorder, *J Chiro Case Rep* 1(1):6, 1993.

41. Araghi HG: Oral apraxia: a case study in chiropractic management. In: *Proceedings of the national conference on chiropractic and pediatrics,* p 34, Arlington, Va, 1994, International Chiropractors Association.

42. Manuele JD, Fysh PN: Acquired verbal aphasia in a 7-year-old female: case report, *J Clin Chiropr Ped* 1:89, 1996.

43. Peet JB: Adjusting the hyperactive/ADD pediatric patient, *Chiro Pediatr* 2(4):12, 1997.

44. Plaugher G, Rowe DJ, Gohl RA: Chiropractic management of spinal fractures and dislocations with closed reduction methods: a report of nine cases. In Wolk S, editor: *Proceedings of the 1992 international conference on spinal manipulation,* p 79, Arlington, Va, 1992, Foundation for Chiropractic Education and Research.

45. Lacunza C, Waldron M, Tarr W: Chiropractic management of a pediatric patient with eczema, *Life Work* 3:20, 1995.

46. Tait CP, Grigg E, Quirk CJ: Brachioradial pruritis and cervical spine manipulation, *Australas J Dermatol* 59:168, 1998.

47. Owens EF, Hoiriis KT, Burd D: Changes in general health status during upper cervical chiropractic care: PBR progress report, *Chiro Res J* 5:9, 1998.

48. Morter T, Schuster TL: Changes in salivary pH and general health status following the clinical application of bio-energetic synchronization, *J Vertebr Sublux Res* 2(1):35, 1998.

49. Blanks RHI, Schuster TL, Dobson M: A retrospective assessment of network care using a survey of self-rated health, wellness and quality of life, *J Vertebr Sublux Res* 1(4):15, 1997.

50. Lauro A, Mouch B: Chiropractic effects on athletic ability, *Chiropr: J Res Chiropr Clin Invest* 6:84, 1991.

51. Schwartzbauer J et al: Athletic performance and physiological measures in baseball players following upper cervical chiropractic care: a pilot study, *J Vertebr Sublux Res* 1(4):33, 1997.

CHAPTER 17

Neurologic Holism: Chiropractic's Scientific Future

Charles S. Masarsky, DC • Marion Todres-Masarsky, DC

Orthodox Health Care: A Culture of Crisis

For today's orthodox clinician, health care is often tantamount to war. A martial orientation to clinical practice and health care policy is exemplified by such phrases as "fighting infection" and "conquering disease" with "magic bullets" and the rest of the "armamentarium" available to "heroic medicine." In this orientation, health care is largely seen as the effort to keep the material body's home turf free of enemy matter. Sontag[1] said the following:

> The military metaphor in medicine first came into wide use in the 1880's, with the identification of bacteria as agents of disease. Bacteria were said to 'invade' or 'infiltrate' . . . With the patient's body considered to be under attack ('invasion'), the only treatment is to counterattack.

Heroics are most likely to be appreciated during a crisis. In the context of today's health care system, third-party reimbursement is always most likely when the clinician is working with a clearly defined "illness" or injury, with a precise date of onset. The most advanced health care technology is available to the practitioner of crisis intervention. In television portrayals of clinical practice the most likely setting is the hospital, trauma center, or MASH unit—the places most likely to generate medical drama.

This cultural orientation creates almost irresistable psychologic and economic incentives to reframe almost any life event in terms of a health care crisis, which demands the martial virtues of speed and authoritative decisiveness from the

practitioner. For example, as obstetrics became a technologically sophisticated specialty, expectant mothers and their unborn children were increasingly subjected to invasive tests and monitoring, as if pregnancy was a dangerous illness, and normal births were exceedingly rare.

Hormone replacement therapy is becoming increasingly routine once women enter "perimenopause." Men are said to suffer from a parallel "male menopause," which may justify interventions ranging from counseling to pharmaceutically induced erections. Parents are urged to have the serum cholesterol of their children tested so that they will not suffer from the "epidemic" of juvenile heart disease.

This emphasis on crisis in health care tends to move control away from the individual. Just as an armed force can only operate with a strict chain of command, a heroic health care system demands obedience to centralized authority. Many real-world examples are apparent to the most casual observer.

For instance, most jurisdictions within the United States do not merely *offer* vaccination; they *mandate* it. If the individual resists this mandate a child may be barred from school or an adult may be removed from military service. These policies ignore recent reappraisals of the risk and benefit ratio of many vaccines, particularly regarding the polio, measles, and pertussis vaccinations.[2] The trend in the biomedical literature has been to encourage clinicians to downplay the hazards of vaccination, and some medical doctors have officially objected to the mere distribution of vaccine information pamphlets in the United States.[3,4] Such flagrant disregard for the principle of informed consent would never be tolerated without the widely accepted notion that mandatory vaccination is necessary in the "war" against disease.

Perhaps the most dangerous aspect of the crisis-centered health care hero is the raw drive to "do something" in situations, which can threaten the patient's well being. Examples in the somatovisceral arena include such uncomfortable and hazardous tests as cardiac catheterization for patients with misdiagnosed cervical angina[5-7] and widespread, inappropriate use of antibiotics and surgery for pediatric otitis media.[8] Browning[9] reported multiple, unnecessary surgeries performed on one patient with pelvic pain and organic disorders related to lower sacral nerve root irritation. Woo[10] reported the induction of iatrogenic Cushing's syndrome resulting from steroid therapy in a patient with posttraumatic myelopathy. Incidents such as these are repeated thousands of times every year, with substantial harmful, regressive, and negative consequences for the public health.

Practical Vitalism: An Emerging Paradigm

Regarding patient visits and money, alternative health care has become a serious competitor to the medical orthodoxy.[11] Some of these alternatives are not radical departures from the crisis-oriented mainstream. For instance, botanical medicine is often a matter of "fighting disease" with cultivated plants rather than the synthetic products of industrial plants.

However, other systems are rising in popularity, which deviate from heroic health care in fundamental ways. These systems adopt a "practical vitalism" approach. Practitioners of these systems do not necessarily believe that living organisms are animated by a nonmaterial spirit or soul, as expressed in many religious beliefs; however, they all acknowledge the immense complexity of the body's inherent recuperative powers and at least the possibility that energic pathways exist that are not fully understood. These powers and pathways are often viewed with an emotional intensity that transcends mere respect, perhaps best described as awe. These practitioners essentially see themselves not as combatants fighting disease, but rather as respectful facilitators of this inherent healing vitality

and practice a pragmatic vitalism. These practitioners would agree with Pasteur's reputed dying words, "The microbe is nothing; the soil is everything." They would also concur with the Hippocratic ethic of first doing no harm to the patient, and only then seeking to beneficially intervene.

As noted in Chapter 2, acupuncture, Ayurveda, and magnetic healing are in this category. Chiropractic, when practiced in the spirit of its founding principles, is also a system of practical vitalism. The importance of this perspective was recently acknowledged by Phillips and others[12]:

> There are expressions of vitalism, not necessarily implying the presence of a supernatural intelligent being. An example is captured by the expression *vis medicatrix naturae* (i.e., the healing power of nature), which describes the inherent capacity of the body to heal itself. This form of vitalism is an important part of contemporary chiropractic insofar as it points the way to a unique conception of the practitioner as a facilitator in the healing process wherein the true locus of health is the patient. It is this philosophical tenet that is shared, implicitly or explicity, by most chiropractors and is the position of the Los Angeles College of Chiropractic.

Vis medicatrix naturae is a close companion to the traditional chiropractic concept of *innate intelligence*. According to some authors the terms are synonymous.[13]

A clinician who sees the patient in a vitalistic way cannot view health as the mere absence of sickness any more than viewing peace as the mere absence of war. The vitalist's most important roles are preheroic (precrisis health care) and postheroic (building human potential). The difference between the heroic and vitalistic approaches to health care are apparent not only in the clinician but also in the scientist.

The research community affiliated with a vitalistic system is apt to be more interested in learning how to assist the body in optimizing global immunocompetence than to search for a "magic bullet" to fight a specific disease. Enhancing the patient's ability to adapt to stress would interest vitalistic scientists more than pharmaceutical containment of specific stress-related symptoms. In other words, research based on a paradigm of practical vitalism strives towards what may be described as a "science of wellness."

Research conducted by practical vitalists also must confront the scientific consequences of the tremendous individuality of the expression of innate intelligence in each of their patients. For this reason the science of wellness is also the science of the individual. In this arena the randomized, controlled trial is not seen as the only way to perform "real science." Case reports, case series, time-series reports, and other descriptive study methods are increasingly valued for their potential to capture the evolution of wellness in all of its individualistic complexity. This type of scientist is a health naturalist first and an experimentalist second. The clinic is a more appropriate setting for this type of science than the laboratory. Recognizing this reality, Keating[14] recommended the deliberate and wide-spread development of chiropractic clinician-researchers:

> The clinician-researcher could be the saving grace for the broad traditions of the chiropractic art. If we were to train our doctors to be bold in generating clinical hypotheses, to be meticulous in documenting observations, to be cautious in what is claimed about the value of chiropractic methods in not-yet-legitimized areas of practice, and to publish what goes on in the clinical setting, we could set in motion a research enterprise fueled by curiosity and pointed at the broad horizons envisioned by the Founder.

An Information-Centered Clinical Logic

An individualistic science of wellness is clearly a paradigm that will attract contributions from nutritionists, Ayurvedic healers, acupuncturists, meditation instructors, and others. In this regard, asking what the unique chiropractic contribution to this emerging concept is worthy.

One of the traditional tenets of chiropractic philosophy is that life is the expression of intelligence through matter.[15] "Intelligence" in this traditional sense refers to innate intelligence. Although the concept of innate intelligence enters philosophic discourse with relative ease, handling it in the scientific context is often difficult.

One aspect of intelligence is information. Information theory has a rich intellectual history, with a well-developed mathematical foundation. Therefore a science-friendly corollary of the traditional chiropractic tenet might be, "Life functions depend upon the free and timely flow of information and the integrity of matter."

A comprehensive health science must recognize material integrity and informational fidelity. In practice, however, most health professions focus on one aspect more than the other. From its beginnings, chiropractic has favored an information-centered clinical logic, while the medical orthodoxy has tended to be matter centered.

An early illustration of this distinction can be found in an often cited anecdote related by D.D. Palmer.[16] A patient, J.M. the farmer, complained of ankle pain. Approximately 3 years previously, he had been kicked by a cow. A number of doctors and remedies had failed to give J.M. any relief.

D.D. Palmer found no local problem in J.M.'s ankle. Nerve tracing from the affected ankle led Palmer to a lumbar vertebra. However, when Palmer proposed an adjustment of the subluxated vertebra, J.M. refused, insisting that the problem was in his ankle not his back. He urged Palmer to treat the ankle and to leave his back alone. Palmer stated, "I refused to touch the ankle, telling him I did not want to rob him of his money nor fool away my time." At a subsequent visit, J.M. finally relented and the lumbar adjustment was followed by a rapid and dramatic improvement in the patient's ankle.

What J.M. and his previous doctors had in common was a matter-centered clinical logic. In this case the assumption was made that ankle pain means that something was wrong with the *matter* in the patient's ankle (e.g., sprained ligaments, strained muscles, inflamed joint capsules). This reductionistic approach to pain is one of the hazards of a matter-centered clinical logic. Much of the time, orthodox health care follows an unspoken (and largely unconscious) axiom: "The locus of a pain is the locus of its cause."

Palmer's focus on the tone of the nervous system centers chiropractic clinical logic on the free and timely flow of information. This information-centered logic provides built-in protection against reductionistic errors in clinical assessment. The integrative nature of the nervous system directs the chiropractic clinician towards a neurological holism. Such a clinician can never assume that the locus of a pain is the locus of its cause. For the chiropractor, pain or any other symptom is an indicator consistent with disturbed

Neurologic Holism: Chiropractic's Scientific Future **227**

tone but not a reliable indicator of where the disturbance originates. A symptom is a good barometer but a poor compass; it may indicate the presence of "stormy weather," but cannot reliably guide you to the center of the storm.

Neurologic holism of chiropractic already serving its research enterprise well is apparent from much of the somatovisceral research reviewed in this text. Considering to what extent this same neurologic holism can generate a significant paradigm shift in the future is tempting. Some tentative speculations from a few years ago are worth revisiting now.[17]

Cost-Effectiveness Research with a "Wide Angle Lens"

In considering whether chiropractic care is more cost effective for musculoskeletal injuries such as work-related injuries or whiplash trauma to the neck than medical care, the research questions usually reveal a matter-centered orientation. How much money is required to restore the injured back or neck to preinjury status under chiropractic versus medical care? What is the best way to treat a specific injury? Although significant, these situations arise from the perspective that the injured area is the site of damaged matter (strain, sprain, etc.) and that the injury somehow occurs in isolation from the rest of the organism. This tends to narrow the research focus to the clinical and economic consequences of localized pain and disability.

For a neurologic holist the injured area is most importantly a site of disrupted information flow. Localized pain and disability is just one aspect of disturbed neurologic tone that can affect the entire organism. The resulting research questions will not merely center on the restoration of local function, but on restoration of the neurological fitness of the whole person. Chiropractors want to know the number of days of work that their patients will lose over a specified period because of cystitis, dysmenorrhea, digestive disorders, asthma or any other health problems that may occur. They also want to know if a significant difference will occur in these statistics when neck or back-injured patients are cared for chiropractically versus medically. When viewing cost-effectiveness

through this wide-angle lens, localized pain is just the beginning.

Researching this may seem unrealistically expensive but does not have to be. A recent British study used the Oswestry questionnaire to follow up at 1 and 3 years.[18,19] This questionnaire was useful in determining whether chiropractic care and hospital-based physical therapy differed in terms of long-term relief of low back pain and related disability. If this research team had been informed by the perspective of neurologic holism, a different questionnaire may have been used. In Chapter 6, information on pencil-and-paper outcome measures related to overall wellness can be found. The funding levels for performing cost-effectiveness research according to the chiropractic (neurologic holism) paradigm would be approximately the same as the funding levels for doing it the orthodox way. The only major difference would be what kind of questionnaire is used.

The Ergonomics of Neurologic Holism

D.D. Palmer believed that subluxation results from "traumatism, poison, and auto-suggestion". Currently, chiropractic purports that the etiology of the vertebral subluxation complex is rooted in mechanical, chemical, and emotional stressors. Analysis of the long-range consequences of these stressors in the work environment could open up new avenues in the science of ergonomics.

For example, research reviewed in Chapter 9, reveals the importance of thoracic subluxation on gastric health. Inhaled chemical irritants might be expected to render workers vulnerable to thoracic subluxation. Whether a link exists between indoor air pollution and gastric ulcer is not known, nor is the way this factor interacts in the over-all picture of a person's alimentary health. Such questions might not occur to an orthodox ergonomic scientist. In the ergonomics of neurologic holism, such questions are obvious.

Vitalistic Gerontology

A number of studies reviewed previously indicated that the VSC may be related to reduced lung volumes, slowed reaction time, increased blood pressure, decreased visual acuity, and depressed immune function. These physiologic changes are also biologic markers of aging. Within the profession, chiropractic adjustments adding "years to your life and life to your years" was claimed. Chiropractic research could offer the science of gerontology new insights by systematically studying the effect of the VSC and adjustment on a wide variety of such biologic markers.

Immunity as a Sensory Function

Interest in the immune system's response to subluxation and adjustment has increased in recent years because of the discovery of neurotransmitter receptor sites on leukocyte membranes, and the ability of some leukocytes to secrete neurotransmitters. This implies two-way communication between the immune system and the nervous system—a great spur to the development of neuroimmunology.

The primal immunologic act is the discrimination between "self" and "nonself." Before neuroimmunology, this act taking place entirely at the level of the leukocyte was widely assumed. Neurologic holists might consider to what extent this ability is a perceptual function. Does an "immune sense," or a full-fledged perceptual system such as vision or hearing exist? How much of the long-term "memory" of the immune system is stored in the nervous system? If subluxation can disturb hearing, vision, balance and touch, chiropractors want to know if it can also disturb what might be described as "immunoception." Research in these areas could be uniquely and decisively helpful to the development of neuroimmunology.

Human Potential

Typically a patient arrives at the chiropractic office with a symptom. The designation of "patient" implies the presence of a symptom. The symptoms prompting chiropractic visits are usually musculoskeletal pain or injury (back pain, neck pain). Some of the studies reviewed in this textbook suggest that certain visceral symptoms may also be caused or exacerbated by subluxa-

tion, making chiropractic participation in their management also clinically reasonable.

However, because the nervous system influences all aspects of physiology in higher animals, a neurologic holist might wonder whether this expanded conception of subluxation-related symptoms is even too limiting, asking the following questions:

Should an accountant seek a chiropractic consultation when concentration is poor?
Should a singer be checked for subluxation when the voice loses power or range?
Should a novelist seek a chiropractic analysis during an episode of writer's block?
Can subluxation reduce the ability of an arbitrator to facilitate the resolution of conflicts?
Can dysponesis related to the VSC interfere with the depth of experience enjoyed by a practitioner of meditation, yoga, or tai chi chuan?

In short, does the practitioner of neurologic holism require a non-traditional symptomatology? The answer has implications throughout the profession, from the director of a chiropractic research department designing next year's investigation to the private clinician updating the practice's case history form.

Chiropractic care improving the lives of the asymptomatic is yet to be known, with preliminary research suggesting that people with no apparent respiratory problems may experience improved lung volumes when subluxation is corrected.[20,21] Two studies have demonstrated an apparent improvement in athletic ability under chiropractic care.[22,23] A recent investigation revealed that visual acuity may improve in people with "normal" vision when subluxation is corrected.[24]

Studying the effect of subluxation in the asymptomatic population may generate entirely new fields of human potential research, with the following questions being asked:

Does the diner's enjoyment of a meal or the theater patron's appreciation of a play suffer in the presence of subluxation?
Can subluxation prevent the person of average intelligence from becoming brighter?
Does an electrophysiologic signature of creativity exist, and if so, does it appear with more frequency when subluxation is corrected?

Summary

Despite generations of scientists dismissing the VSC as insignificant, chiropractic research has already made impressive improvements. The ancient Chinese philosopher Lao Tsu said the following about subjects considered insignificant by the majority[25]:

> The Wise want the unwanted; they set no high value on things which are hard to get. They study what others neglect, and restore to the world what multitudes have passed by.

STUDY GUIDE

1. What did Sontag[1] mean by the "military metaphor" in medicine? Discuss this "crisis concept" in terms of increasing stress for the patient and for the health care practitioner.
2. What is the logical outcome of a populace being convinced that no amount of personal education and research can qualify them to make their own health care decisions? Technology can do amazing things for society. How do we determine what technologic developments should be pursued and when they should be used?
3. Discuss the concept of the DC as a "respectful facilitator" of inherent healing vitality.
4. Compare and contrast the concepts of *vis medicatrix naturae* and "innate intelligence."
5. Health is more than the absence of disease. Where in this concept does dis-ease fit? Discuss this in terms of the Nansel and Slezak paper mentioned in the referred pain chapter.
6. According to Keating,[14] what is the fuel on which the ideal chiropractic research paradigm would run? For the clinician-researcher to achieve optimal usefulness to the profession, what skills must be honed?
7. In the story of J.M. the farmer, why was he having so much trouble understanding his problem? What is meant by reductionism?
8. "A symptom is a good barometer, but a poor compass." What does this mean? Is the VSC a symptom? Explain your answer.
9. How does cost effectiveness with a wide angle lens return chiropractic to the basic chiropractic paradigm?
10. Lack of funding has often been a serious impediment to certain kinds of chiropractic research. Discuss how the appropriate pencil-and-paper instrument can make any clinician-researcher engaging in a retrospective "wellness" study on a very limited budget possible.
11. Write the beginning of a grant proposal in which you suggest studying the effects of workplace "poisons" and "autosuggestion" on the workers' nervous systems and general health presentations through a chiropractic lens.
12. How might research based on the fullness of the chiropractic paradigm provide useful information on aging gracefully and healthfully?
13. What is the primary immunologic act? Where in the living organism does this occur?
14. Has current, mainstream health care possibly accepted too low a standard in terms of human potential? What social forces would encourage acceptance of unnaturally low expectations? In one paragraph, propose a basic experiment, preferably one that could be performed in a chiropractic office, that would examine a commonly accepted limitation and disprove it. Explain your hypothesis.

REFERENCES

1. Sontag S: *Illness as metaphor,* p 65, New York, 1978, Farrar, Straus and Giroux.
2. Lanfranchi R, Alcantara J, Plaugher G: Vaccination issues. In Anrig CA, Plaugher G, editors: *Pediatric chiropractic,* p 24, Baltimore, 1998, Williams & Wilkins.
3. Goldsmith MF: Vaccine information pamphlets are here, but some physicians react strongly, *JAMA* 267:2005, 1992.
4. Crozier K: Vaccine information pamphlets: just another barrier to vaccination? *Infect Dis Child* 6:12, 1993.
5. Booth RE, Rothman RH: Cervical angina, *Spine* 1:28, 1976.

6. Jacobs B: Cervical angina, *NY Sta J Med:* 90:8, 1990.
7. Wells P: Cervical angina, *Am Fam Physician* 55:2262, 1997.
8. Agency for Health Care Policy and Research: *Clinical practice guideline #12: otitis media with effusion in young children,* Rockville, Md, 1994, U.S. Department of Health and Human Services.
9. Browning JE: Mechanically induced pelvic pain and organic dysfunction in a patient without low back pain, *J Manipulative Physiol Ther* 13:406, 1990.
10. Woo CC: Post-traumatic myelopathy following flopping high jump: a pilot case of spinal manipulation, *J Manipulative Physiol Ther* 16:336, 1993.
11. Eisenberg DM et al: Unconventional medicine in the United States: prevalence, costs, and patterns of use, *New England J Med* 328:246, 1993.
12. Phillips RB et al: A contemporary philosophy of chiropractic for the Los Angeles College of Chiropractic, *J Chiropr Humanities* 4(1):20, 1994.
13. Hildebrandt RW: Editorial: vis medicatrix naturae—the innate therapeutic force, *J Manipulative Physiol Ther* 3:135, 1980.
14. Keating JC: *Toward a philosophy of the science of chiropractic: a primer for clinicians,* p 91, Stockton, Calif, 1992, Stockton Foundation for Chiropractic Research.
15. Stephenson RW: *Chiropractic textbook,* Davenport, Iowa, 1948, Palmer School of Chiropractic.
16. Palmer DD: *The science, art and philosophy of chiropractic,* p 647, Portland, Ore, 1910, Portland Printing House.
17. Masarsky CS, Weber M: Stop paradigm erosion, *J Manipulative Physiol Ther* 14:323, 1991.
18. Meade TW et al: Low back pain of mechanical origin: randomized comparison of chiropractic and hospital outpatient treatment, *BMJ* 300:1431, 1990.
19. Meade TW et al: Randomized comparison of chiropractic and hospital outpatient management for low back pain: results from extended follow-up, *BMJ* 11:349, 1995.
20. Masarsky CS, Weber M: Chiropractic and lung volumes—a retrospective study, *ACA J Chiro* 20(9):67, 1986.
21. Kessinger R: Changes in pulmonary function associated with upper cervical specific chiropractic care, *J Vertebr Sublux Res* 1(3):43, 1997.
22. Lauro A, Mouch B: Chiropractic effects on athletic ability, *Chiropr: J Res Chiropr Clin Invest* 6:84, 1991.
23. Schwartzbauer M, Hart J, Zhang J: Athletic performance and physiological measures in baseball players following upper cervical chiropractic care: a pilot study, *J Vertebr Sublux Res* 1(4):33, 1997.
24. Kessinger R, Boneva D: Changes in visual acuity in patients receiving upper cervical specific chiropractic care, *J Vertebr Sublux Res* 2(1):43, 1998.
25. Lao Tzu: Tao Te Ching. Quote adapted from Blakney RB: *The way of life: Lao Tzu,* p 117, New York, 1955, Mentor Books.

GLOSSARY

This glossary is intended to facilitate the study of chiropractic literature in general, and that literature dealing with the somatovisceral aspects of chiropractic in particular. In most cases the definitions provided were derived from the published sources cited. Definitions that are not specifically referenced were developed by one or more of the authors of this textbook.

Activator technique A chiropractic system in which analysis is guided by the assessment of functional leg length inequality under various test conditions and in which minimum-force adjustments are accomplished by a hand-held spring-activated instrument that delivers a controlled impulse. This system was developed by Arlan W. Fuhr, D.C. and W.C. Lee, D.C.[1]

Adjustment A maneuver specific in vector, velocity, intensity of force, and point of application that is intended to assist the body in restoring normal tone by correcting subluxation in whole or in part.[2]

Antidromic Opposite the normal direction. This term is generally used to describe neural impulse conduction.

Applied Kinesiology A system in which the results of manual muscle testing serve as indicators of the somatic, visceral, emotional, and biochemical aspects of health; these indicators are held to be especially valuable in the assessment of health problems that have not yet reached the level of pathology. This system was originated in 1964 by George Goodheart, D.C.[3]

Autonome A cutaneous area innervated by autonomic nerves originating from a particular segmental level. Such an area can often be visualized with thermographic methods.[4]

Carver, Willard (1866-1943) Chiropractic practitioner, technique developer, politician, educator, and author, Carver began his professional life as an attorney in 1891. After graduating from the Parker School of Chiropractic in Ottumwa, Iowa, he opened a school in Oklahoma City with L.L. and Myrtle V. Denny in 1906. Carver was incarcerated for contempt of the Senate on March 3, 1917, after publishing a newspaper article critical of the Oklahoma Senate's recent actions on chiropractic legislation. He considered "correct auto-suggestion" an important factor in health.[5]

Case report A descriptive study of an individual patient presented in narrative form. Details included in such a study generally contain the patient's health history and presenting complaints, any relevant examination findings, diagnostic or analytical conclusions, intervention protocols, and outcomes assessment.

Case series A descriptive study of two or more patients with significant clinical similarities.

Causalgia See *reflex sympathetic dystrophy.*

Cervical angina A pseudoangina resulting from referred pain from cervical dysfunction. Costly and hazardous cardiologic workups are often fruitlessly endured by patients with this disorder.[6]

Cervical migraine A syndrome characterized by headache, neck pain, vertigo, and loss of cervical range of motion at the gross and segmental levels, particularly in rotation.[7]

Cervicogenic headache A headache with the site of origin in the cervical spine.[2]

Cervicogenic vertigo Dizziness provoked by movement or digital pressure at the cervical spine. It is generally accompanied by subluxation of the upper three cervical motion segments and is sometimes accompanied by nystagmus.[8]

Chapman's reflexes Tender zones at various locations on the body surface, correlated by Frank Chapman, D.O., with lymphatic stasis in various internal organs, and more recently correlated by George Goodheart, D.C., with lymphatic stasis in various skeletal muscles. (A synonym is neurolymphatic reflexes.)[1]

Chiropractic analysis The clinical assessment of a patient's state of biomechanical and neurologic integrity, primarily for the purpose of characterizing subluxation.[2]

Chiropractic Biophysics Technique (CBP) A full-spine technique in which postural analysis and other physical examination findings are correlated with x-ray signs. The patient is positioned in the mirror image of the postural distortion during adjustment.

Chiropractic philosophy A conceptual framework in health care characterized by a profound respect for the organism's adaptive vitality and by an emphasis on removing interference to the organism's ability to sense its internal and external environment.[9]

Chiropractic science The science concerned with the relationship between structure (primarily of the spine) and function (primarily of the nervous system) because that relationship may affect the restoration and preservation of health. The study of the vertebral subluxation complex is a special concern of this science.[10]

Clear View Sanitarium Institution founded in 1926 in Davenport, Iowa by John Baker, D.C. and Harvey Fennerm, D.C. to care for the mentally ill using only chiropractic care. Initial evaluation included physical examination, x-ray, blood work, and urinalysis. Heat-reading instrumentation (neurocalograph) was an important component of the chiropractic analysis performed at this facility. A number of Palmer School of Chiropractic faculty members, including A.B. Hender, D.C., were associated with this institution. After its purchase in 1951 by B.J. Palmer, D.C., it was incorporated into the Palmer Clinics and provided a specialized rotation for interns under the directorship of W.H. Quigley, D.C. It was closed in 1961.[11]

Clear View Sanitarium A sister institution to the Davenport, Iowa facility by the same name. It was founded by Harvey Fennerm, D.C. in 1930 in Gardena, California and closed in 1933.[11]

Cleveland, Carl S., Jr. (1918-1995) A 1942 graduate of the Cleveland College of Chiropractic in Kansas City, Mo, Dr. Cleveland served as president of this college from 1967 to 1981, president of the Los Angeles campus from 1982 to 1992, and chancellor of the Cleveland College system from 1993 to his death. He pioneered animal experimentation in chiropractic research. He was the son of Drs. Carl and Ruth Cleveland, who founded the Central Chiropractic College (later named Cleveland Chiropractic College, Kansas City, Mo) in 1922.[12]

Descriptive study A research report used to illustrate, initiate, disconfirm, or support a clinical hypothesis; included are nonexperimental research designs (e.g., case reports and case series) and quasiexperimental approaches (e.g., time-series reports).[2]

Diagnosis The scrutiny of clinical information for the purpose of characterizing a patient's health status. Also, the conclusion reached after such scrutiny. (A synonym is clinical assessment.)

Diagnosis, differential The recognition of a specific disease, syndrome, injury, or condition based on the scrutiny of clinical information, including data from a patient's history, physical examination, laboratory testing, and response to treatment.

Disease A process in which the normal state of living tissue is altered; it may affect the whole organism or any of its constituent parts.[2]

Dis-ease A disruption of physiologic coordination by the nervous system; aberrant tone; dysponesis.[2]

Diversified technique Adjustive technique designed to correct vertebral and extravertebral subluxations. In general, each college teaches its own version of diversified technique.[10]

Dysafferentation Abnormal afferent input as a result of joint restriction, involving a functional decrease in the activity of large-diameter mechanoreceptor afferent fibers and a simultaneous functional increase in activity of nociceptive afferent nerve fibers.[2]

Dysponesis A reversible physiopathologic state consisting of unnoticed, misdirected neurophysiologic reactions to various agents (environmental events, bodily sensations, emotions, and thoughts) and the repercussions of these reactions throughout the organism. These errors in energy expenditure, which are capable of producing functional disorders, consist mainly in covert errors in action-potential output from the motor and premotor areas of the cortex and the consequences of that output.[13]

Ergotropic function The adjusting of circulatory, metabolic, and visceral activity according to musculoskeletal energy demands. These physiologic adjustments are controlled by the sympathetic nervous system. Disturbed ergotrophic function resulting from aberrant kinesthetic information is a potential feature of the state of dysponesis generated by the vertebral subluxation complex.[14]

Facilitation Lowered threshold for firing in a spinal cord segment, resulting from afferent bombardment associated with spinal dysfunction.[2]

Fixation A dysfunctional state of decreased mobility within an articulation's normal physiologic range of motion. This state is often a feature of subluxation in general and the vertebral subluxation complex in particular.[2]

Flexion-distraction A long-lever, low-velocity, low-amplitude adjustment technique administered with the assistance of a specialized table. Its application is intended to create a negative intradiscal pressure and facet joint gapping. Variations of this technique are used to correct intervertebral disc lesions, facet joint dysfunction, spinal stenosis, spondylolisthesis, scoliosis, and mechanically induced pelvic pain and organic dysfunction. This procedure was introduced to the chiropractic profession mainly through the efforts of James M. Cox, D.C.[15]

Foundation for Chiropractic Education and Research (FCER) Organization founded in 1944 for the funding and support of scientifically sound chiropractic research. In addition to its research activities the foundation also offers educational fellowships and many other programs and materials for doctor and patient education.

Ganglion, dorsal nerve root Enlargement of the dorsal root of the spinal nerve located at or just medial to the junction of the ventral and dorsal spinal roots. It contains the cell bodies of the afferent neurons, including visceral afferents, entering the spinal cord by the dorsal root.

Ganglion, middle cervical Sympathetic ganglion located anterolateral to the C5-6 vertebral bodies that receives preganglionic fibers primarily from the T1-T5 spinal nerve levels. Postganglionic fibers project to the heart, thyroid gland, parathyroid gland, trachea, and esophagus. Disturbance of this ganglion may be suspected in the presence of middle cervical subluxation.

Ganglion, stellate The structure formed by the fusion of the sympathetic chain ganglia of C7-T1 in most people. Preganglionic fibers from spinal nerves T1 to as low as T10 synapse at this ganglion. Postganglionic fibers project to the heart, some blood vessels of the face and cranium, and the upper extremities. Dysfunction of this ganglion may contribute to reflex sympathetic dystrophy of the upper extremity. Disturbance of this ganglion may be suspected in the presence of subluxation of the intervertebral or costovertebral joints of the cervicothoracic junction.

Ganglion, superior cervical The largest of the three cervical sympathetic ganglia, located between the occiput and C3. It receives preganglionic fibers from spinal nerves T1-T5. Postganglionic fibers project to the heart, pupils, salivary glands, pharynx, and most of the cranial blood vessels. It also provides gray rami to the first four cervical spinal nerves. Disturbance of this ganglion may be suspected in the presence of upper cervical subluxation.

Ganglion, sympathetic chain A connected series of sympathetic ganglia located anterolateral to either side of the vertebral column from the upper cervical region to the coccyx. At the coccyx the left and right chains are joined, forming the ganglion impar. The superior cervical, middle cervical, and stellate ganglia are located within the sympathetic chain ganglia.

Gonstead technique A chiropractic method developed by Clarence S. Gonstead, D.C. of Wisconsin (1898-1978), in which x-ray analysis, paraspinal temperature readings, static palpation, and motion palpation are used to characterize subluxation.[16]

Grostic technique A technique developed by John D. Grostic, Sr., D.C., which uses x-ray analysis and supine leg checks to characterize the upper cervical subluxation. A manually directed apparatus is used to deliver a minimal-force adjustment.

Holism In health care, holism is an approach that attempts to comprehend the unique interaction of physiologic, psychosocial, and environmental factors in an individual's life, and to apply this understanding to the promotion of the well being or wholeness of that individual. In chiropractic clinical work, the appreciation of mechanical, emotional, and chemical stressors as etiologic factors in the vertebral subluxation complex and the recognition of the consequences of the resulting dysponesis for the whole person are traditional holistic tenets.[2]

Homewood, A. Earl (1916-1990) Chiropractic clinician and scholar, Homewood served as President of Canadian Memorial Chiropractic College and Los Angeles Chiropractic College. He was also the author of *The Neurodynamics of the Vertebral Subluxation,* in which he made a detailed case for the importance of the somatovisceral aspects of chiropractic.[17]

Horner syndrome Constriction of the pupil, partial ptosis of the eyelid, recession of the eyeball into the orbit, and sometimes ipsilateral loss of facial sweating. This is generally related to cervical sympathetic hypotonia, which can result from cervical or cervicothoracic subluxation.[18]

Innate intelligence The inborn capacity of an organism to heal itself and adapt to the dynamics of the external and internal environment; roughly synonymous with *vis medicatrix naturae.* (This term is sometimes capitalized in chiropractic literature. Abbreviating the term to "innate" is also common practice.)[9]

Intervertebral canal The canal that originates in the evagination of the dural sac to form the sheath of the spinal nerve roots. It terminates at the intervertebral foramen. The dorsal nerve root ganglion is particularly vulnerable to compressive forces in this region in the presence of the vertebral subluxation complex, especially when the ligamentum flavum undergoes hypertrophy or buckling at the canal's posterior border.[19]

Intervertebral foramen (IVF) Opening that forms the intervertebral canal's lateral border. It is formed anteriorly by the intervertebral disc, the lower portion of the vertebral body above, and the upper portion of the vertebral body below. It is formed posteriorly by the posterior zygapophyseal joint and ligamentum flavum and superiorly and inferiorly by the vertebral pedicle.

Ischemic penumbra A state of decreased blood flow to a neural structure that is low enough to bring about electrical silence without causing cellular death. This phenomenon may underlie apparent functional hibernation of portions of the brain or other neural structures. This state can be reversed once adequate blood flow is restored. Furthermore, some deleterious effects of the vertebral subluxation complex may result from the creation of such hibernation states.[20]

Kentuckiana Children's Center A nonprofit organization founded in 1957 by Lorraine M. Golden, D.C. in Louisville, Kentucky to provide special education and health care to multihandicapped children without charge. Chiropractic is the primary form of care in this multidisciplinary facility, which also provides nutritional therapy, counseling, visual and speech therapy, Doman-Delacato patterning, and dental and medical care.[21]

L'Hermitte's sign A test for myelopathy resulting from conditions such as stenosis, tumor, disc herniation, and multiple sclerosis. The patient's head is passively flexed by the examiner. A positive test is indicated by a sharp, electric-like pain radiating down the spine and into one or more extremities.[21]

Lillard, Harvey (1856-1925) Patient described by D.D. Palmer as the recipient of the first chiropractic adjustment on September 18, 1895. Mr. Lillard's primary presenting complaint was longstanding hearing loss that was reportedly resolved by correction of a T4 subluxation.

Logan Basic Technique Adjusting procedure developed by Hugh B. Logan, D.C. of Missouri (1881-1944). This technique emphasizes the importance of sacroiliac integrity to optimize spinal biomechanics and uses x-ray analysis, palpation, and bilateral scales to characterize the vertebral subluxation complex. Minimal-force manual adjusting is used.[1]

Manipulation A manual procedure that involves a directed thrust to move a joint past its physiologic range of motion without exceeding the boundaries of anatomic integrity. Audible joint cavitation noise is commonly produced by this procedure.[22]

Manual therapy Procedures by which the hands directly contact the body to treat the articulations and/or soft tissues.[22]

Mechanism The metaphysical point of view that living organisms are essentially complex electrochemical machines and are not animated by nonmaterial forces or spirits. In clinical work it is the conception that healing results from repair of the patient's *machinery* rather than from the patient's innate healing vitality.

Meric technique A chiropractic system in which a clinical problem is considered in terms of which *zone*, or body segment innervated by a pair of spinal nerves, it occurs. All tissue of one type within a zone is considered a *mere* (e.g., all of a zone's nerve tissue constitutes its *neuromere*, all of its visceral tissue constitutes its *viscemere*).[2]

Morikubo trial Trial of Shegatoro Morikubo, Ph.D., D.C. in July 1907 in La Crosse, Wisconsin. He was charged with the unlicensed practice of medicine, surgery, and osteopathy. Arguing that chiropractic was based on a philosophy distinct from medicine, osteopathy or surgery, defense attorney Thomas Morris won the case.[23]

Motion palpation Assessment technique in which an examiner monitors the degree and quality of joint motion through the sense of touch while a joint is in active or passive motion. This process is a widely used technique in chiropractic analysis.[24]

Motion segment A functional unit made up of two adjacent articulating surfaces and the connecting tissues binding them to each other. In the past this entity was often referred to as a *motor unit*. This created considerable confusion because the term "motor unit" also denotes a motor neuron and the muscle fibers innervated by it.[22]

Nerve energy Information transmitted by neural signals that results in contraction or relaxation of muscle (skeletal, cardiac, or smooth), promotion or inhibition of glandular activity, the conscious or unconscious registration of sensory stimuli, or the acceleration or deceleration of any function coordinated by the nervous system. (A synonym is nerve force.)[9]

Nerve tracing The use of digital pressure to follow a line of tenderness from a painful body part to the spine or vice versa. Nerve tracing is the earliest recorded method of chiropractic analysis, first described by D.D. Palmer. These lines of hyperpathia often do not correspond to named nerves.[2]

Network Spinal Analysis A method of chiropractic analysis developed by Donald Epstein, D.C. of Colorado. It places primary importance on cervical and sacrococcygeal subluxations (referred to as *facilitated subluxations* in this system), due to the whole-body implications of the resulting dura mater distortion. Thoracic and lumbar dysfunctions (referred to as *structural subluxations* in this system) are considered after facilitated subluxations have been addressed.

Neuro Emotional Technique A chiropractic system developed by Scott Walker, D.C. that emphasizes the identification of chronic or recurrent subluxations in relation to unresolved emotional material (fixations of emotions or neuro emotional complex) and the administration of the adjustment while the patient recalls this material. This is done to explicitly address the emotional etiology of the vertebral subluxation complex without practicing psychotherapy.

Neurological fitness The state of physiologic efficiency of a nerve or group of nerves, a nerve structure or group of nerve structures, or the nervous system as a whole; the degree of freedom from dysponesis.[25]

NINCDS conference An interdisciplinary scientific conference on spinal manipulation that was one of the first to bring doctors of chiropractic, medical doctors, doctors of osteopathy, and researchers together. The conference was held at the National Institutes of Health campus in Bethesda, Maryland from February 2-4, 1975, sponsored by the National Institute of Neurological and Communicative Disorders and Stroke (NINCDS). Proceedings were edited by Murray Goldstein, D.O., M.P.H. and titled *The Research Status of Spinal Manipulative Therapy.*[26]

Nociceptor A receptor preferentially sensitive to a noxious stimulus or a stimulus that would become noxious if prolonged. Such a noxious or potentially noxious stimulus may be mechanical, chemical, thermal, or electric. A nociceptor generally takes the form of a free nerve ending. Pain is a conscious perception commonly associated with sensory input from nociceptors.

Office of Alternative Medicine Established as part of the National Institutes of Health by a 1992 congressional mandate. The purpose of the Office of Alternative Medicine is to facilitate the evaluation of alternative health care methods and to help integrate such methods into mainstream health care. It has funded research projects involving various nonallopathic methods, including chiropractic.[2]

Outcome measure A quantitative or qualitative record of the effect of a clinical intervention on one or more aspects of a patient's health.[2]

Outcomes assessment The use of one or more outcome measures to assess the effect of a clinical intervention.

Outcomes assessment, patient-based Assessment using self-rated records of pain, disability, and other patient-based measures. This type of assessment is widely used to monitor patient satisfaction with care, perception of improvement, quality of life, and general health status.

Palmer, Bartlett Joshua (1882-1962) Son of Daniel David Palmer, B.J. was president of the Palmer School of Chiropractic (1906-1962). He is widely considered one of the most important early

developers of chiropractic and was a staunch advocate of chiropractic as a distinct profession. His many writings include *The Bigness of the Fellow Within* and *The Subluxation Specific, The Adjustment Specific.* He was the husband of Mabel Heath Palmer.

Palmer, Daniel David (1845-1913) Educator, farmer, grocer, and magnetic healer born in the province of Ontario, Canada. Administered the first chiropractic adjustment to Harvey Lillard in Davenport, Iowa, reportedly on September 18, 1895. Founder of the first chiropractic school. Author of *The Chiropractor's Adjustor: The Science, Art, and Philosophy of Chiropractic.*

Palmer, Mabel Heath (1881-1949) A 1905 graduate of the Palmer School of Chiropractic. She was a chiropractic educator and author. Her writings include the books *Chiropractic Anatomy* (1918) and *Stepping Stones* (1942). She was the wife of B.J. Palmer.

Palmer trial Trial in Davenport, Iowa in which D.D. Palmer was found guilty of the unlicensed practice of medicine. He was sentenced on March 28, 1906. Refusing to pay a $350 fine, he was imprisoned at Scott County Jail, thus becoming the first of several thousand chiropractic prisoners of conscience in the United States from 1906 to 1974.[23]

Palmer Upper Cervical technique A chiropractic technique developed by B.J. Palmer, D.C. that uses x-ray and heat-reading instrumentation as analytic tools. Also known as *HIO (hole in one)* technique, reflecting Palmer's belief that all other vertebral subluxations are secondary to the upper cervical subluxation.

Paradigm A model that helps to clarify a complex process.[2]

Paradigm shift A revolutionary alteration in the explanatory model that forms the basis of an entire discipline.[2]

Randomized controlled trial (RCT) An experimental study for assessing the effects of a particular health intervention, in which each subject is randomly assigned to an experimental or control group; the subjects in the experimental group receive the intervention and the subjects in the control group do not. Ideally the experimental and control groups should be identical in all significant respects, with the exception of the application or nonapplication of the intervention under study.[2]

Receptive field A region of the body where stimulation excites or inhibits activity of a particular sensory neuron or group of sensory neurons. The smaller the receptive field, or the more dense the receptive fields, the greater the topographic discrimination. Conversely, as receptive fields become larger and more diffuse, topographic discrimination becomes less accurate. For example the neurons responsive to touch at the fingertips have smaller and denser receptive fields than those at the upper arm.

Referred pain Pain experienced at a site distant from the locus of its cause. This phenomenon is a source of frequent confusion in clinical assessment.

Reflex sympathetic dystrophy (RSD) Burning pain, usually felt in a traumatized extremity, and often accompanied by symptoms and signs consistent with sympathetic hypertonia such as increased sweat gland activity, reduced temperature, muscle weakness, edema, and degeneration of skin and bone in the affected body part. (The synonym is causalgia.)[27]

Risk factor A category of behavior, environmental component, genetic trait, or any other factor that increases the probability of the development of a particular health problem.

Sacro-occipital technique (SOT) A chiropractic system developed by Major Bertrand DeJarnette, D.C. that emphasizes the importance of cerebrospinal fluid flow as it is affected by pelvic and cranial dysfunction. Postural assessment, palpation of soft-tissue fibers in the trapezius muscle, along the occiput and along the temporosphenoidal line, and manual muscle testing are all part of this system's analysis.[1]

Schwartz, Herman S. (1894-1976) A 1922 graduate of the Carver Chiropractic Institute in New York, he was an advocate of the role of chiropractic in mental health. He edited the 1973 text, *Mental Health and Chiropractic.*

Scotoma An area of impaired perception in the visual field.

Sensory nerve fibers, type I Myelinated sensory nerve fibers with a diameter of 12-22 micrometers and a conduction velocity of 65-130 m per second. They are the most rapidly conducting of the peripheral sensory nerve fibers. (The synonym is type Aa fibers.)

Sensory nerve fibers, type II Myelinated sensory nerve fibers with a diameter of 5-15 micrometers and a conduction velocity of 20-90 m per second. (The synonyms is type Ab or Ac fibers.)

Sensory nerve fibers, type III Myelinated sensory nerve fibers with a diameter of 2-10 micrometers and a conduction velocity of 12-45 m per second. Some nociceptive signals are carried by such fibers. (A synonym is type Ad fibers.)

Sensory nerve fibers, type IV Unmyelinated sensory nerve fibers with a diameter of 0.2-1.5 micro-

meters and a conduction velocity of 0.2-2.0 m per second. Some nociceptive signals are carried by such fibers. (A synonym is type C fibers.)

Somatic dysfunction Impaired or altered function of the skeletal, arthrodial, myofascial, vascular, lymphatic, or neuronal components of one or more motion segments. This impaired or altered somatic function can result in visceral disturbance and musculoskeletal pain. This term was introduced in 1970 to replace *osteopathic lesion.*[28]

Somatic dyspnea Difficulty in breathing or air hunger related to the vertebral subluxation complex or other somatic dysfunction.[2]

Somatovisceral reflex Alteration in the tone of smooth or cardiac muscle or glandular activity in response to a somatic stimulus. The provocative somatic stimulus can result from injury to or dysfunction of somatic structures, including subluxation. Under such circumstances the response may create a disturbance of visceral tone. (A synonym is somatoautonomic reflex.)[2]

Spears, Leo (1894-1956) A 1921 graduate of the Palmer School of Chiropractic, he opened the Spears Hospital in 1943 in Denver, Colorado. After a long legal battle the Colorado Supreme Court ordered the State Health Department to license Spears Hospital in 1950. This institution admitted more than 151,000 patients and provided more than 8 million dollars of free interdisciplinary health care between 1943 and its closing in 1984.[12]

Subluxation A complex of functional and/or structural and/or pathologic articular changes that compromise neural integrity and may influence organ system function and general health.[29]

T4 syndrome Pain or numbness in the hand and/or forearm in a glove-like distribution associated with upper thoracic subluxation in general and subluxation of the T3-4 or T4-5 motion segments in particular. Concomitant symptoms may include headache, chest pain, and interscapular pain or stiffness. Risk factors include a forward posture of the head and disturbed tone in the muscles of the shoulder girdle. Patients suffering from this disorder are often dismissed as hysterics because of the glove-like distribution of symptoms.[30]

Thermatome Area of cutaneous vasomotor disturbance most commonly related to dysfunction at a particular nerve root level. Thermatomes often overlap with dermatomes but do not have identical boundaries.[4]

Thompson technique A chiropractic system developed by J. Clay Thompson, D.C. that uses palpation and the observation of functional leg length inequality as analysis procedures. Specialized tables incorporate drop pieces for cervical, thoracolumbar, and pelvic adjusting. Dr. Thompson maintained that subluxation correction occurs when the drop table piece stops moving—the "terminal point."[31]

Time-series study A type of descriptive study that incorporates quasiexperimental elements. In the most basic type of time-series study, one or more outcome measures are recorded during a period of observation or sham intervention (baseline); these measures continue to be recorded once intervention begins. In effect, subjects serve as their own control group. The time-series study is particularly favored when investigators wish to avoid the artificiality, financial strains, or ethical conflicts usually raised by the randomized controlled trial.

Toftness technique A system of minimal-force adjusting developed by I.M. Toftness, D.C. A basic tenet of this system is that subluxation can be located by detecting the emission of microwaves of a certain frequency.[10]

Tone The rate or intensity of function of any tissue or organ, reflecting the neurologic integrity of that tissue or organ.[2]

Tone, vasomotor The amount of smooth muscle contraction in a blood vessel, especially during its neutral resting state, when it is neither fully constricted nor dilated. Control of vasomotor tone is a combined function of sympathetic innervation and local chemical mediators.

Trophic nerve function The function of nerves related to nutrition and growth. Trophic substances produced by nerves have been found to be essential for the maintenance of proper tissue structure and function.[2]

Vertebral subluxation complex (VSC) Subluxation at one or more spinal levels resulting from mechanical, chemical, or emotional stressors, and resulting in functional and eventual pathologic changes in the constituent tissues of the involved motion segments. Functional and eventual pathologic changes may also occur in distant tissues influenced by the resultant neural disturbance.[2]

Viscerosomatic reflex Altered tone of musculoskeletal structures in response to stimuli originating in visceral tissues. Referred visceral pain is one possible consequence of such a reflex.[2]

Vis medicatrix naturae The organism's natural healing vitality. The body's ability to heal itself is a fundamental tenet of most holistic health methods, including chiropractic.[9]

Vitalism The metaphysical point of view that each living organism is animated by a nonmaterial force or spirit. In classic chiropractic philosophy the theory that the life of an organism depends on the expression of innate intelligence through matter. In holistic health care systems generally the conception that health comes from the natural vitality (*vis medicatrix naturae*) of the organism. The practitioner's role in such systems is not to be an invasive agent of therapeutic intervention, but to respectfully facilitate the patient's natural healing vitality.[9]

Wilk Trial Trial that ended in August 1987, after an 11-year antitrust suit by Chester A. Wilk, D.C. and 4 other doctors of chiropractic against the American Medical Association (AMA) and 15 other defendants. The AMA was found guilty of conspiring to "contain and eliminate" the chiropractic profession by disrupting chiropractic education, third-party reimbursement, media and governmental relations, interprofessional referral, and other boycott activities in violation of the Sherman Antitrust Act. The AMA was permanently enjoined by Judge Susan Getzendanner of Chicago's Seventh Federal District Court to refrain from such boycott activities in the future.

REFERENCES

1. Bergmann TF: Chiropractic reflex techniques. In Gatterman MI, editor: *Foundations of chiropractic: subluxation,* p 105, St Louis, 1995, Mosby.
2. Redwood D: *Contemporary chiropractic,* p 333, New York, 1997, Churchill Livingstone.
3. Perle SM: Applied kinesiology (AK), *Chiro Technique* 7:103, 1995.
4. Ben-Eliyahu DJ, Silber BA: Thermography and MRI in patients with cervical disc protrusion, *Am J Chiropr Med* 3:57, 1990.
5. Jackson RB: Willard Carver, LL.B., D.C., 1866-1943: doctor lawyer, Indian chief, prisoner and more, *Chiro Hist* 14:13, 1994.
6. Jacobs B: Cervical angina, *NY Sta J Med* 90:8, 1990.
7. Stodolny J, Chmielewski H: Manual therapy in the treatment of patients with cervical migraine, *J Man Med* 4:49, 1989.
8. Cote P, Mior SA, Fitz-Ritson D: Cervicogenic vertigo: a report of three cases, *J Can Chiro Assoc* 35:89, 1991.
9. Masarsky CS: A language of our own: some observations and practical hints for chiropractic lexicographers, *Dynamic Chiro* 13(21):20, 1995.
10. Christensen MG, editor: *Job analysis of chiropractic by state,* Greeley, Colo, National Board of Chiropractic Examiners.
11. Palmer BJ: *Clear View Sanitarium: chiropractic care for mental and nervous disorders (pamphlet),* Davenport, Iowa, 1951, B.J. Palmer Chiropractic Clinic.
12. Rehm WS: The pathfinders. In Peterson D, Wiese G, editors: *Chiropractic: an illustrated history,* St Louis, 1995, Mosby.
13. Friel JP, editor: *Dorland's illustrated medical dictionary: twenty-eighth edition,* Philadelphia, 1994, W.B. Saunders.

14. Korr IM: Sustained sympatheticotonia as a factor in disease. In Korr IM, editor: *The neurobiologic mechanisms in manipulative therapy,* New York, 1977, Plenum Press.

15. Cox JM: *Low back pain: mechanism, diagnosis and treatment,* ed 5, Baltimore, 1990, Williams & Wilkins.

16. Plaugher G, editor: *Textbook of clinical chiropractic: a specific biomechanical approach,* Baltimore, 1993, Williams & Wilkins.

17. Homewood AE: *The neurodynamics of the vertebral subluxation,* St Petersburg, Fla, 1977, Valkyrie Press.

18. Fitz-Ritson D: Cervicogenic sympathetic syndromes: etiology, treatment and rehabilitation. In Gatterman MI, editor: *Foundations of chiropractic: subluxation,* p 319, St Louis, 1995, Mosby.

19. Giles LGF: A histological investigation of human lower lumbar intervertebral canal dimensions, *J Manipulative Physiol Ther* 17:4, 1994.

20. Terrett AGJ: Cerebral dysfunction: a theory to explain some of the effects of chiropractic manipulation, *Chiro Technique* 5:168, 1993.

21. Masarsky C, Weber M: Visceral disorders research. In Redwood D, editor: *Contemporary chiropractic,* p 189, New York, 1997, Churchill Livingstone.

22. Gatterman MI, Hansen DT: Development of chiropractic nomenclature through consensus, *J Manipulative Physiol Ther* 17:302, 1994.

23. Gibbons RW: Go to jail for chiro, *J Chiropr Humanities* 4:61, 1994.

24. Scaringe JG, Sikorski D: The art of manual palpation and adjustment. In Redwood D, editor: *Contemporary chiropractic,* p 111, New York, 1997, Churchill Livingstone.

25. Masarsky CS, Weber M: Stop paradigm erosion, *J Manipulative Physiol Ther* 14:323, 1991.

26. Goldstein M, editor: *The research status of spinal manipulative therapy,* Bethesda, Md, 1975, National Institute of Neurological and Communicative Disorders and Stroke.

27. Langenweiler MJ, Febbo TA: Reflex sympathetic dystrophy syndrome: a case report, *J Neuromusculoskel Syst* 1:69, 1993.

28. Northup GW: History of the development of osteopathic concepts: osteopathic terminology. In Goldstein M, editor: *The research status of spinal manipulative therapy,* Bethesda, Md, 1975, National Institute of Neurological and Communicative Disorders and Stroke.

29. Association of Chiropractic Colleges: *Issues in chiropractic, position paper #1: the ACC chiropractic paradigm,* Chicago, Ill, July 1, 1996, Association of Chiropractic Colleges.

30. DeFranca GG, Levine LJ: The T4 syndrome, *J Manipulative Physiol Ther* 18:34, 1995.

31. Cooperstein R: Thompson technique, *Chiro Technique* 7:60, 1995.

INDEX

Page numbers followed by *f* indicate illustrations, page numbers followed by *t* indicate tables, and page numbers followed by *b* indicate boxes.